Virtual Endoscopy and 3D Reconstruction in the Airways

Nabil A. Shallik • Abbas H. Moustafa
Marco A. E. Marcus

Editors

Virtual Endoscopy and 3D Reconstruction in the Airways

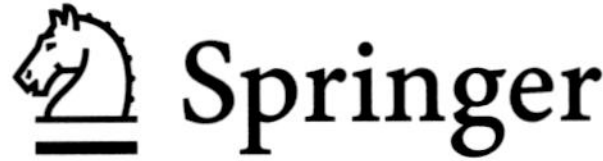

Springer

Editors
Nabil A. Shallik
Department of Clinical Anesthesiology
Weill Cornell Medical College in Qatar
Doha
Qatar

Department of Anesthesiology
ICU and Perioperative Medicine
Hamad Medical Corporation
Doha
Qatar

Department of Anesthesiology
and Surgical Intensive Care
Faculty of Medicine
Tanta University
Tanta
Egypt

Marco A. E. Marcus
Department of Anesthesiology
ICU and Perioperative Medicine
Hamad Medical Corporation
Doha
Qatar

Department of Clinical Anesthesiology
Weill Cornell Medical College in Qatar
Doha
Qatar

Department of Clinical Anesthesiology
Qatar University
Doha
Qatar

Abbas H. Moustafa
Clinical Radiology and Medical Imaging
Department
Hamad Medical Corporation
Doha
Qatar

Diagnostic Radiology and Medical
Imaging
El Minia University
El Minia
Egypt

ISBN 978-3-030-23252-8   ISBN 978-3-030-23253-5   (eBook)
https://doi.org/10.1007/978-3-030-23253-5

This Springer imprint is published by the registered company Springer Nature Switzerland AG
The registered company address is: Gewerbestrasse 11, 6330 Cham, Switzerland

Preface

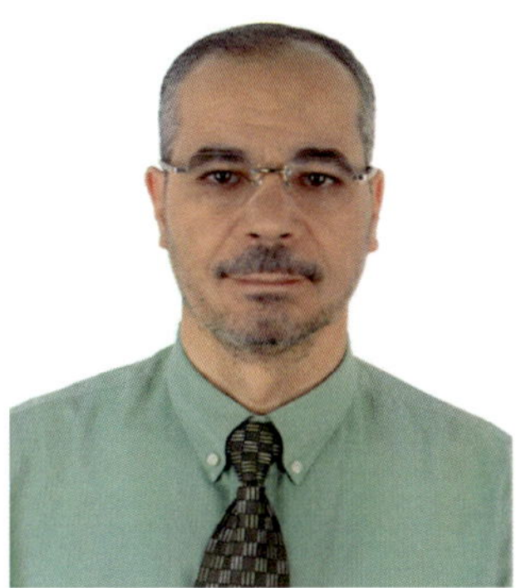

New technologies in airway management never cease to amaze me, and it is especially wonderful to be existed in a period when rapid medical advances are changing the clinical practice landscape with reassuring certainty and frequency—having seen the world around me slowly transition from 2D to 3D imaging and even 4D in certain cases! It was only a matter of time before clinicians would find themselves needing 3D imaging on a regular basis.

In less than 10 years, virtual endoscopy and 3D reconstruction have spread all around the world, and the diffusion of this technique may be traced through the increasing number of published papers in the literature. I have personally kept in touch with the major advances in the field and have used virtual endoscopy for many of my patients. Having been in the field of airway management for 20 years, I can confidently attest to its robustness and efficacy in managing hitherto impossible to intubate patients.

From my experience and those of my colleagues, we have gathered a lot of knowledge and wisdom on the subject, and I am delighted to present the first edition of our book *Virtual Endoscopy and 3D Reconstruction in the Airways.*

While this book is mainly intended for anesthesia trainees and consultants, we believe it would be well suited for intensive care physicians, emergency physicians, radiologists, ORL-HNS surgeons, maxillofacial surgeons , pulmonologists, paramedical staff, and medical students.

The content includes a brief review of the fundamental airway anatomy and moves onto radiologic and virtual 3D evaluation of normal and diseased airways. The discussion also deals with the use of this technology in oral, nasal, maxillofacial, and skull base surgeries. We also discuss about 3D virtual endoscopy in ICU settings, augmented reality visualization in pulmonary interventions, and implications of 3D printing on airway management. There is a section on challenging cases derived from real patient experiences in our hospital. The book ends with future perspectives and recommendations.

While we did our best to prevent any misinformation of any form, we would urge our readers to inform us of any such error, including spelling or contextual errors. We also would advise that this book certainly does not replace professional or expert guidance and consultation.

I am much thankful to my wife, sons, and daughter for their continuous help in all stages of this book.

I would also like to thank Dr. Hanan Mawlana for her constant support while editing this unique book and to all the participating authors for their contribution.

Thank you and enjoy your book!

Doha, Qatar   Nabil A. Shallik

Preface

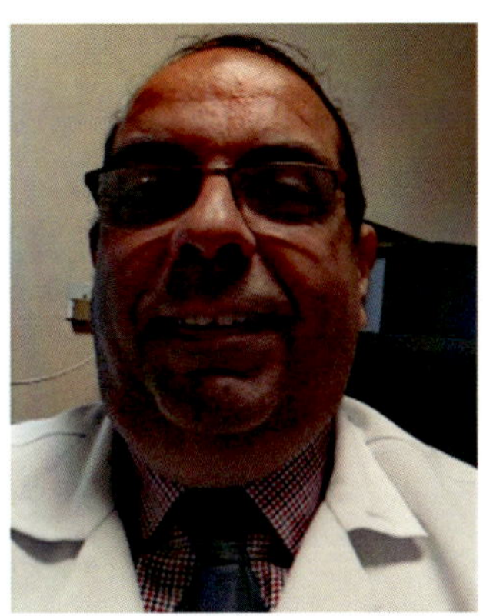

Ever since the dawn of time, mankind has brought forth innumerable innovations, and the medical field is a prime example. As a radiologist, I firmly believe that an image is worth a thousand words, as the saying goes, and this could not be more true with the advent of 3D reconstructions, volume rendering techniques, and virtual endoscopy (VE). In today's world, it is difficult to imagine living without technology. Some of the newest innovations today were either in the realm of fiction years ago or were just a seed in someone's mind, ready to evolve into something far greater.

Computer-aided diagnosis (CAD), coupled with VE, can inevitably aid in providing better healthcare.

3D printing can be done for difficult and complicated cases, as surgeons will have a physical model of the pathology to have a clear approach to proceed with the surgery, and can be a great tool to use when teaching junior colleagues.

Many people consider 3D imaging and VE as difficult tasks; however, when well practiced, it is considered a great asset with limitless clinical value.

In some respects, the workstation of a radiologist is their own high-end video games console, just like Sony's PlayStation 4 capable of rendering millions of high-fidelity imaging metadata, as well as providing aesthetically pleasing and clear information.

I am inviting all our colleagues to practice the 3D imaging and VRT techniques which are considered fun with great clinical impact and value; please enjoy.

Doha, Qatar   Abbas H. Moustafa

Preface

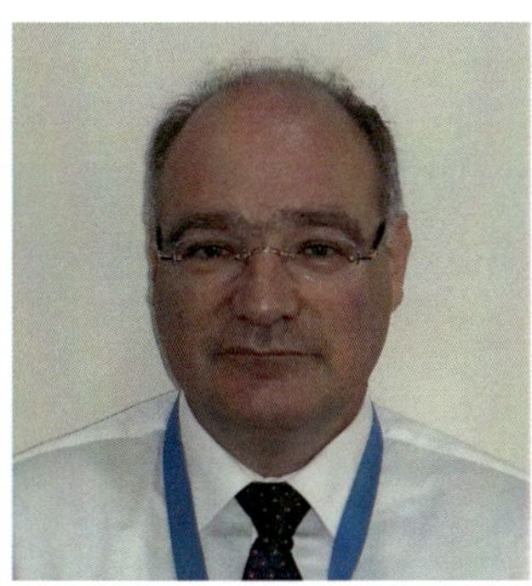

Within a fast-changing world like ours, very detailed descriptions are often important. To get autonomous cars running perfectly, you need detailed maps and instructions to navigate the cars through a jungle of obstacles.

So too, the future of surgery lies with automatization; through automatization, we seek to get a safe and stable product free of human error. Automatization provides potential to extract consistent and standardized information from patients, such as genetic profiles for pharmacokinetic modelling and dexterous robots as surgeons and anesthesiologists to be handled by experts of course! However, for automatization in anesthesiology, absolute accuracy and meticulous detail of anatomy are needed, which would have to be even more precise than the detailed maps we need to drive autonomous cars. To make robots that intubate patients, we first need even more precise understanding and detail of the anatomy of the airway. This book can bring us to that future of automatization!

Let us start first by minimizing dangerous situations, such as "cannot intubate/cannot ventilate," which can be accomplished through better training programs, better tools, and better understanding of the airway.

Different angles from different specialists give us better understanding about the airway. A book about the anatomy of the airway is therefore essential.

Hopefully, all will read this book with pleasure. I congratulate every author for the effort they put in and the other editors especially Dr. Nabil for their patience and endurance.

Happy reading.

Doha, Qatar   Marco A. E. Marcus

Acknowledgments

The preparation of the *Virtual Endoscopy and 3D Reconstruction in the Airways* book has required the help and cooperation of many. To each individual, we acknowledge our debt of gratitude. It has been both an honor and a privilege to have worked with all of the authors who are expert anesthesiologists, radiologists, surgeons, and technologists from across the world.

First and foremost, we would like to extend our gratitude to Mr. Samir R. Khiste, a radiology technologist who did a great job in 3-D reconstruction of our clinical cases. Also, we would like to thank Dr. Serag Kamel for editing the diagrams and photos for normal anatomy chapter and to Dr. Abderrazak Sahraoui for his talent in photography of our 3-D printed projects.

The staff at Springer have contributed in countless ways, with competence, patience, and hard work, particularly Ms. Reshmi Rema and Mr. Andrea Ridolfi who kept us on task and played a pivotal role in the quality of the final written text.

We especially wish to express our deep appreciation to the Anesthesia, ICU, and Perioperative Medicine Department and Clinical Radiology & Medical Imaging Department, both at Hamad Medical Corporation, Doha, Qatar; without their relationships, we would not have become the editors of this book.

Lastly, we would like to thank from the bottom of our hearts our God for helping us make this work feasible and our families whose understanding, forbearance, and support made this book possible.

Contents

1 Introduction... 1
Nabil A. Shallik

2 Review of Upper Airway Anatomy
and Its Clinical Application 3
Ahmed Zaghw, Nabil A. Shallik, Ahmed Fayed El Geziry, and
Amr Elhakeem

3 Radiological Evaluation of the Airway: One-Stop Shop....... 15
Abbas H. Moustafa and Nabil A. Shallik

4 Evaluation of the Normal Airway Using Virtual Endoscopy
and Three-Dimensional Reconstruction.................... 31
Nabil A. Shallik, Abbas H. Moustafa, and Yasser Hammad

5 Virtual Endoscopy and 3-D Reconstruction in
Patients with Airway Pathology.......................... 39
Imran Ahmad, Britta Millhoff, Sarah Muldoon, and Kayathrie
Jeyarajah

6 Virtual Endoscopy and 3-D Reconstruction in the Nose,
Paranasal Sinuses, and Skull Base Surgery: New Frontiers...... 53
Shanmugam Ganesan, Hamad Al Saey, Natarajan
Saravanappa, Prathamesh Pai, Surjith Vattoth,
and Michael Stewart

7 Computer-Assisted 3D Reconstruction in Oral
and Maxillofacial Surgery 67
Mathias Martinez Coronel, Ismail Farag, and Nabil A. Shallik

8 Virtual Endoscopy and 3-D Reconstruction/Prototyping
in Head and Neck Surgeries............................. 85
Hassan Mohammed, Hassan Haidar, Nabil A. Shallik,
Amr Elhakeem, Majid Al Abdulla, and Zenyel Dogan

9 Perspectives in the Current and Future Use of Augmented
Reality Visualization in Thoracic Surgery
and Pulmonary Interventions 101
Mohamed A. Elarref, Ahmed Aljabary, Nabil A. Shallik,
Mohamed Abbas, and Noran Elarif

10 Role of Virtual Endoscopy and 3-D Reconstruction in Airway Assessment of Critically Ill Patients 117
Adel E. Ahmed Ganaw, Moad Ehfeda, Nissar Shaikh,
Marcus Lance, Arshad Hussain Chanda, Ali O. Mohamed
Belkair, Muhammad Zubair Labathkhan, and Gamal Abdullah

11 Three-Dimensional Printing and Its Implication on Airway Management 129
Yasser Al-Hamidi, Abdulla Baobeid, and Nabil A. Shallik

12 Challenging Clinical Cases Discussion 143
Nabil A. Shallik, Abbas H. Moustafa, and Amr Elhakeem

Abbreviations

2-D	Two-dimensional
2-D MPR	Two-dimensional multi-planar reconstructions
3-D	Three-dimensional
4-D	Four-dimensional
A & E	Accident and emergency
ABS	Acrylonitrile butadiene styrene
AD	Arytenoid dislocation
AP	Anteroposterior
AR	Augmented reality
AS	Aortic stenosis
AS	Arytenoid subluxation
ASA	American Society of Anesthesiologists
ATLS	Advanced trauma life support
BI	Bronchus intermedius
BMI	Body mass index
BPF	Bronchopleural fistula
C-MPR	Curved multi-planar reconstruction protocol
CAD	Computer-aided design
CAS	Computer-assisted surgery
CFD	Computational fluid dynamics
CMF	Cranio-maxillofacial surgery
CN	Cranial nerve
CoCr	Cobalt chromium
CPAP	Continuous positive airway pressure
CSF	Cerebrospinal fluid
CT	Computed tomography
CTM	Cricothyroid membrane
CV	Cervical vertebrae
DED	Directed energy deposition
DICOM	Digital imaging and communications in medicine
DISH	Diffuse idiopathic skeletal hyperostosis
DLP	Direct light processing
DO	Distraction osteogenesis
DOD	Drop on demand
EBM	Electron beam melting
FBA	Foreign body aspiration
FDM	Fused deposition material

FESS	Functional endoscopic sinus surgery
FOB	Fiber-optic bronchoscopy
FT	Flexible tracheobronchoscopy
GE	General electric
HU	Hounsfield units
IGS	Image-guided surgery
IIG	Inter-incisor gap
IJV	Internal jugular vein
IV	Intravenous
IVS	Interactive virtual simulation
LMA	Laryngeal mask airway
MDCT	Multi-detector computed tomography
MDCT (VB)	Multi-detector computed tomography virtual bronchoscopy
MinIPs	Minimum intensity projections
MIP	Maximum intensity projection
MPR	Multi-planar reformations
MPR	Multi-planar reconstruction
MPRs	Multi-planar reformations
MRI	Magnetic resonance imaging
NAP4	The Fourth National Audit Project
NiTi	Nickle titanium
OAP	Obstructing airway pathology
OPG	Orthopantomogram
OR	Operating room
OSA	Obstructive sleep apnea
PACS	Patient archive and communication system
PBF	Powder bed fusion
PEEK	Polyether ether ketone
PET/CT	Positron emission tomography-computed tomography
PFR	PaO_2-to-FiO_2 ratios
PLA	Polylactic acid
SARI	Simplified airway risk index
SGD	Supraglottic device
SHS	Selective heat sintering
SII	Smoke inhalation injury
SLA	Stereolithography apparatus
SLS	Selective laser sintering
SSD	Shaded surface display
STL	Standard tessellation language
T-B	Tracheal-bronchial
TBI	Tracheobronchial injury
TEF	Tracheoesophageal fistula
TM	Tympanic membrane
TMD	Thyro-mental distance
TMJ	Temporomandibular joint
TMJA	Temporomandibular joint ankylosis
TMVR	Transcatheter mitral valve repair
TEF/TOF	Tracheo-osophageal Fistula

TPN	Total parenteral nutrition
TTP	Tissue transparent projection/Tissue transition projection
US	Ultrasound
UV	Ultraviolet
VB	Virtual bronchoscopy
VE	Virtual endoscopy
VPI	Velopharyngeal insufficiency
VR	Virtual reality
VRT	Volume rendering techniques
VSP	Virtual surgical planning
WHO	World Health Organization

List of Videos

Movie 3.1 Reconstructed images resembling orthopantomogram-like images (OPG—panoramic view) using curved MPR technique

Movie 3.2 The resultant 3-D images can be demonstrated and displayed along any axis freely at 360°, features that give more perspectives and hidden relations that cannot be appreciated by any other modalities

Movie 3.3 Normal virtual endoscopy of the airway totally resembling the conventional endoscopic images

Movie 3.4 Virtual endoscopy fly-through technique showing normal finding of VE from nose to carina

Movie 3.5 Detailed VRT and post-processing techniques for full and detailed evaluation of the airway

Movie 3.6 Detailed VRT and post-processing techniques for full and detailed evaluation of the airway

Movie 3.7 Detailed VRT and post-processing techniques for full and detailed evaluation of the airway

Movie 4.1 Normal VE video series from nose to carina

Movie 4.2 Normal VE video series from nose to carina

Movie 4.3 Normal VE video series from nose to carina

Movie 4.4 VRT reconstruction image of the skin contour as well as the cartilaginous framework of the nose is demonstrated clearly using the VRT model

Movie 5.1 Real-time assessment of the upper airway obtained by flexible naso-endoscopy (the main editor is the one appearing in the video)

Movie 5.2 Volume-rendering technique TTP showing the level and extent of the trans-glottic indentation and displacement of the airway by the mass lesion

Movie 5.3 Glottic tumour involving the arytenoid cartilages seen by VE movie

Movie 5.4 Large supraglottic obstructing airway pathology arising from the right vallecula and pushing the epiglottis over to the left proved by VE movie

Movie 5.5	VE of a patient with a base of tongue tumour and the abnormally shaped epiglottis
Video 7.1	Reconstructed images resembling orthopantomogram-like images (OPG—panoramic view) using curved MPR technique
Movie 8.1	3-D reconstruction of foreign body ingestion using different series and reconstruction methodology to accurately delineate the metallic FB (needle) and its relation to the different adjacent structures
Movie 8.2	3-D reconstruction of foreign body ingestion using different series and reconstruction methodology to accurately delineate the faint FB (fish bone) and its relation to the different adjacent structures
Movie 8.3	3-D reconstruction of foreign body ingestion using different series and reconstruction methodology to accurately delineate the faint FB (fish bone) and its relation to the different adjacent structures
Movie 8.4	Virtual endoscopy evaluation inside the trachea showing no extension of the FB into the tracheal lumen
Movie 8.5	Preoperative naso-endoscopic evaluation revealed the presence of abnormal mucosal lined drumstick-shaped structure of odd presentation, yet with no signs of malignancy or hyper-vascularity
Movie 8.6	3-D reconstruction video shows displaced blade of the hyoid bone, in which the thyroid mass lesion was clearly visualized
Movie 8.7	Naso-endoscopic assessment revealed a web formation at the level of the glottis extending from the anterior commissure to the junction between the anterior two-thirds and posterior one-third of the vocal cord
Movie 8.8	Virtual endoscopic evaluation was done which showed the web to be at a supraglottic region, while the glottic region was clear
Movie 8.9	Virtual endoscopic evaluation was done which showed the web to be at a supraglottic region, while the glottic region was clear
Movie 9.1	Virtual bronchoscopy and VRT movies as a non-invasive method that allows accurate grading of tracheobronchial stenosis
Movie 9.2	MDCT scan reveals absent left lung, obliterated left main bronchus with nippling, absent left pulmonary artery and significant hyperinflation of the right lung crossing to the left through the anterior mediastinum
Movie 9.3	MDCT scan reveals absent left lung, obliterated left main bronchus with nippling, absent left pulmonary artery and significant hyperinflation of the right lung crossing to the left through the anterior mediastinum

Movie 9.4	MDCT scan reveals absent left lung, obliterated left main bronchus with nippling, absent left pulmonary artery and significant hyperinflation of the right lung crossing to the left through the anterior mediastinum
Movie 9.5	MDCT scan reveals absent left lung, obliterated left main bronchus with nippling, absent left pulmonary artery and significant hyperinflation of the right lung crossing to the left through the anterior mediastinum
Movie 10.1	VB shows external nonmucosal compressions on the bronchial wall that cause indentation upon the related part of the trachea with subsequent reduction of its AP dimension
Movie 10.2	VB shows external compressions caused by normal anatomic structure (esophagus)
Movie 10.3	Virtual endoscopy for a case of tracheal stenosis demonstrating the level and extent
Movie 10.4	Conventional flexible endoscopic evaluation for a case of TOF
Movie 11.1	Shows 3-D printed prototype and develop new medical tools of video-laryngoscopy (Shalliscope) for endotracheal intubation
Movie 12.1	TTP of the airway showing significant reduction of the airway caliber
Movie 12.2	Circular hyoid bone demonstrated in the VRT images which is rotated 360 degrees. Note that the superior cornu of the thyroid cartilage is sharing in the same process
Movie 12.3	CA right side maxilla with right-sided sizable highly vascular metastatic neck lymphadenopathy mass lesion
Movie 12.4	CA right side maxilla with right-sided sizable highly vascular metastatic neck lymphadenopathy mass lesion

Electronic Supplementary Material is available in the online version of the related chapter on SpringerLink: http://link.springer.com/

Introduction

Nabil A. Shallik

Medicine is an everyday progressing science, where health-care providers continue to enhance their knowledge and develop their skills. Moreover, technology has made the application of medical knowledge more versatile and widely available.

The combined use of knowledge and technology has the power to improve health-care services, which is not achieved by using the best technology but achieved by the excellent use of technology (Fig. 1.1).

The quote, "a picture is worth a thousand words," refers to the notion that a complex idea can be conveyed with a single image, as it illustrates these meanings more effectively than any description can.

The goal of this book is to utilize all these concepts to emulate the above, to produce a textbook that simplifies complex topics and makes it relevant to students, trainees, anesthetists, radiologists, intensivists, surgeons, and physicians.

1.1 Book Overview

The book adopts a concise, practical, and simple approach to all topics of discussion. Care has been taken to confirm the accuracy of the information presented and to describe generally accepted practices.

The chapters in the virtual endoscopy (VE) and three-dimensional (3-D) sections were specifically written to simplify complex topics, extrapolate them to real processes, and apply them to relevant perioperative clinical situations.

Each chapter provides a list of additional complementary topics that are available within the book, giving readers the opportunity to supplement their knowledge of any given topic.

I strongly believe that this will appeal to all anesthetists seeking a practical guide in the management of airway. I sincerely hope that the practical nature and quality of this text will contribute to your learning and benefit patients in the ever-growing field of anesthesia.

N. A. Shallik (✉)
Department of Clinical Anesthesiology, Weill Cornell Medical College in Qatar, Doha, Qatar

Department of Anesthesiology, ICU and Perioperative Medicine, Hamad Medical Corporation, Doha, Qatar

Department of Anesthesiology and Surgical Intensive Care, Faculty of Medicine, Tanta University, Tanta, Egypt
e-mail: Nshallik@hamad.qa

© Springer Nature Switzerland AG 2019
N. A. Shallik et al. (eds.), *Virtual Endoscopy and 3D Reconstruction in the Airways*,
https://doi.org/10.1007/978-3-030-23253-5_1

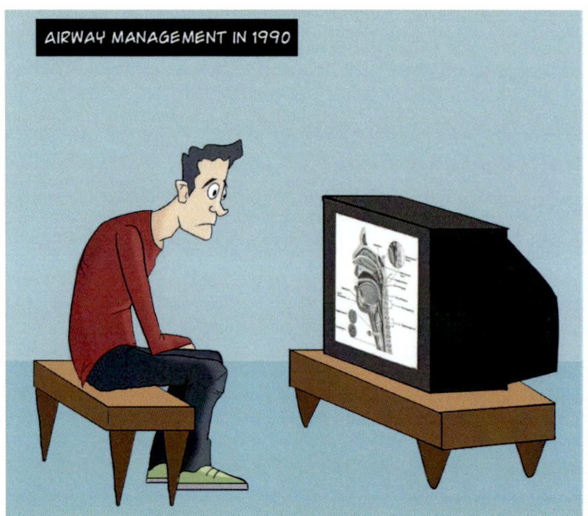

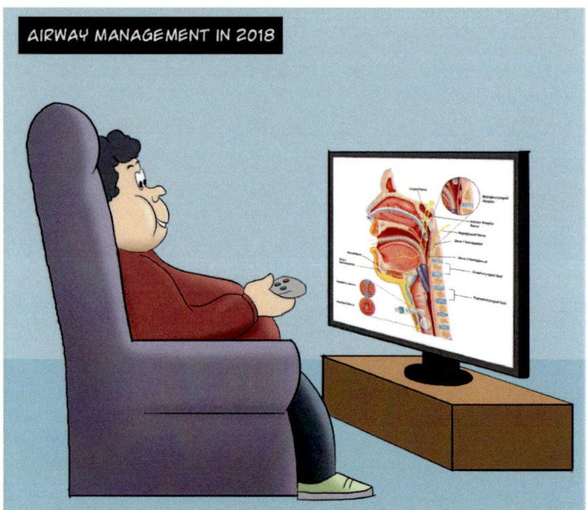

Fig. 1.1 Left sided image (thin man reviewing black and white TV for an airway image); the right one allowed him fat due to mind relaxation by the couuoured LED TV supererb same image giving more detialed information; thanks for the techonology (picture is worth a thousand words)

1.2 How to Move Inside the Book

The initial chapters cover the review of the normal airway anatomy and normal airway evaluation by 3-D and VE, including its radiology.

The core of the book addresses virtual endoscopy (VE) and 3-D computer-assisted reconstruction of airway pathology. Additionally, it addresses nasal, skull base, oral, maxillofacial, and prototyping in head and neck surgeries. This book also highlights the perspectives of using augmented reality visualization in pulmonary interventions, complications, and interactive virtual endoscopy and 3-D reconstruction in ICU settings.

In the chapter dedicated to discussions of challenging and interesting cases, there is special emphasis on the appropriate use of technology to provide a better and safer way to diagnose and manage these conditions.

The last chapters describe 3-D printing and its implication in airway management. Research and future perspectives will help to guide the advancement of this subject.

Each chapter is described by leading experts in their field, making this book an essential tool for every anesthesiologist, radiologist, surgeon, intensivist, chest physician, and other specialists concerned with airway management.

Application of this information in any particular situation remains the professional responsibility of the practitioner.

1.3 In Conclusion

The authors, editors, and publisher have exerted every effort to ensure that technique selections and reconstruction procedures in this text are in accordance with current recommendations and practice at the time of publication. However, with ongoing research, many changes will continue to happen.

We would like to finish our book with a quote: "knowledge sharing is the one the best thing a man can do for humanity."

Review of Upper Airway Anatomy and Its Clinical Application

Ahmed Zaghw, Nabil A. Shallik, Ahmed Fayed El Geziry, and Amr Elhakeem

2.1 Introduction

Airway management requires sound knowledge of the anatomy of the airway and its related structures. Understanding of the functional anatomy and the airway physiology under different clinical conditions, is necessary to avoid catastrophic airway events. Multidimensional anatomical orientation is essential when anesthetists or other health care providers are in the process of handling the airway. This chapter will cover the general airway anatomy, however detailed surgical anatomy is beyond the scope of this chapter.

A. Zaghw (✉) · A. F. El Geziry
Department of Anesthesiology, ICU and Perioperative Medicine, Hamad Medical Corporation, Doha, Qatar
e-mail: azaghw@hamad.qa

N. A. Shallik
Department of Anesthesiology, ICU and Perioperative Medicine, Hamad Medical Corporation, Doha, Qatar

Department of Clinical Anesthesiology, Weill Cornell Medical College in Qatar (WCMQ), Doha, Qatar

Department of Anesthesiology and Surgical Intensive Care, Faculty of Medicine, Tanta University, Tanta, Egypt
e-mail: Nshallik@hamad.qa

A. Elhakeem
(ORL-HNS) Department, Hamad Medical Corporation, Doha, Qatar

2.2 Structural Anatomy

The upper airway anatomy from an anesthetist's point of view can be described as two cavities. The nasal cavity and the oral cavity, which is separated by the hard-bony palate anteriorly and soft palate posteriorly. These two cavities unite posteriorly and inferiorly to form a common pharyngeal tube, which then further downward encompasses the laryngeo-tracheal and the pharyngeo-esophageal tubes.

2.2.1 Nasal Cavity

The nasal cavity refers to each of the two sides of the nose or the two sides as one. The front of the nasal cavity is the nasal vestibule and external opening (the nares) while the back blends, through the *choanae*, into the nasopharynx. The nasal cavity has *two walls* (lateral and medial), a *roof* and a *floor*. The lateral wall is formed of three mucosal coverings, horizontal, bony outgrowths called nasal *conchae* or turbinates (superior, middle, and inferior), under which three meatus are formed respectively. Lateral wall contains the sphenoethmoidal recess, which lies above the superior concha and receives the sphenoidal sinus opening. The ethmoidal sinus opens under the superior conchae. The frontonasal duct and maxillary sinus open

© Springer Nature Switzerland AG 2019
N. A. Shallik et al. (eds.), *Virtual Endoscopy and 3D Reconstruction in the Airways*,
https://doi.org/10.1007/978-3-030-23253-5_2

under the middle conchae. The naso-lacrimal duct opens under the inferior conchae.

- The *medial* wall forms the nasal septum, which is made of a number of cartilages anteriorly and bones posteriorly, which are mucosal covered.
- The *roof* of each nasal cavity is formed in its upper third by the nasal bone superiorly and inferiorly by the junctions of the upper lateral cartilage and nasal septum. The connective tissue and skin cover the bony and cartilaginous components of the dorsum of the nose.
- The *floor*, which also forms the roof of the mouth, is made up of the bones of the hard palate; the horizontal plate of the palatine bone posteriorly and the palatine process of the maxilla anteriorly.

The nasal cavity is lined by mucosa of pseudostratified columnar epithelium with the exception of the vestibule, which is covered by skin. The nasal cavity is functionally divided into two different segments; the olfactory segment and the respiratory segment. The olfactory segment occupies the upper one-third and is lined by a specialized type of pseudostratified columnar epithelium, known as olfactory epithelium, which contains receptors for sense of smell. This segment is located in and beneath the mucosa of the roof of each nasal cavity and the medial side of each middle turbinate. The respiratory segment occupies the lower two-third and is lined by the respiratory epithelium, whose functions are filtration, humidification, and thermoregulation.

The nasal cavity walls are supplied by five arteries, namely, the sphenopalatine, greater palatine, superior labial, facial, and anterior ethmoidal (branches of the external carotid artery) and posterior ethmoidal (branch of the internal carotid artery).

These branches of arteries anastomose with each other on the same side and on the contralateral side, the most common site where they communicate is in the anterior part of the septum forming the Kiesselbach plexus, the most common site for nasal bleeding.

Nerve supply: The innervation of the septum and lateral wall originates from the Ophthalmic branch of the trigeminal nerve (V1) in the antero-superior part and maxillary branch of trigeminal (V2) in the posteroinferior part.

2.2.2 Oral Cavity

The oral cavity spans between the oral fissure (opening between the lips) anteriorly and the oropharyngeal isthmus (opening to the oropharynx) posteriorly. The teeth and their bony scaffolding forms the upper and lower dental arches that divides the oral cavity into the vestibule and the oral cavity proper. The vestibule is a horseshoe space bounded by the teeth and gingiva posteriorly and the lips and cheeks anteriorly. It communicates with the mouth proper through the space behind the third molar tooth.

The oral cavity proper starts internal to dental arches, from the maxillary and mandibular dental arches to end at the oropharyngeal isthmus, where the oropharynx starts. The oral cavity has two borders, a roof and a floor, with the tongue filling a large proportion of it. The oropharyngeal isthmus is formed by the soft palate superiorly, the palatoglossal arch laterally, and the posterior one-third of the tongue inferiorly. The roof of the oral cavity proper consists of the hard palate anteriorly and soft palate posteriorly. The floor of the mouth is formed of muscles including the tongue, which is the main muscular organ of the oral cavity. The sulcus terminalis is a V-shaped shallow groove between the anterior two-thirds and posterior one-third of the tongue, delineating the boundary between the oral cavity and oropharynx. Muscles of the tongue are Styloglossus, Hyoglossus, Genioglossus and Palatoglossus known as extrinsic group in addition to overlapping vertical, longitudinal and transverse muscles known as intrinsic group. The floor of the mouth is formed by a group of four suprahyoid muscles; *Mylohyoid*, *Geniohyoid*, *Stylohyoid*, and *Digastric* muscles (Fig. 2.1).

The *arterial* supply originates from the infra-orbital arteries for upper lips and facial artery

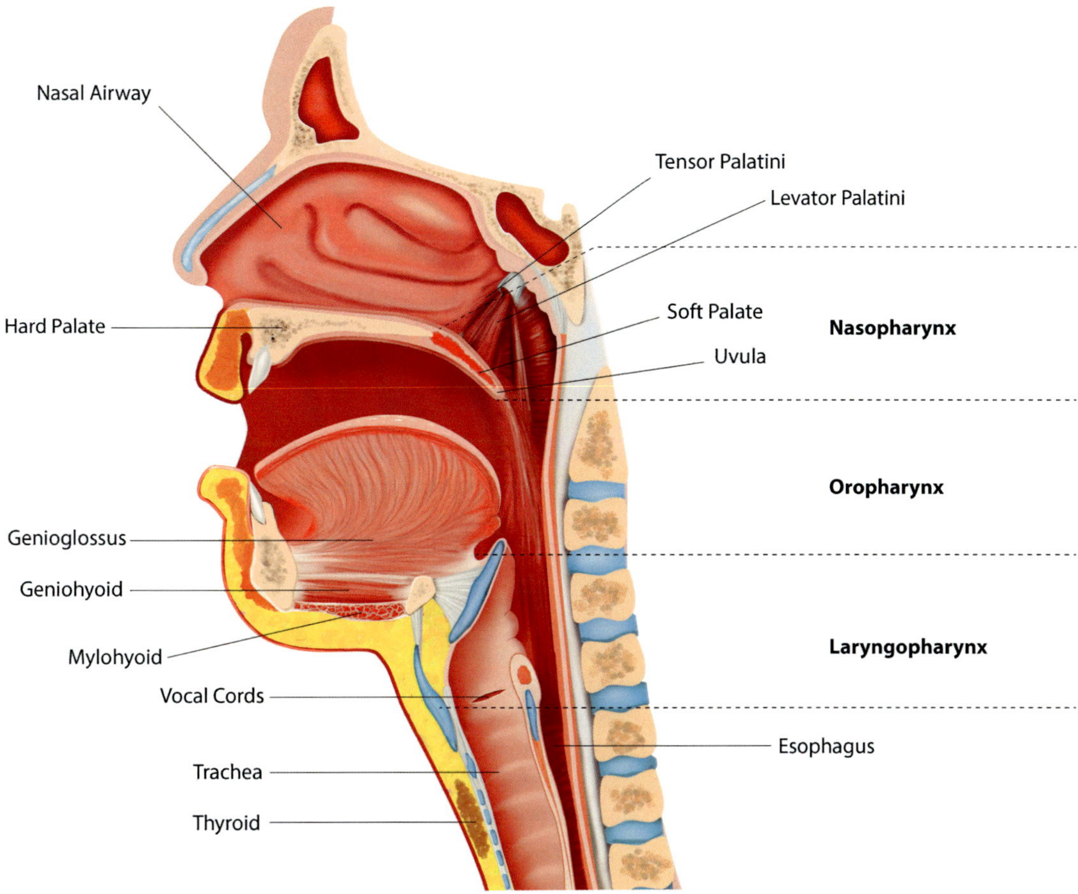

Fig. 2.1 Anatomical sagittal section for the major anatomical landmarks for the airway with delineation among the three parts of the pharynx "Naso—Oro—Laryngo pharynx." The important muscles that hold airway patent are shown as those who hold the soft palate and tongue, thus keeping the retropalatal and retroglossal space patent

branches for both upper and lower lips. The sensory innervation is mainly trigeminal origin, as the upper lip is supplied by the infra-orbital nerves of the maxillary branches (CN V2) and the lower lip is supplied by the inferior labial nerves of the mandibular branches (CN V3). All tongue muscles are supplied by the Hypoglossal nerve (CN XI), except Palatoglossus muscle which is supplied by the Vagus nerve (CN X). The sensory supply for the anterior 2/3 and posterior 1/3 is lingual branches from Trigeminal (V3) and Glossopharyngeal nerve (IX), respectively. The taste sensation is supplied in the same manner by facial nerve (CN VII) for the anterior 2/3 and Glossopharyngeal nerve for the posterior 1/3.

2.2.3 Pharynx

The pharynx is a U-shaped fibromuscular tube that makes up the part of the throat situated immediately behind the nasal cavity, the mouth, and above the esophagus. It starts from the base of the skull and ends at the level of the *sixth cervical* vertebrae "*C6*" (opposite to the lower end of the cricoid cartilage). It is divided into three parts, namely *nasopharynx, oropharynx,* and *hypopharynx (laryngopharynx)* (Fig. 2.1).

- *Anteriorly,* the pharynx has no complete anterior wall, as it communicates with nasal cavity (choana), oral cavity (oropharyngeal isthmus), and laryngeal inlet.

- *Posteriorly*, the constrictor muscles merge to form the *pharyngeal raphe*, a longitudinal fibrous band on the posterior wall of the pharynx. It is related to the first six cervical vertebrae, and it overlies both the prevertebral and deep cervical fasciae.
- *Laterally*, the pharynx is fixed by the medial pterygoid plate, pterygomandibular raphe, mandible, lateral aspect of the tongue, hyoid bone, and thyroid and cricoid cartilages.

The *pharyngeal wall* is formed of four layers; inner mucosal layer, submucosal layer, muscular layer, and outer fascial layer.

1. The *mucosal* layer starts from the ciliated columnar epithelium in the nasopharynx, then turns to a stratified squamous epithelium at oropharynx. The pharyngeal mucosa reflects over different muscular structures to form either arches "folds" or pouches "recesses".
2. The *submucosa* is a thin fibrous layer, except superiorly where it get thick, when it merges with the pharyngobasilar fascia and in the oropharynx, to form the sheath surrounding the tonsils (palatine tonsils). The *Waldeyer* ring is a group of lymphoid tissues across different parts of the pharynx, starting from the most superior nasopharyngeal tonsil known as adenoids, then oropharyngeal palatine tonsils, to lingual tonsils at the base of the tongue.
3. The *muscular layer* constitutes two main groups of pharyngeal muscles; *longitudinal* and *circular* groups. The three circular pharyngeal constrictor muscles the *superior, middle,* and *inferior pharyngeal constrictors.* They stack like glasses to form an incomplete muscular circle as they attach anteriorly to structures in the neck. The circular muscles contract sequentially from superior to inferior to constrict the lumen and propel food into the esophagus. All pharyngeal constrictors are innervated by the vagus nerve (CN X). The three longitudinal muscles are the *stylopharyngeus, palatopharyngeus,* and *salpingopharyngeus.* They shorten, widen the pharynx and elevate the larynx during swallowing. All the six pharyngeal muscles decussate and unite with the muscles of the opposite side posteriorly to form the pharyngeal raphe. All together, they control swallowing and contribute to voice formation.
4. The *fascial layer* is the most external fascial layer, that holds the pharynx to the pharyngobasilar fascia of the base of the skull "occipital and sphenoid bones".

The motor innervation of the muscles of the upper airway including the palate, pharynx, and larynx may seem confusing because the terminology and nomenclature of the nerve supply are different in various textbooks of anatomy. All muscles of palate, pharynx, and larynx are supplied by the vagus nerve (CN X) either by direct branches or by indirect branches from the pharyngeal plexus. With the exception of the tensor veli palatini and the stylopharyngeus muscle that are supplied by motor branches of trigeminal nerve (CN V) and the glossopharyngeal nerve (CN IX), respectively. The pharyngeal neural plexus is formed in the posterior pharyngeal wall at the level of the middle pharyngeal constrictor, by contributions from motor branches of the vagus nerve, sensory branches of glossopharyngeal nerve, and vasomotor branches of cervical sympathetic ganglion. It should be known that the motor fibers in the vagus nerve to the upper airway muscles are from the cranial root of the accessory nerve (CN XI) that joined the vagus nerve before exiting the cranium.

The *sensory* supply of the nasopharynx and oropharynx is mainly innervated by the Trigeminal nerve (CN V) the Glossopharyngeal nerve (CN IX) however, the hypopharynx is innervated by the vagus nerve. The overlapping zones of the palatine tonsil's pillars are innervated by branches of the greater petrosal nerve of the facial nerve (CN VII).

The *arterial* supply for the pharynx is mainly from the pharyngeal branches of the external carotid artery, maxillary artery, and the facial arteries. The caudal portion of the pharynx is supplied by the superior and inferior thyroid arteries. The *venous* drainage is through the pharyngeal venous plexus, which eventually ends in the internal jugular vein.

2.2.3.1 Nasopharynx

It's the superior part of the pharynx, which starts at base of the skull and ends at the level of soft palate opposite the first cervical vertebrae C1. At C1, the buccopharyngeal fascia merges with pharyngobasilar fascia to fill the space between the superior constrictor and the base of the skull.

It continues anteriorly with the nasal cavity through the choanae and inferiorly with the oropharynx through the pharyngeal isthmus. The isthmus is the space between the posterior wall of the pharynx and the free border of the soft palate, whereas the other lateral, superior, and posterior walls are rigid fibromuscular wall. The posterior wall contains the nasopharygneal tonsils as called "Adenoids". The lateral wall contains the cartilaginous lip of the Eustachian tube. The salpingopharyngeus muscle merges with the pharyngeal wall behind the lip of the auditory tube to form a mucosal reflection over the fossa of Rosenmuller. It is lined with the respiratory mucosal of ciliated pseudostratified columnar epithelium with goblet cells. Kindly review (Fig. 2.1).

2.2.3.2 Oropharynx

It is the middle part of the pharynx with mainly swallowing function. It starts from the soft palate at the level of C1 (pharyngeal isthmus) till it ends at the hyoid bone at the level of C3, where the hypopharynx starts inferiorly. The rigid posterior and lateral walls are continuation of the pharyngobasilar fascia and the superior constrictor muscle. The anterior and lateral walls are covered by a mucosal fold over the palatopharyngeus muscle (palatopharyngeal fold), which arises from the soft palate superiorly to form the oropharyngeal isthmus. Palatine tonsils are lymphoid tissue located in the tonsillar fossa (between the palatoglossal and palatopharyngeal arches of the oral cavity). The remaining of the anterior wall is formed by the posterior one-third of the tongue with the lingual tonsils (lymphoid tissue at the base of the tongue) (Fig. 2.1).

2.2.3.3 Hypopharynx

The hypopharynx is the inferior and narrowest part of the pharynx. It starts at the level of C3 to end at the esophageal inlet opposite the lower border of the cricoid bone at the level of C6. At that level, the mucosa folds to form pyriform fossa on each side of the esophageal inlet.

Pharynx is a common site for airway collapse under different conditions. The *retropalatal, retroglossal,* and *retroepiglottic are* among the most vulnerable spaces for volume reduction. In the awake state, the airway patency relies on the pharyngeal dilator muscles; a group of muscles that antagonizes the airway collapsing forces. The dilator muscles include the *tensor palatine muscle,* which opens the retropalatal space by pulling the soft palate away from the posterior pharyngeal wall. The *genioglossus* opens the retroglossal space by moving the tongue anteriorly. The muscles that open retroepiglottic space by moving the hyoid bone forward, including; the *Geniohyoid, Sternohyoid,* and *Thyrohyoid* muscles. The negative intraluminal pressure during inspiration in a spontaneously breathing adult could lead to airway collapse especialy if the nasal passages is blocked or the upper airway is obstructed. Kindly refer to (Fig. 2.1).

2.2.4 Larynx

The larynx is a fibrocartilagenous tube in the anterior compartment of the neck. Anchored superiorly by the hyoid bone (free standing bone), allowing a wide range of movements and functions. It extends between C3 and C6, continues inferiorly with the trachea, and opens superiorly into the hypopharynx. All parts of the larynx are lined with ciliated pseudostratified epithelium except for the vocal folds, which are lined by nonkeratinized squamous epithelium.

The boundaries of the laryngeal inlet include the following:

- *Anteriorly* by the *Epiglottis* and the posterior wall of thyroid cartilage down to the cricoid cartilage
- *Posteriorly* by *hypopharynx* (laryngopharynx)
- *Superiorly* by the *interarytenoid* folds, that forms the posterior commissures until the posterior lamina of cricoid cartilage
- *Laterally* by *Aryepiglottic fold* until the inner side of cricoid cartilage
- The *floor* is formed by the *Conus elasticus* (the extension of lateral cricothyroid ligaments from the inner surface of the cricoid cartilage to the vocal ligaments)

Clinically, the larynx is divided into three regions: Kindly refer to (Fig. 2.2), that shows open posterior view of the larynx.

- *Supraglottic* region from the inferior surface of the epiglottis to the vestibular folds (false vocal cords)
- *Glottis* region contains vocal cords and is 1 cm below them. The opening or space between the vocal cords is known as *Rima Glottidis*, the size of which is altered by the muscles of phonation
- *Subglottic* region from the inferior border of the glottis to the inferior border of the cricoid cartilage

2.2.4.1 Cartilaginous Frameworks

It is made of six (*6*) cartilages, which are held together by a series of ligaments, membranes, and muscles. The cartilages are as follows:

- Three single cartilages, namely; *Thyroid, Cricoid,* and *Epiglottis*
- Three paired cartilages, namely; *Arytenoids, Corniculates,* and *Cuneiforms*

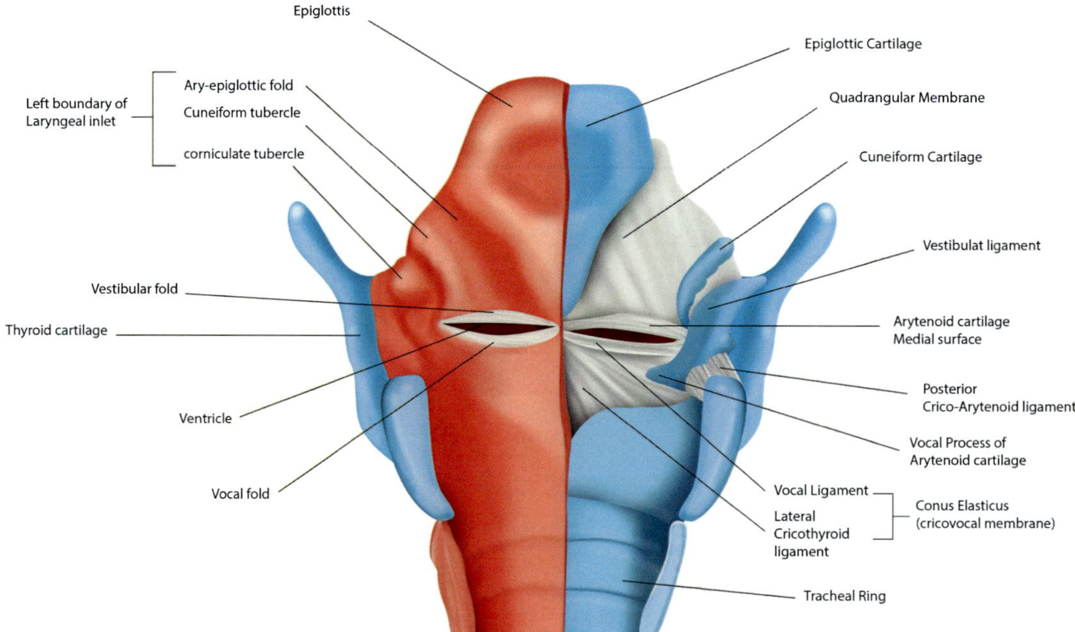

Fig. 2.2 Anatomical sagittal section for the major anatomical landmarks for the laryngeal cavity starting from laryngeal inlet to tracheal rings. The right side (blue) shows the inner laryngeal cartilages connected by ligaments. The left side (red) shows the mucosal coverings over the laryngeal cartilages, ligaments, and membranes, forming different folds

Thyroid Cartilage

It is the largest cartilage made of two laminae, two borders, two notches (superior and inferior), and two posterior horns (superior and inferior). The laryngeal prominence is formed by the anterior fusion of the two laminae in the median plane. Internally, it is connected to the other laryngeal cartilages by membranes that get thickened to form ligaments. The inner lamina is also connected to the anterior wall and vocal process of the arytenoid cartilage to form vestibular ligament and vocal ligament, respectively. It is connected superiorly to the hyoid bone and inferiorly to the *cricoid* cartilage by *thyrohyoid* membrane and median *cricothyroid* ligament, respectively. The thyrohyoid membrane condenses medially to form the *median thyrohyoid ligament* and laterally to form the *lateral thyrohyoid ligament.*

Cricoid Cartilage

It is a signet-shaped cartilagenous ring and the only complete ring of the larynx. The posterior lamina thicker and longer than the anterior one. It provides attachment for intrinsic laryngeal muscles and articulates with the arytenoid cartilage by cricoarytenoid joint. The anterior lamina is attached to the thyroid cartilage with cricothyroid membrane (CTM), an important landmark for emergency access to the airway by cricothyroidotomy. The control of the cricothyroid joint offers gliding, rocking, and rotational changes of the vocal cord length.

Epiglottis Cartilage

It is a leaf-shaped cartilage that acts as a guard for the laryngeal inlet. As it is a movable flap-like cartilage, it becomes stabilized by ligamentous attachments to the surrounding structures. It is attached to the pharyngeal root "base" of the tongue, hyoid bone, thyroid, and arytenoid cartilage by glosso-epiglottic ligament, hyo-epiglottic ligament, thyro-epiglottic ligament, and ayro-epiglottic ligament, respectively. The *Valleculae* are formed by a mucosal recess between the median and lateral glosso-epiglottic ligament. During direct laryngoscopy, the *Valleculae* is the site of the laryngeal lift by the direct laryngoscopes.

Arytenoid Cartilage

It is two pyramidal-shaped cartilages with one apex, two processes, and three walls. The processes include lateral muscular process and the anteromedial vocal process as an attachment for the vocal cords. The arytenoid cartilage lies on the posterior part of the larynx and articulates with the superior border of the lateral surface of the posterior lamina of the cricoid cartilage. The ayro-epiglottic fold is formed by *quadrangular* ligament attaching the apex of arytenoid cartilage to the epiglottis. In the *ayro-epiglottic* fold, the *corniculate* cartilage is articulating with the apex of the arytenoid cartilage.

Corniculate Cartilage (Cartilages of Santorini)

It's a horn-shaped elastic cartilage, located at the apex of each arytenoid cartilage.

Cuneiform Cartilage (Cartilages of Wrisberg)

These are two small, wedge-shaped elastic cartilage, placed on either side, in the aryepiglottic fold anterior to corniculate cartilages.

2.2.4.2 Laryngeal Muscles and Ligaments

Muscles

There are two groups of muscles: extrinsic and intrinsic. The extrinsic passes between the larynx and the surrounding parts, and the intrinsic is confined entirely.

Extrinsic Group

They connect the laryngeal cartilages with the surrounding structures. They support the position of the larynx within the mid-cervical region and aid axial movements of the larynx and hyoid.

- Depressors of the larynx include *Sternothyroid, Omohyoid, Sternohyoid,* and *Inferior constrictor muscles*
- Elevators of the larynx include *Thyrohyoid, Stylohyoid, Mylohyoid, Geniohyoid,*

Hyoglossus, Genioglossus, and *Digastric muscles*

Intrinsic Group

They internally connect the laryngeal cartilages together, thus having respiratory and phonatory functions. It mainly changes the length and tension of the vocal cords as well as sizes and shapes of the Rima Glottidis. It includes the following; *Cricothyroid, Thyroarytenoid, Posterior Cricoarytenoid, Lateral Cricoarytenoid, Transverse Arytenoid*, and *Oblique Arytenoid* muscles. Most of the intrinsic muscles are attached to the arytenoid cartilage for its complex articulation and its critical attachment to the false and true vocal cord, except the *Cricothyroid* muscle, the only intrinsic muscle that lies outside the laryngeal cavity has not attachment with arytenoid cartilage. The *Cricothyroid* lengthens and tenses the vocal folds. The *Posterior Cricoarytenoid* abducts and externally rotates the arytenoid cartilages, resulting in abducted vocal folds, and it is the only muscle to do that function. The *Lateral Cricoarytenoid* muscle adducts and internally rotates the arytenoid cartilages, increasing medial compression. The *Transverse Arytenoid muscle* adducts the arytenoid cartilages, resulting in adducted vocal folds; oblique arytenoid, which narrows the laryngeal inlet by constricting the distance between the arytenoid cartilages. The *Thyroarytenoid* muscle "sphincter of vestibule" narrows the laryngeal inlet and shortening the vocal folds and lowering voice pitch. All muscles are innervated by branches of the *Vagus* nerve (CN X). All intrinsic muscles are innervated by the *recurrent laryngeal nerve* expect *Cricothyroid* muscle by external branch of the superior laryngeal nerve.

Ligaments

The *vestibular* fold "false cord" is formed by vestibular ligament, which attaches the anterior wall of the arytenoid cartilage to the thyroid cartilage. The vocal fold "true cord" is formed by vocal ligament, which attaches the vocal process of the arytenoid cartilage to the laminal junction of the thyroid cartilage. The laryngeal ventricle is a mucosal recess formed between the vocal fold and the vestibular fold. The *fibroelastic* membrane of the larynx is formed by the quadrangular ligament superiorly and vestibular ligament inferiorly.

2.2.4.3 Neurovascular Supply

All motor supply of the muscles is by the recurrent laryngeal branch of the vagus (CN X) except for the cricothyroid muscle.

The *superior laryngeal nerve is a* branch of the vagus (CN X) divides into two branches as follows:

- The *internal laryngeal nerve* (sensory and autonomic): along with the superior laryngeal artery penetrates the thyrohyoid membrane to supply the sensory fibers to the laryngeal mucosa from the laryngeal vestibule until the superior surface of the conus elasticus and the vocal folds.
- The *external laryngeal nerve* (motor): descends posterior to the sternothyroid muscle along with the superior thyroid artery. It then pierces the inferior pharyngeal constrictor to contribute to the pharyngeal plexus and continues to supply the cricothyroid muscle (the only muscle it supplies).

The *recurrent laryngeal nerve* injury will paralyze all laryngeal muscles it supplies, but the final positions of the vocal folds depend on its predominant site of injury.

- When the abductor muscles are affected, then it leads to a medial position, which affects breathing, necessitating an emergency airway access.
- When the adductor group of muscles is affected, it will end on a lateral position affecting phonation.
- If the injury affects abductor and adductor muscles equally, then the fold will end on an intermediate position affecting both breathing and phonation.

2.2.4.4 Vascular Supply

The *arterial supply* of the upper portion is supplied by the pharyngeal branches of the external carotid artery, the maxillary artery, and the facial artery "palatine and tonsillar." The superior thyroid and the inferior thyroid arteries supply the caudal portion of the pharynx.

The *venous drainage* is by the pharyngeal venous plexus that lies between the prevertebral fascia and the constrictor muscles and drains by the pterygoid venous plexus and the internal jugular and facial veins. Excessive neck anteflexion and tight neck straps for ETT have been reported to cause laryngeal edema, necessitating intubation and respiratory support in the postoperative period.

2.2.5 Hyoid Bone

It is a U-shaped bone with a body and two horns, namely greater and lesser horns. With no bony articulation, it is anchored by the stylohyoid ligament to styloid processes and by the thyrohyoid membrane to the thyroid cartilage. It offers the origin for the intrinsic tongue muscles and the attachment to the pharyngeal constrictors.

Clinical Pearls:

- The *airway patency* is a common term in airway management that refers to the ability of the airway passages to stay open so that ventilation and oxygenation could be carried on. The airway patency is an interaction of collapsing forces and the protective dilatory mechanism including the structural and neuroprotective reflexes. The *Retropalatal* space *"velopharyngeal space"* has been proven by MRI studies to be the main common site for airway obstruction under anesthesia/sedation in normal healthy adults' images. The base of the tongue and epiglottis are the other sources of airway obstruction. Historically, the base of the tongue was thought to be the main reason for the obstruction of the airway under sleep, sedation, and anesthesia (kindly refer to Fig. 2.1).
- The *Genioglossus* muscle plays a major role in decreasing the tendency of airway to collapse in obstructive sleep apnea (OSA) patients during the awake state. Electromyographical studies showed that OSA patients have significantly greater basal genioglossal muscle activity than age and body mass index (BMI) matched non-OSA subjects during wakefulness, suggesting that the compensatory mechanism to open the airway is exaggerated during awake state and is being lost during sleep, leading to oropharyngeal collapse [1, 2].
- In patients with *Obstructive Sleep Apnea (OSA)*, the pharyngeal volumes change due to either local factors such as mucosal edema and fat deposition in the lateral pharyngeal wall or depressed protective mechanisms as proven by CT and MRI studies [3–5]. The compressive effects of deposited fatty tissue around the pharynx therefore may increase upper airway collapsibility and possibly offset the effects of dilator muscles that maintain airway patency [6, 7]. The anteroposterior (AP) diameter in OSA patients is more prominent than the transverse diameter, contrary to the normal condition. The continuous positive airway pressure (CPAP) is expected to increase the pharyngeal volume by increasing the transverse diameter.
- *Deglutition* "swallowing" is a very complex mechanism that necessitates a lot of neuromuscular coordination. The pharyngeal isthmus closes by elevation of the soft palate to the posterior pharyngeal wall. The *velopharyngeal insufficiency* (VPI) is a disorder in the closing mechanism of palatopharyngeal isthmus during phonation and deglutition due to either structural or neuromuscular disorders, which leads to nasal resonance phonation and nasal regurgitation.
- *Laryngospasm* is a protective glottic closure reflex that starts initially due to stimulation of the internal branch of the superior laryngeal nerve in the supraglottic region; however, repetitive stimulations could induce focal seizure in the laryngeal adductors innervated by recurrent laryngeal nerve. Other nerves have also been reported but with a lesser degree of closure, such as trigeminal and glossopharyngeal, can produce

a lesser degree of reflex glottic closure [8]. The reflex could be initiated by different stimuli such as saline, secretion, suctioning, or a foreign body. The reflex could be either transient or persistent, but usually it is aborted by developing hypoxia. Removal of the stimulus, deepening the anesthetic depth, or using even short-acting muscle relaxants are the most common techniques to abort the spasm.

- Supraglottic devices (*SGDs*) or laryngeal mask airways (LMA) are commonly used in modern anesthesia instead of classical tracheal intubation. The properly inserted LMA cuff is positioned over the inferior pharyngeal constrictor, and the tip is placed against the upper esophageal sphincter at the lower border of the hypopharynx (vertebral level of C6) (Fig. 2.3). However, because of its popularity and reliability, malposition after insertion has been documented by many manikin and human studies, reaching around 50–80% of patients [9]. The tip of epiglottis has been confirmed to be displaced over the bowl of the SGD in 50% in

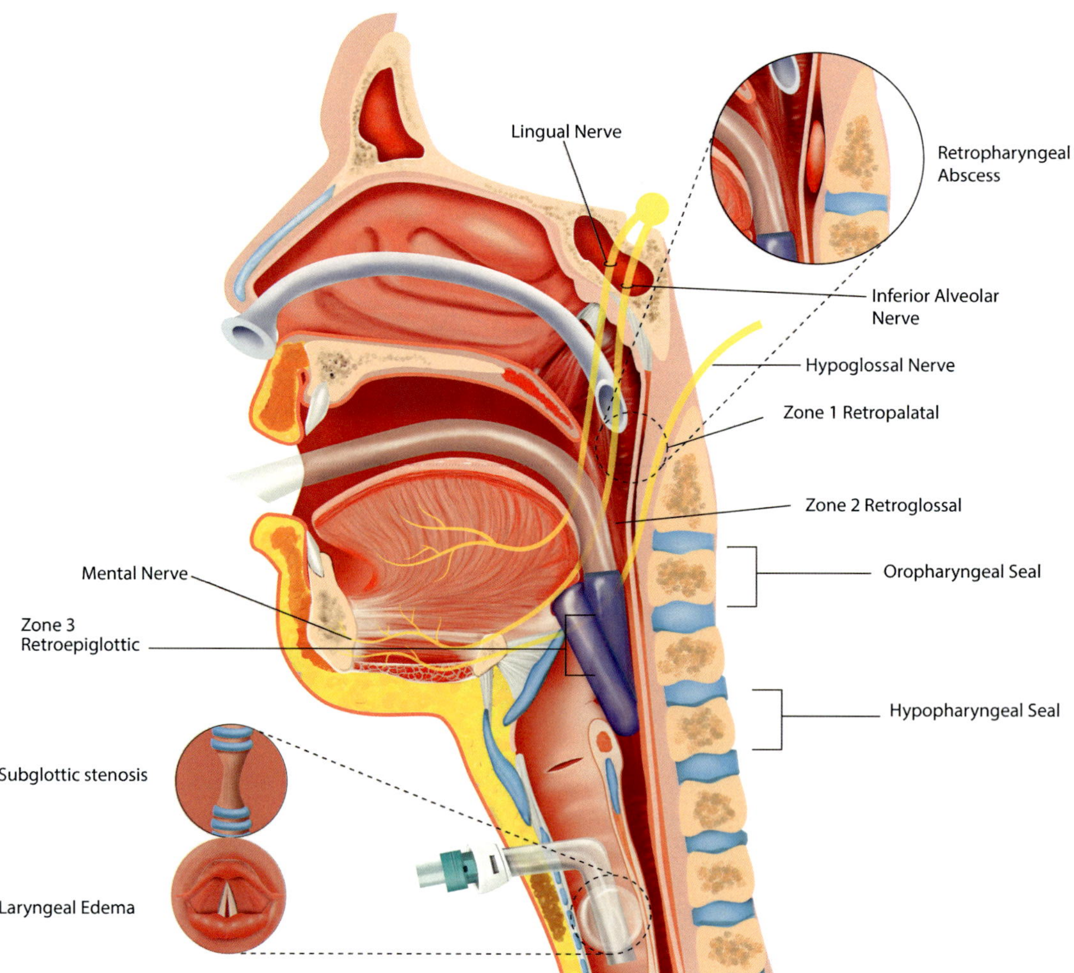

Fig. 2.3 Anatomical sagittal section for the most commonly used airway devices with its related anatomical landmarks. The three potential spaces for airway collapse are highlighted, namely retropalatal, retroglossal, and retroepiglottic. Nasal airway and LMA could play a role to prevent the sedation-induced airway collapse. It also shows a diagram for a properly positioned LMA, facing the laryngeal inlet and sealing the esophageal entry. Serious and life-threatening airway problems such as retropharyngeal abscess, subglottic stenosis, laryngeal edema, and rare LMA-induced neuropathy are demonstrated

fiber-optic studies or deflected in 80% to posterior pharynx in CT studies [10, 11]. A malpositioned SGDs could be clinically tolerated for short procedures; however, they can be a cause for significant leakage, airway trauma, obstruction, regurgitation, or gastric distension with mechanical ventilation (kindly refer to Fig. 2.3).

- Inappropriate *LMA* usage has been attributed to cranial nerve palsy, most commonly the recurrent laryngeal nerve, then the lingual nerve, a mandibular branch from the trigeminal nerve, and then a hypoglossal nerve. Excessive cuff inflation, >60 cm H_2O, failure to measure and adjust the cuff pressure, and inappropriate size selection were all reported as leading causes for complications (refer to Fig. 2.3).

- *Arytenoid subluxation (AS) and arytenoid dislocation (AD)* are disorders of the cricothyroid joint that occurs mainly from traumatic intubation; however, other less common etiologies have been reported, such as a blunt external neck trauma, chronic joint disorders, and congenital musculoskeletal disorders. Both could be misdiagnosed with recurrent laryngeal nerve injury.

2.3 Summary and Conclusion

A profound knowledge of the airway is necessary for anesthesiologists to deliver safe anesthetic practice and manage better complicated airway. This chapter reviewed the airway anatomy, with main focus on the clinical relevance and its applied usefulness in airway management.

References

1. Mezzanotte WS, Tangel DJ, White DP. Waking genioglossal electromyogram in sleep apnea patients versus normal controls (a neuromuscular compensatory mechanism). J Clin Invest. 1992;89(5):1571–9. http://www.ncbi.nlm.nih.gov/pubmed/1569196

2. Mezzanotte WS, Tangel DJ, White DP. Influence of sleep onset on upper-airway muscle activity in apnea patients versus normal controls. Am J Respir Crit Care Med. 1996;153(6 Pt 1):1880–7.. http://www.ncbi.nlm.nih.gov/pubmed/8665050

3. Haponik EF, Smith PL, Bohlman ME, Allen RP, Goldman SM, Bleecker ER. Computerized tomography in obstructive sleep apnea. Correlation of airway size with physiology during sleep and wakefulness. Am Rev Respir Dis. 1983;127(2):221–6.. http://www.ncbi.nlm.nih.gov/pubmed/6830039

4. Schwab RJ, Gupta KB, Gefter WB, Metzger LJ, Hoffman EA, Pack AI. Upper airway and soft tissue anatomy in normal subjects and patients with sleep-disordered breathing. Significance of the lateral pharyngeal walls. Am J Respir Crit Care Med. 1995;152(5 Pt 1):1673–89.. http://www.ncbi.nlm.nih.gov/pubmed/7582313

5. Trudo FJ, Gefter WB, Welch KC, Gupta KB, Maislin G, Schwab RJ. State-related changes in upper airway caliber and surrounding soft-tissue structures in normal subjects. Am J Respir Crit Care Med. 1998;158(4):1259–70.. http://www.ncbi.nlm.nih.gov/pubmed/9769290

6. Patil SP, Schneider H, Schwartz AR, Smith PL. Adult obstructive sleep apnea: pathophysiology and diagnosis. Chest. 2007;132(1):325–37.. http://www.ncbi.nlm.nih.gov/pubmed/17625094

7. Isono S. Obstructive sleep apnea of obese adults: pathophysiology and perioperative airway management. Anesthesiology. 2009;110(4):908–21. https://doi.org/10.1097/ALN.0b013e31819c74be.

8. Sasaki CT, Suzuki M. Laryngeal spasm: a neurophysiologic redefinition. Ann Otol Rhinol Laryngol. 2018;86(2 pt. 1):150–7.. http://www.ncbi.nlm.nih.gov/pubmed/848825

9. Aoyama K, Takenaka I, Sata T, Shigematsu A. The triple airway manoeuvre for insertion of the laryngeal mask airway in paralyzed patients. Can J Anaesth. 1995;42(11):1010–6.. http://www.ncbi.nlm.nih.gov/pubmed/8590489

10. Joshi S, Sciacca RR, Solanki DR, Young WL, Mathru MM. A prospective evaluation of clinical tests for placement of laryngeal mask airways. Anesthesiology. 1998;89(5):1141–6.. http://www.ncbi.nlm.nih.gov/pubmed/9822002

11. Payne J. The use of the fibreoptic laryngoscope to confirm the position of the laryngeal mask. Anaesthesia. 1989;44(10):865. https://doi.org/10.1111/j.1365-2044.1989.tb09121.x.

Radiological Evaluation of the Airway: One-Stop Shop

3

Abbas H. Moustafa and Nabil A. Shallik

3.1 Introduction

The airway, which is an inherent curved anatomical complex matrix, makes the evaluation of its distensibility and the potential collapse a great obstacle and challenge for proper assessment. The aero-digestive airway is unique regarding its anatomical and functional perspectives. It is a common pathway for respiratory and digestive systems and composed of potentially collapsible air-filled space (especially its proximal portion) with epithelial lined musculocutaneous components [1, 2].

Due to its wide range of anatomical variations, it is crucial to be fully aware of the detailed radiological anatomy of the distinguished anatomical part of the body with many variants for better interpretation [3–5].

Electronic Supplementary Material The online version of this chapter (https://doi.org/10.1007/978-3-030-23253-5_3) contains supplementary material, which is available to authorized users.

A. H. Moustafa (✉)
Department of Clinical Radiology and Medical Imaging, Hamad Medical Corporation, Doha, Qatar

Department of Diagnostic Radiology and Medical Imaging, El Minia University, El Minia, Egypt
e-mail: AMoustafa4@hamad.qa

N. A. Shallik
Department of Anesthesiology, ICU and Perioperative Medicine, Hamad Medical Corporation, Doha, Qatar

3.2 History

Before the era of computed tomography (CT), plain radiography, conventional tomography, and barium studies, as well as laryngography using water-soluble contrast have been employed for several years with numerous constraints in their clinical impact. First of all, the superimposition effect of the different anatomical structures in the plain radiography hinders the proper visualization of the airway-related structures. This issue was partially solved by the introduction of the conventional tomography techniques at the expense of more radiation dosage given to the patient [1, 6, 7].

For decades, evaluation of the airways was extremely limited and was resorted to by plain radiography in both anteroposterior and lateral views. It was quite limited due to the effect of superimposition of the overlying osseous, cartilaginous, and soft tissues. Laryngo-graphic evaluation using the positive contrast agent "Hytrast" was introduced into clinical practice for evaluation of the airways.

Department of Clinical Anesthesiology, Weill Cornell Medical College in Qatar (WCMQ), Doha, Qatar

Department of Anesthesiology and Surgical Intensive Care, Faculty of Medicine, Tanta University, Tanta, Egypt
e-mail: Nshallik@hamad.qa

© Springer Nature Switzerland AG 2019
N. A. Shallik et al. (eds.), *Virtual Endoscopy and 3D Reconstruction in the Airways*,
https://doi.org/10.1007/978-3-030-23253-5_3

It was a relatively difficult examination for the patient in particular; local anesthetic is to be sprayed profusely into the larynx and pharynx in order to overcome the gag reflex, with potential risk of aspiration during the procedure and frequent cough that interferes with the quality of the examination and the patient welfare [6, 7] (Fig. 3.1).

Shortly after the advent of the conventional tomography procedure, the case became relatively better. However, it entails the higher radiation dose given to the patient in this particular precious part of the body containing several radiosensitive structures including the eye globes, eye lens, salivary glands, and thyroid gland [8].

After the introduction of the computed tomography (CT) in 1979 by Sir Alan McCormick and Godfrey into the medical field and radiological evaluation, the situation has tremendously changed with better evaluation of the different segments of the airway; the surrounding soft tissues and vascular structures became more distinct and better evaluated. The evolution of computed tomography (CT) generations starting from the first generation, where the scanning time and the reconstruction time were significantly prolonged, passing through the slip-ring technology, and lastly with spiral/helical and multidetector computed tomography (MDCT) further improved the status, and introduction of the mega computers with more and more storage capacity made evaluation of the airway even easier and more elaborative [9].

Historically, CT scanning of paranasal sinuses and the neck region was done using separate direct axial and coronal scan acquisitions. But nowadays, these are acquired volumetrically using multi-detector CT scan machines (or spiral CT scan if multi-detector scanners are not available). Unenhanced thin volumetric axial images are

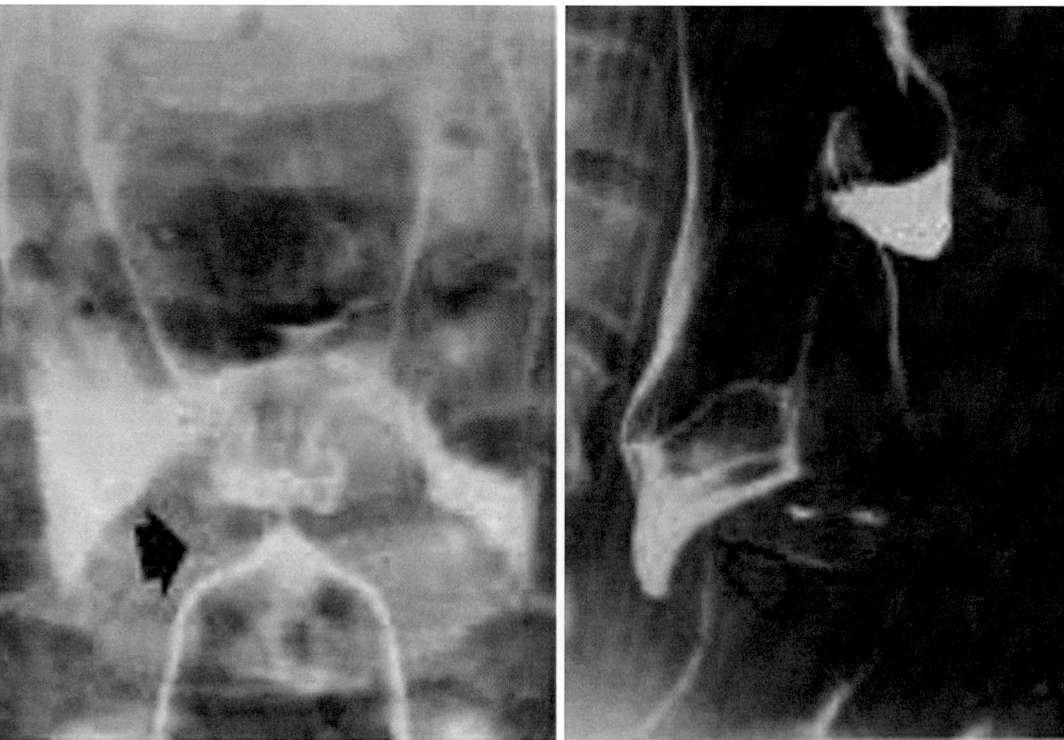

Fig. 3.1 AP and lateral views of the larynx showing well delineation by Hytrast (positive contrast). This procedure (laryngogram) is now obsolete after the advent of CT. Arrow is pointing to the vocal cord level

acquired and reconstructed to thinner 0.625 mm axial images. From these axial images, multi-planar reconstructions (MPR) are done in sagittal and coronal planes at 1–2 mm intervals. Both high-resolution bone and soft tissue algorithm reconstructions in all three planes can be made to analyze the images. The imaging is performed with the patient in the supine position without any CT gantry tilt, and the field of view includes ears, entire maxilla, tip of nose, chin, and frontal sinuses to ensure compatibility with functional endoscopic sinus surgery (FESS) navigation software. A flat depiction of the 3-D data set called maximum intensity projection (MIP) can also be done by highlighting selected threshold limits [10].

This was accompanied by state-of-the art technology in computers and mega storage that opened the gate toward the era of three-dimensional imaging field as well as virtual endoscopic studies. David Vining was the first person worldwide who introduced virtual bronchoscopy into clinical practice, and he presented his first presentation about virtual bronchoscopy at the radiological society of North America RSNA 1993 Chicago, USA, and after that, it was followed by the introduction of virtual colonoscopy, virtual angioscopy, etc., and lastly, the effect of virtual osteoscopy, which was introduced by the author with navigation into the

compact bone substance and ended with the discovery of the "calvarial butterfly" within the occipital bone between the internal and external occipital protuberance, which is considered as a "fingerprint" with unique criteria and features distinct for every individual adding to the criteria of Forensic Medicine and Anthropology [11–14] (Fig.3.2).

Evaluation of the airways is an extremely difficult task, and for several decades, it was heavily dependent on the clinical evaluation, which is extremely subjective, and Mallampati scoring and different measurement, which is beyond the scope of this chapter; so, it will be discussed in full detail in another chapter (V) within the context of this book.

It is extremely important to evaluate the airways, especially for those patients with suspected or anticipated difficult intubation, for instance, Mallampati score 3 or 4, and previous history of difficult intubation due to any reason, for instance, short neck with limited mobility or patients with severe facial trauma. Any congenital anomalies within the head and neck, limiting the opening of the mouth, probably due to lesions within the temporomandibular joint including dislocation or traumatic fractures, will also interfere with the easy intubation maneuver [15].

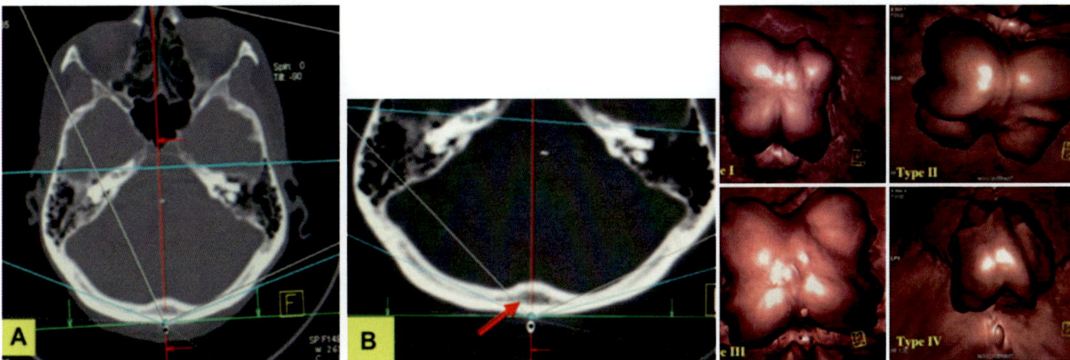

Fig. 3.2 (**a**) Virtual osteoscopy technique showing axial MDCT slice at the level of the occipital protuberance with the virtual endoscope in place. (**b**) Bone window setting of the bony calvarium (occipital bone) showing marrow within diploic space at the occipital region (orange arrow). The colored platen shows the four types of calvarial butterfly

3.3 Multi-detector CT Evaluation of the Airway

Multi-detector CT scans of the head and neck proved to be of significant value and great impact in the evaluation of the airway from inside and outside perspectives.

Criteria and parameters of the airway MDCT evaluation include the following:

3.3.1 Coverage

The coverage area of the examination should be between the skull base superiorly down to the level of the tracheal bifurcation (Carina level) [16].

3.3.2 Radiation Dose and Potential Hazards and Dose Modulation

There is a large debate regarding the radiation hazards from using the CT in this vital and crucial part of the body that contains many radiosensitive organs and structures including the eye lens with potential hazards of early cataract, the thyroid gland as well as the salivary glands including the submandibular and parotids with deterministic effects. The risk/benefit ratio should be the decision maker in such circumstances; besides, the modern technology in recent days with the development of many dose regulation and modification (radiation dose modulation) techniques helped a lot in reducing the radiation dosage without compromise upon the diagnostic quality of the resultant images [8, 17–21].

3.3.3 Special Instruction

3.3.3.1 Modified Valsalva Maneuver

As described above regarding the potential partially collapsible airway track during rest and normal breathing, the simple trick of asking the patient to do a "modified Valsalva maneuver" is by asking him/her to have a very deep inspiration, hold it inside, and to get it exhaled slowly through a slit-like orifice from the lips with buffed cheeks. This will help in increasing intrathoracic pressure to as much as 80 mmHg and subsequently result in full distension of the collapsed airway fully and open the potentially under-filled different segments with air. The patient has to be trained for this maneuver prior to the CT exposure and make sure that he will obey the commands perfectly during the exposure time, which usually lasts for around 20–25 s at the maximum. It has a great impact to distend the potentially collapsible fibromuscular airways structures for better evaluation (Fig. 3.3). It will distend the valleculae, pyriform sinuses, the vocal cords, and the different segments of the airways, including the nasopharynx, oropharynx, and hypopharynx for better evaluation and to depict any subtle or trivial pathologies, as well as obtain nice comprehensive (three-dimensional) 3-D images in the reconstructions as well as the virtual endoscopy (VE). Not only that, but also it will prevent the patient from swallowing, coughing, or deglutition, which may result in unavoidable motion artifacts that ultimately degrade the resultant 3-D images and VRT models as well as the VE [22, 23].

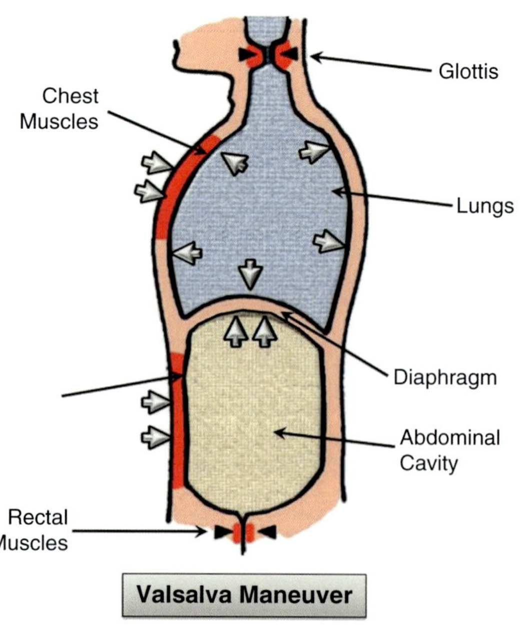

Fig. 3.3 Shows Valsalva maneuver and increased pressure inside different body cavities (hand-drawn by the author)

3.3.3.2 Gentle Neck Extension

A considerable neck extension is mandatory during the patient's intubation. Subsequently, it is important to evaluate the cervical spine integrity, alignment, presence or absence of fractures or subluxations and any pathology to give the anesthesiologist colleague a comprehensive data prior to the anesthesia procedure.

3.3.4   Evaluation of the Cervical Spine

Special attention should be paid to the patients with severe polytrauma for proper assessment of their cervical spine integrity. It is extremely difficult to clinically assess the cervical spine in a comatose or agitated post-traumatic patient with the potential risk of grave injury including atlanto-axial subluxation or dislocation, presence of cord compression with severe implication of the spinal canal due to traumatic pathology, etc. Not only that, but also the limited mobility which might be encountered due to associated ankylosing spondylitis of DISH syndromes (diffuse idiopathic skeletal hyperostosis) of extensive ligamentous calcification, which might alter the manipulation of the head extension to open the airway during the intubation procedure (Fig. 3.4). The presence of instability of the cervical and proximal dorsal spine can be evaluated easily, especially by the application of the curved multiplanar reconstruction protocol (C-MPR) as a post-processing procedure, and subsequently, evaluation of the level and extent of the pathology can be easily depicted. The presence of exuberant osteophyte complexes can also be evaluated [24].

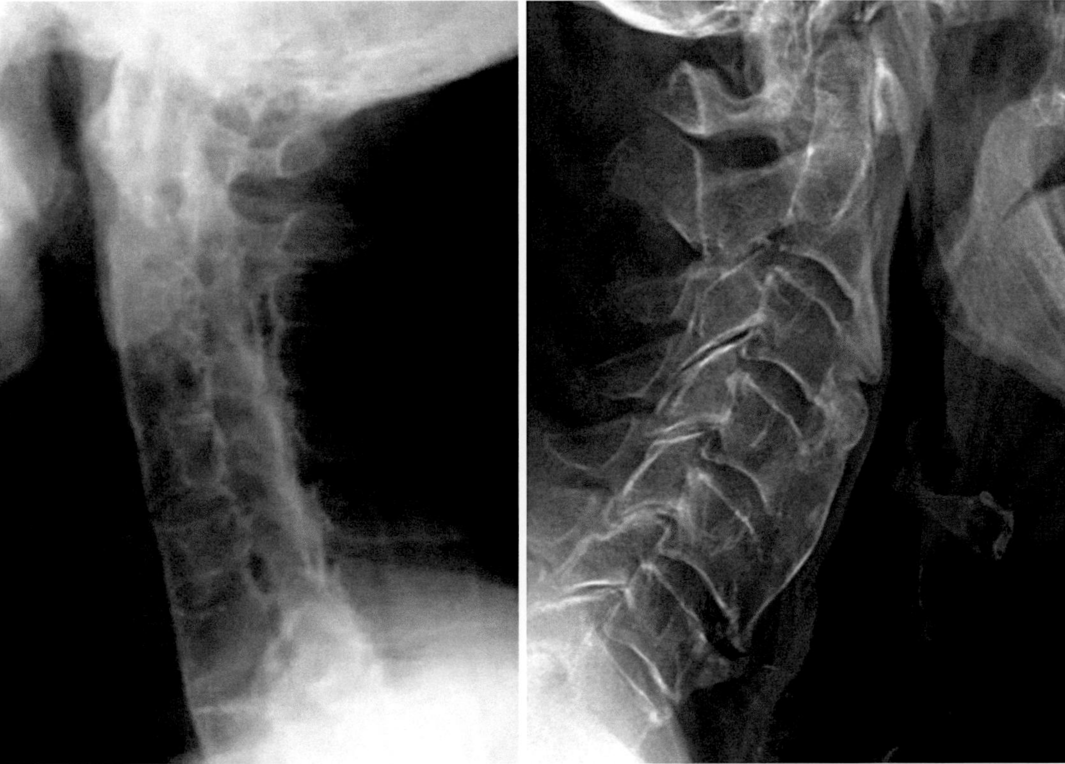

Fig. 3.4 Lateral views for the cervical spine; the left one showing radiographic evidence of ankylosing spondylitis and the right one showing DISH changes

3.3.5 Teeth, Maxillary, and Mandibular Arches Evaluation

Evaluation of the Maxillary Arch and the Mandible Evaluation:

From the medicolegal point of view, it is very essential to assess the condition of the teeth prior to anesthesia maneuvers of tracheal intubation procedures; any loss of teeth, aspiration, or fracture will be counted on the anesthesiologist or the attending Accident and Emergency (A&E) or the intensive care unit (ICU) physician. So, and from this point of view, curved MPR reconstructions of the maxillary arch as well as the mandible are done by obtaining orthopantomogram-like images (OPG-panoramic view) (Fig.3.5) (Movie 3.1), and the details of the teeth integrity, lost ones, fractures or loss of the lamina dura, and integrity of the temporomandibular joints are obtained to check whether there is an element of dislocation or subluxation. All this valuable information can be obtained in a single-shot reconstructed image and subsequently will enrich the data provided to the physician colleagues and prevent any potential medico-legal negligence issues, which might supervene [25].

3.4 Post-processing Techniques

Evaluation of the airway using 3-D reconstruction with the resultant images will give more comprehensive evaluation for our colleagues in the other subspecialties, especially those dealing with the head and neck regions including the ENT, head and neck surgeons, and maxillofacial subspecialties, not only that but also our colleagues from ICU, anesthesia, and emergency departments. The anatomy of the resultant images

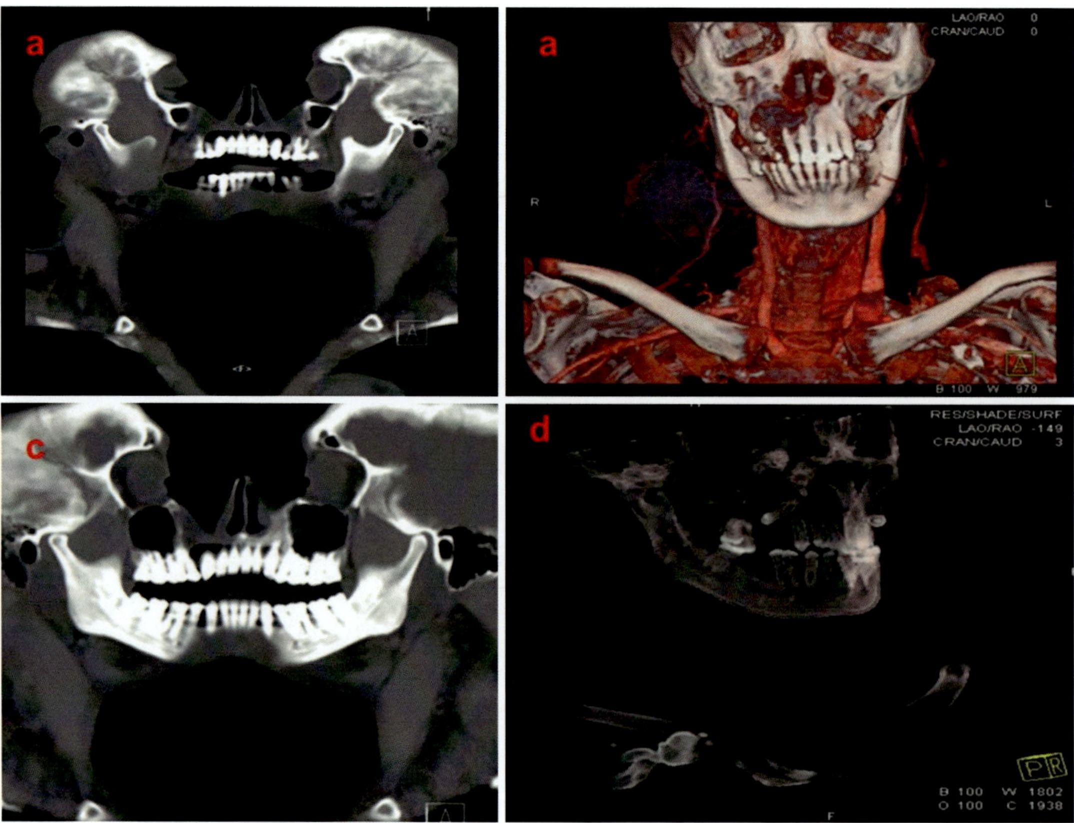

Fig. 3.5 Shows orthopantomogram (left sided images) and OPG-panoramic views and VRT reconstruction (right sided images) from CT volumetric study MDCT

is far easier to comprehend compared to those of cross section or the reconstructed coronal or axial images. Easy understanding of the magnitude and extent of the pathological entity will greatly impact the management with resultant better clinical outcome.

It is crucial to be familiar with the 3-D reconstructed image anatomy in order to read the images faster and more precisely.

This includes the evaluation of the airway proper using tissue transparent projection (TTP) and volume-rendering techniques (VRT) protocols. These techniques are preset in most of the commercially available workstations and could be even manipulated and modulated according to the clinical scenarios and situation pre-requisite. The generated VRT and TTP models can elaborate the inner and outer surfaces of the reconstructed image. The surrounding osseous, soft tissue, muscular, and vascular structures are well demonstrated and subsequently better perception of the anatomical relationship for the clinicians will help in better judgment and decision-making [10] (Fig. 3.6).

3.4.1 Evaluation of the 3-D Models in 360° Along Any Axis Freely

The resultant 3-D images can be demonstrated and displayed along any axis freely at 360°, features that give more perspectives and hidden relations that cannot be appreciated by any other modalities (Movie 3.2).

3.5 Surface Rendering

Surface rendering provides a three-dimensional view of the surface structures by defining thresholds to determine the inclusion or exclusion of pixels, which are the tiny elements forming a two-dimensional image. Voxel is an individual volume element or the smallest distinguishable volume part of a 3-D space, which merge to create the 3-D model, analogous to a 2-D image formed by pixels [26]. The 3-D model is created by linking the contours of objects from one CT scan section to those in

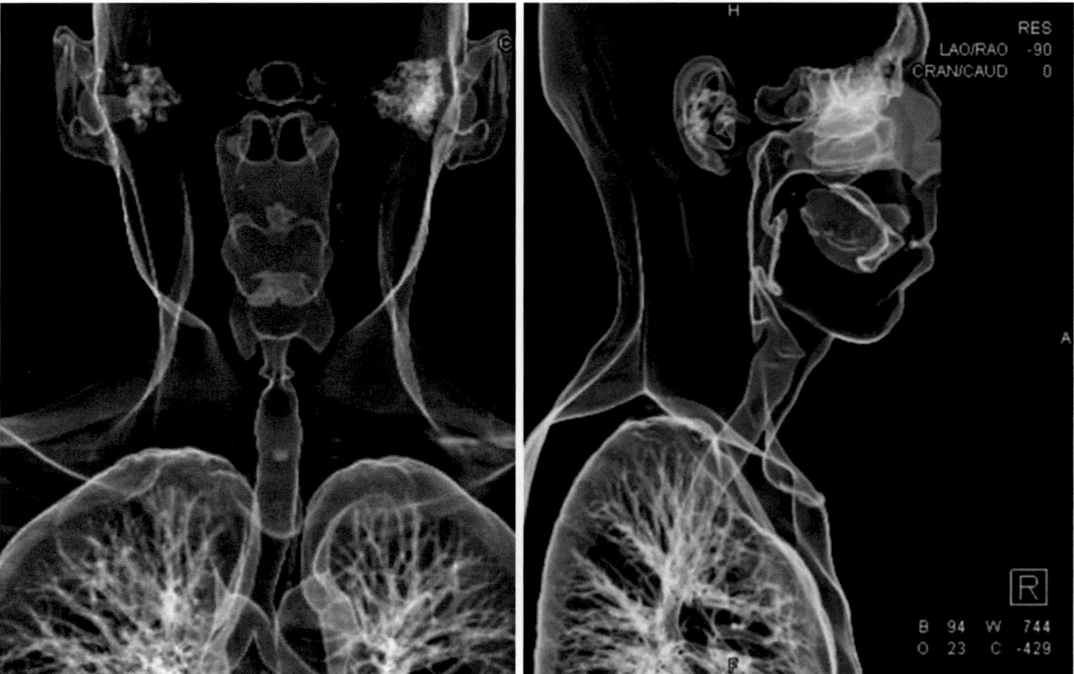

Fig. 3.6 TTP VRT tissue transparent projection of the airway AP and lateral projections; however, these reconstruction models can be projected easily and freely with 360°

adjacent slices [27]. Segmentation is an intermediate step in the process to transform the volume into a mesh of polygons, which are then transformed into the 3-D model by software [26]. The complex segmentation steps are usually semiautomatic [26, 27].

Surface-rendered structures can be subjected to shading techniques to highlight them further, and this is called surface shaded display (SSD) (Fig.3.7). Surface shading can be based on the orientation of the surface or the distance of the surface from the observer and can aid in the appreciation of the position of one structure relative to another [28]. Threshold ranges from −520 to −200 Hounsfield units (HU) are used to avoid voxels denser than −500 HU. The thresholds of −250 and −400 HU can be used to optimally view the various sinonasal structures in healthy controls and those with sinonasal disease. Surface rendering has reduced definition and accuracy, as there could be data loss regarding the inner aspects of the objects under display [28–30].

3.6   Volume Rendering (VR)

Volume rendering is performed by software by casting rays from an observation point through the remaining part of the volume being visualized. This observation point can be either outside the volume or from within it. Unlike the surface-rendering technique, which focuses solely on surface features, the volume-rendering technique also displays more 3-D information of the structures as if they are partially transparent by modifying the percentage of light ray within a voxel [26]. While the surface-rendering technique uses a set threshold, all the pixels are kept in memory in volume rendering and allows the acquisition of more information and increased detail [27]. The volume data itself is analyzed without the surface representation step of surface rendering. The quality of the final volume-rendered images depends on the quality of the original axial images like thinner slices and greater pixel image matrix [29] (Fig. 3.8).

Fig. 3.7 TTP-VRT frontal and lateral projection of the entire airway down to the tracheal bifurcation

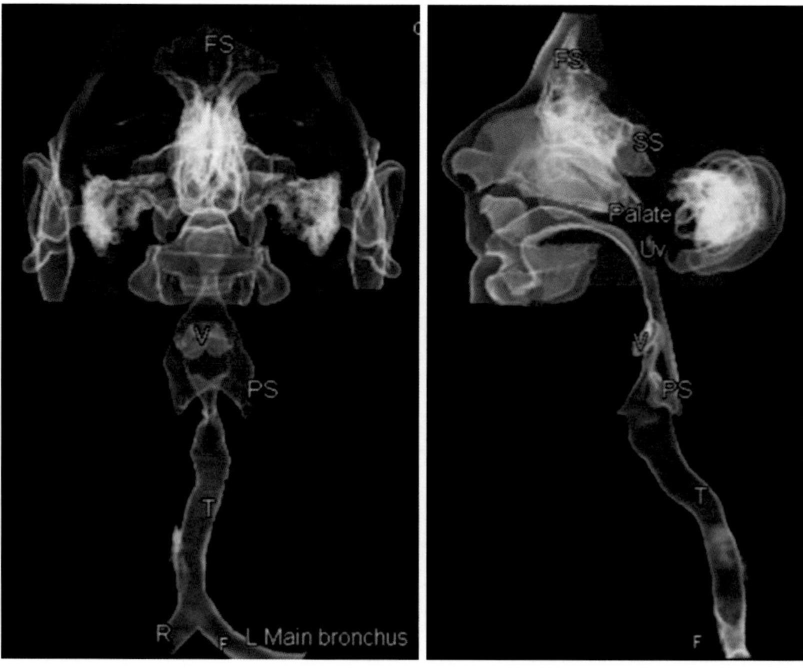

3.7 Vascular Evaluation

Evaluation of the related vessels, presence or absence of violation, displacement, or invasion is very essential. As their integrity, tear, partial injury, or leakage can be easily assessed by the CT and the advent of the reconstruction post-processing facilities even get the job more easily to depict and characterize VRT images and virtual angioscopy can give more details and precise diagnosis.

Sometimes the mystery of some cases can be easily solved, for instance, the abnormal congenital medial retropharyngeal course of the internal carotid artery presenting itself clinically as pulsating retropharyngeal mass lesion, which is well demonstrated on the reconstructed VRT image model (Fig.3.9).

The vascularity of lesions and presence of malignant circulation, arteriovenous malformation can also be easily judged [26–30].

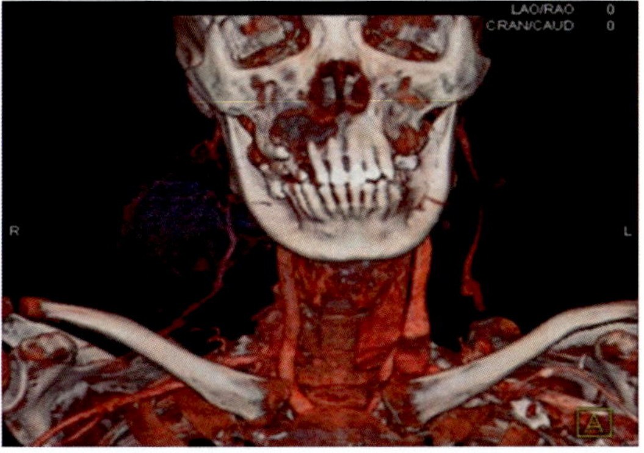

Fig. 3.8 Volume rendering techniques (VRT) or shaded surface display (SSD) for a patient with destructive mass lesion within the right of the maxilla with related floating teeth. Soft tissue right sided neck swelling with related bizzare-shaped vessels is also noted

3.8 Bone Subtraction Technique

Subtraction of the osseous bony framework helped much in more delineation of the underlying and related visceral structures and hollow organs notably the airway. However, fusion of the 3-D images for both the reconstructed airway and the bones will give added value to the diagnosis as it will give information about the extent of

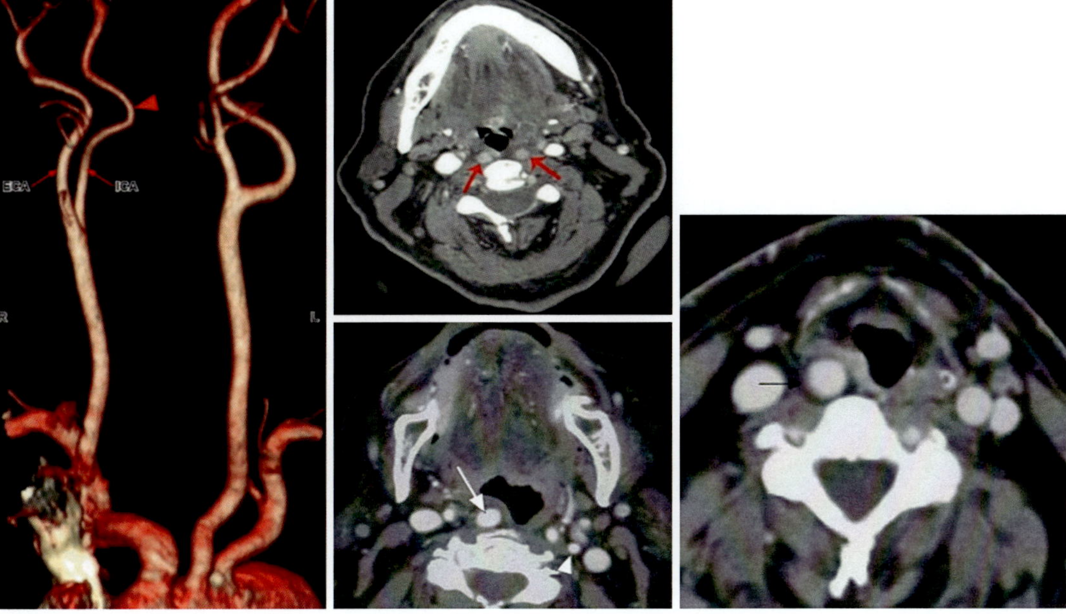

Fig. 3.9 Neck vessels including the common carotids and their bifurcation with retropharyngeal course of the internal carotid artery indenting and violating the airway (arrows)

the lesions/pathology against a fixed anatomical landmark, that is, bony structure [26, 28, 30].

3.9 Virtual Endoscopy

Noninvasive imaging of the airways has made remarkable progress and impact in the past decade. The introduction of multi-row detector CT scanners has made it possible to acquire high-resolution images of the upper, central, and segmental airways within a short time. The CT data can subsequently be reconstructed into elegant and distinguished two-dimensional (2-D) reformation and three-dimensional (3-D) images, including internal virtual endoscopic (VE) renderings that closely simulate images from conventional endoscopy. Virtual endoscopy (VE) is performed by reformatting the thin volumetric axial CT images into a 3-D model using any commercially available VE software, usually provided along with the CT scanner like in GE Advantage or Siemens *syngo* fast View workstations (most of our cases were carried out on that workstation) or even the open source commercially available ones including the RadiAnt® or Osirix®. The two principal methods of post-processing this 3-D volumetric data are surface rendering and volume rendering [26, 27, 29] (Fig.3.10) (Movie 3.3).

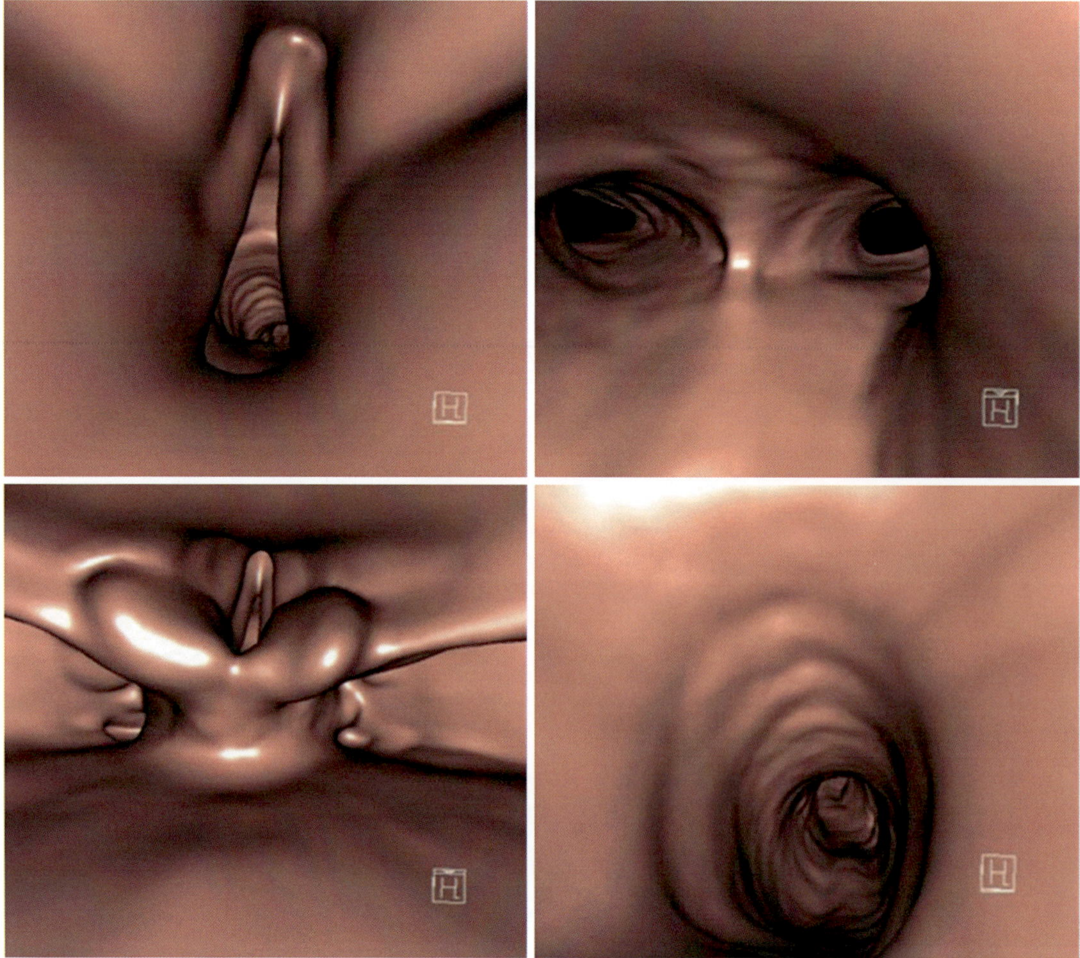

Fig. 3.10 Virtual endoscopic projections at the level of the vocal cords showing the anterior commissure and true and false cords. Tracheal bifurcation is nicely demonstrated. Supraglottic region with the aryepiglottic folds, pyriform sinuses, and the vocal cord are demonstrated. Tracheal view

3.9.1 Flight Path Generation

Commercial VE software provides a navigation tool, the virtual endoscope, which is an optical electronic apparatus to dynamically navigate an organ lumen. The virtual endoscope allows the operator to "fly through" or "sail through" along different directions and positions within the 3-D anatomy of sinonasal cavities and its path demonstrated on the computer screen simultaneously in axial, sagittal, and coronal MPR images to make the orientation easier [13] (Movie 3.4).

3.9.2 Why Virtual Endoscopy?

It has more advantages compared to the conventional one. It uses no local anesthetics; the resultant images are comparable to that of the live one, no patient's discomfort, gag reflex of vomiting and potential aspirations or laryngeal edema and spasm.

There are potential hazards of conventional endoscopy including bleeding, pneumothorax, hypoxemia, and aspiration until the effects of sedatives are alleviated. The risk of conventional endoscopy opens the gates for attempts to locate a new diagnostic risk-free tool, and VE is one of the developments in this field, which is considered a breakthrough, as it is giving similar findings using minimally invasive and far safer techniques [12].

The following table summarizes the potential hazards of conventional endoscopy.

1. Systemic complications	1. Procedure related (vasovagal syncope, nausea/vomiting, aspiration, hypoxia, hypercarbia) 2. Medication related (sedative, nonsedative medications) 3. Comorbid illness (myocardial dysfunction/arrhythmia, pulmonary insufficiency, elevated intracranial pressure, death)
2. Mechanical complications	1. Trauma (oropharyngeal, nasopharyngeal, glottic structure, vocal cord) 2. Bronchospasm/laryngospasm 3. Infection 4. Atelectasis/decruitment 5. Elevated airway pressure 6. Hemorrhage

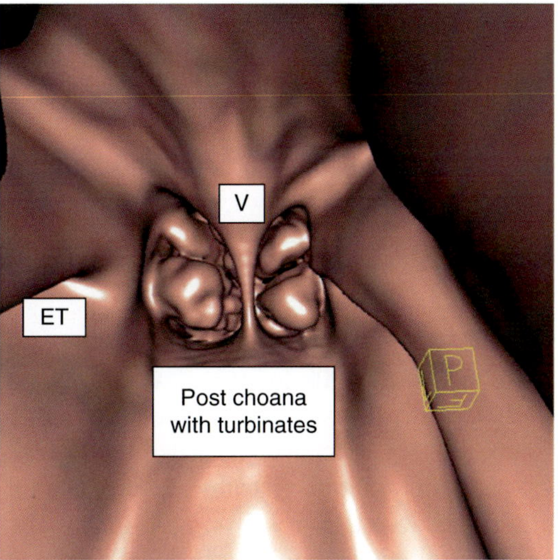

Fig. 3.11 Unique virtual endoscopy view showing the posterior nares, vomer (V), nasal turbinates, and the Eustachian tube (ET) orifices. A projection that cannot be physically duplicated with the conventional endoscope

The virtual endoscopy has more advantages in getting perspectives that cannot be duplicated by any other means, for instance, visualization of the posterior nares and the Eustachian tube orifices (Fig. 3.11), visualization of the subglottic regions, and it can navigate and flythrough narrow segment areas where the conventional endoscopy cannot pass through it and subsequently give more valuable informative data that usually and ultimately change the management of the patients [13] (Fig. 3.11).

There are many techniques for generating the flight path during virtual endoscopy, including manual camera movement, semi-automatic path planning, and automatic path planning. In manual camera movement, the position, field of view, and focal point of the camera are interactively changed by the operator, with software providing collision detection to keep the camera within the potential cavity of the lumen. In semiautomatic path generation (also known as key-framing), the operator specifies key path points having unique special and directional coordinates and field of view, which are connected by cubic splines. The computer generates a continuous interpolated flight path connecting the key views at the rate of 25-30 frames per second. In automatic path planning, the flight path is automatically computed by software once an initial and one or more end points are specified by the operator, by computing the centerline of the imaged structure. The software program records the voxel coordinates of each key point in the specified shortest path to the goal end point and smoothens the path, avoiding the obstacles like sinonasal, nasopharyngeal, oropharyngeal, or laryngeal walls identifying those using ranges of threshold values. A typical flight path is planned through the air containing nostrils, nasal cavities, and natural drainage pathway and ostia of paranasal sinuses, like entering the maxillary sinus through hiatus semilunaris and the frontal sinus through frontal recess and then navigating to the oropharynx down to the trachea, passing through different segments of the airway. The soft tissue could be made transparent so as to visualize the underlying bony anatomy and pre-operatively evaluate critical structures like carotid artery and optic nerve canals while demonstrating the partially transparent nasopharyngeal margins. A nasopharyngeal reconnaissance could be included with the camera panning around the nasopharynx, turbinates and nares could be visualized much better than the clinical and indirect mirror examination by viewing from the posterior aspect of nasal septum and turbinates, and various views of structures not amenable to view in conventional endoscopy can be achieved. Furthermore, evaluation of the base of the tongue, uvula, tonsillar fossa, vallecula, pyriform sinuses, and laryngeal structures including the vocal chords, trachea, and carina is clear and more precise [31]. Automatic flight planning may not be always possible, and manual techniques will have to be used if mucosal swelling

prevents easily entering a sinus cavity [13] (Movie 3.4).

Commercial VE software come equipped with a navigation tool and a virtual endoscope. The VE allows an operator to "journey" through different directions and positions within the 3-D anatomy of the sinonasal cavities and visually demonstrated in axial, sagittal, and coronal MPR images simultaneously to make the orientation simpler [30, 32].

3.9.3 Limitations of VB

However, virtual endoscopy is less sensitive (till now) to visualize any superficial lesions. Also, there are few important limitations of VB; presence of retained mucus or blood can falsely be reported as tracheobronchial stenosis or foreign body; furthermore, the diameter of airway on the CT depends on the respiratory cycle; therefore, stenosis of tracheobronchial tree may be underestimated on inspiration, and it is very important to perform VB during expiration to assess stenosis of tracheobronchial tree, or in some cases such as tracheomalacia during both inspiration and expiration. Obtaining images during both inspiration and expiration can be very challenging in examinations of infants and children. Moreover, VB cannot be used to assess mucosa, perform biopsies, and therapeutic maneuvers. Additionally, VB does not show segmental and subsegmental part of tracheobronchial tree. Finally, it can be difficult or impossible to detect some dynamic airway lesions, such as immobile vocal cords.

3.10 Time Consuming

A great debate regarding the time required to obtain the 3-D reconstructed images and the VRT as well as the virtual endoscopy. I can say confidentially in less than 10 min all the 3-D images can be obtained with a high quality, and of course, it will be less timed if practiced regularly that may reach maximum 5 min (kindly refer to Movies 3.5–3.7 for different techniques), which is real-time video recording from some of our cases.

Siemens Definition 64 Slice MDCT Protocols: Head : Neck Routine (Adult)										
Source: Scanner default										
Protocol	Range	Series Description	kV	Quality Ref. mAs	(Eff.) mAs	CAREDose/CAREDose 4D	CAREDoseType	CTDIvol	RotTime	Pitch
NeckRoutine (Adult)	Topogram	Topogram 0.6 T20s	100	0	168	off	CAREDose	0	0.500	1.0000000
	Neck		120	165	165	on	CAREDose4D	11.9366	1.000	0.90
		Neck 5.0 B31s								
		Neck 1.0 B20s								

Coll.	Slice	Recon increment	Images	Kernel	Window	API	Comment1
0.60	0.60		1	T20s	Topogram Body	None	
0.60						None	
	5.00	5.0	37	B31s	Larynx		
	1.00	0.7	258	B20s	Larynx		

The examination was carried out on Siemens scanner 64 slice MDCT as per the attached above-mentioned protocol.

Software post-processing programs used in our series are as follows:

1. Osirix® version 9.0 release for DICOM from Pixmeo for Mac OS
2. RadiAnt® 4.6.9 free software available
3. Advantage workstation for diagnostic imaging from general electric (GE)
4. The most commonly used one in our series was from Siemens GMBH Syngo fast View

3.11 Conclusion

Indications that need to be evaluated in the airway by the multi-detector CT technique should include the following:

1. Prior to anesthesia procedures, especially when difficult intubation is anticipated
2. History of difficult intubation patients
3. Laryngeal masses and the related airway evaluation
4. Cases with dysphagia
5. Trauma especially with facial implication as well as head and neck injuries including LeForte fractures
6. Oropharyngeal/nasopharyngeal masses
7. Stridor
8. Choking
9. Aspiration
10. Suspected choanal atresia

After performing the MDCT examination as well as the post processing techniques, the following points should be addressed and thoroughly commented upon:

1. Airway (caliber, narrow segments including thorough evaluation of its sites, level, and quantitative assessment in mm regarding its caliber and length for those which is persistent following the application of modified Valsalva maneuver)
2. Nasal septum, deviation, spur, masses, Chonecha bullosa, or significant mucosal thickening, antro-choanal polyp, or inverted papilloma
3. Posterior choana/nares (in children assess choanal atresia) whether it is primarily bony or membranous
4. Dental assessment (panoramic-like view) using curved MPR to create Orthopantomogram (OPG) absent teeth, loosening or loss of the normal lamina dura. Denture artificial teeth or loose implant/prosthesis
5. Temporomandibular Joint (TMJ) (ankyloses, dislocation, osteoarthrosis, osteomyelitis, or fractures)
6. Cervical spine assessment (C-MPR, Ankylosis, DISH, etc.)

 7. Abnormal elongated styloid process (Eagle syndrome)
 8. Vessels (abnormal variants) and tumor vascularity
 9. Goiter and retrosternal extension and its effect on the trachea whether it is compressed or displaced
10. Tracheal caliber and deviation down to the carina and assessment for trachea-malacia if any
11. Laryngeal airway and position of vocal cords
12. Masses (soft tissue displacing/invading the airway)
13. Correlation with Mallampati score and suggestion of the oral versus nasal route for intubation

After fulfilling all the above-mentioned diagnostic criteria points, the MDCT scan of the airway is considered a "one-stop shop."

3.12 Future Application

Using volumetric assessment of the airway, we were able to quantitatively and precisely evaluate the volume of air in cubic centimeters within both lungs, bronchi, and bronchioles, as well as the trachea, and it is to be compared to the tidal volume obtained from spirometry. However, this is still an ongoing research process. Moreover, a trial of obtaining pulmonary cast using the native air within the trachea and main bronchi is also ongoing.

References

 1. Schwab RJ. Upper airway imaging. Clin Chest Med. 1998;19:33–54.
 2. Aygun N, Zinreich J. Diagnostic imaging of the adult airway. Oper Tech Otolaryngol. 2007;18:77–84.
 3. Sittitavornwong S, Waite PD. Imaging the upper airway in patients with sleep disordered breathing. Oral Maxillofac Surg Clin North Am. 2009;21:389–402.
 4. Ahmed MM, Schwab RJ. Upper airway imaging in obstructive sleep apnea. Curr Opin Pulm Med. 2006;12:397–401.
 5. Yucel A, Unlu M, Haktanir A, Acar M, Fidan F. Evaluation of the upper airway cross-sectional area changes in different degrees of severity of obstructive sleep apnea syndrome: cephalometric and dynamic CT study. AJNR Am J Neuroradiol. 2005;26:2624–9.
 6. Kuo GP, Torok CM, Aygun N, James Zinreich S. Diagnostic imaging of the upper airway. Proc Am Thorac Soc. 2011;8:40–5.
 7. Becker M, Burkhardt K, Dulguerov P, Allal A. Imaging of the larynx and hypopharynx. Eur J Radiol. 2008;66:460–79.
 8. Lee CH, Goo JM, Lee HJ, et al. Radiation dose modulation techniques in the multidetector CT era: from basics to practice. Radiographics. 2008;28:1451–9.
 9. Clreniak R. X-ray computed tomography in biomedical engineering. In: Some words about the history of computed tomography, vol. 2; 2011. p. 7–19.
10. Beigelman-Aubry, et al. Multi–detector row CT and postprocessing techniques in the assessment of diffuse lung disease. Radiographics. 2005;25:1639–52.
11. Moustafa AHMN, Megahed HM. "Calvarial butterfly" new multidetector computed tomography (MDCT) virtual osteoscopic (VO) fingerprint for identification. Egyptian J Radiol Nucl Med. 2012;43(2):211–7.
12. Vining DJ. Virtual endoscopy: is it reality. Radiology. 1996;200(1):30–1.
13. Vining, D. J., Stelts, D. R., Ahn, D. K., Hemler, P. F., Ge, Y., Hunt, G. W., Ferretti, G. R. (1997). Freeflight: a virtual endoscopy system. In CVRMed-MRCAS 1997—1st joint conference computer vision, virtual reality and robotics in medicine and medical robotics and computer-assisted surgery, proceedings (Vol. 1205, pp. 413-416). (lecture notes in computer science (including subseries lecture notes in artificial intelligence and lecture notes in bioinformatics); Vol. 1205). Springer Verlag.
14. Benazzi S, Bertelli P, Lippi B, Bedini E, Caudana R, Gruppioni G, et al. Virtual anthropology and forensic arts: the facial reconstruction of Ferrante Gonzaga. J Archaeol Sci. 2010;37:1572–8.
15. Nuckton TJ, Glidden DV, Browner WS, Claman DM. Physical examination: mallampati score as an independent predictor of obstructive sleep apnea. Sleep. 2006;29(7):903–8.
16. de Jong PA, Müller NL, Paré PD, Coxson HO. Computed tomographic imaging of the airways: relationship to structure and function. Eur Respir J. 2005;26:140–52.
17. Amis ES Jr, Butler PF, Applegate KE, et al. American College of Radiology white paper on radiation dose in medicine. J Am Coll Radiol. 2007;4:272–84.
18. Hara AK, Johnson CD, Reed JE, Ahlquist DA, Nelson H, Ehman RL, Harmsen WS. Reducing data size and radiation dose for CT colonography. Am J Roentgenol. 1997;168(5):1181–4.
19. Mulkens TH, Bellinck P, Baeyaert M, et al. Use of an automatic exposure control mechanism for dose optimization in multi–detector row CT examinations: clinical evaluation. Radiology. 2005;237:213–23.
20. Golding SJ, Shrimpton PC. Commentary. Radiation dose in CT: are we meeting the challenge? Br J Radiol. 2002;75:1–4.

21. Kalender WA, Wolf H, Suess C. Dose reduction in CT by anatomically adapted tube current modulation: phantom measurements. Med Phys. 1999;26:2248–53.
22. Çorbacıoğlu ŞK, et al. Comparing the success rates of standard and modified Valsalva maneuvers to terminate PSVT: a randomized controlled trial. Am J Emerg Med. 2017;35(11):1662–5.
23. Elisberg E, Singian E, Miller G, Katz LN. The Effect of the Valsalva Maneuver on the Circulation; Circulation. vol. 7; III. In: The Influence of Heart Disease on the Expected Poststraining Overshoot; 1953. pp. 880-889.
24. Taljanovic MS, Hunter TB, Wisneski RJ, Seeger JF, Friend CJ, Schwartz SA, Rogers LF. Imaging characteristics of diffuse idiopathic skeletal hyperostosis with an emphasis on acute spinal fractures: review. AJR. 2009;193:S10–9.
25. Vaseemuddin S. Incidental findings on panoramic radiograph: a clinical study. J Adv Med Dent Scie Res. 2016;4(6):223–6.
26. Perandini S, Faccioli N, Zaccarella A, Re TJ, Pozzi Mucelli R. The diagnostic contribution of CT volumetric rendering techniques in routine practice. Indian J Radiol Imaging. 2010;20(2):92–7.
27. Kuszyk BS, Heath DG, Bliss DF, Fishman EK. Skeletal 3-D CT: advantages of volume rendering over surface rendering. Skelet Radiol. 1996;25(3):207–14.
28. Todd JT, Egan EJL, Phillips F. Is the perception of 3-D shape from shading based on assumed reflectance and illumination? Iperception. 2014;5(6):497–514.
29. Flohr TG, Schaller S, et al. Multi-detector row CT systems and image reconstruction techniques. Radiology. 2005;235:756–73.
30. Nam T-K, et al. Use of three-dimensional curved-multiplanar reconstruction images for sylvian dissection in microsurgery of middle cerebral artery aneurysms. Yonsei Med J. 2017;58(1):241–7.
31. Bisdas S, Verink M, Burmeister HP, Stieve M, Becker H. Depth perception in translucent volumes. IEEE Trans Vis Comput Graph. 2004;12:1117–23.
32. Anand SM, Frenkiel S, Le BQH, Glikstein R. Virtual endoscopy: our next major investigative modality? J Otolaryngol Head Neck Surg. 2009;38(6):642–5.

Evaluation of the Normal Airway Using Virtual Endoscopy and Three-Dimensional Reconstruction

4

Nabil A. Shallik, Abbas H. Moustafa, and Yasser Hammad

4.1 Introduction

Virtual endoscopy (VE) is a technique for creating computer simulations of anatomy from radiological image data and viewing those simulations in a way that is analogous to conventional endoscopy. Progress in computer technology has generated many advances in noninvasive diagnostic imaging. For example, the advent of helical computed tomography (CT) has permitted the acquisition of volumes of CT data from which three-dimensional (3-D) images can accurately be extracted. VE utilizes such 3-D images in real time to simulate the views obtained during real endoscopy [1].

The semitransparent, color-coded volume reconstruction offers the advantage that in addition to the endoluminal representation, the surrounding structures can also be assessed. Other major advantages of the virtual versus the fiber-optic endoscopy are their noninvasiveness, the possibility of passage of subtotal stenosis with assessment of the downstream airways, and navigational aids and retrograde view. Disadvantages are the lack of color rendering, lack of proper evaluation of the superficial mucosal lesions, and intervention possibilities. Compared to other forms of CT imaging, a virtual-endoscopically more realistic assessment of tracheobronchial stenosis is possible than with axial sectional images or multiplanar reformation. As a complementary method to fiber-optic endoscopy, virtual endoscopy of the respiratory tract can be used preoperatively, prior to tracheostomy, stenting, or resection, as well as in the postoperative course assessment. Virtual endoscopy will increasingly be used as an assistant in bronchoscopic and surgical procedures on the airways [2].

It is helpful to orient the image to correspond with a conventional endoscopic view. For example, nasal endoscopy is performed in a

Electronic Supplementary Material The online version of this chapter (https://doi.org/10.1007/978-3-030-23253-5_4) contains supplementary material, which is available to authorized users.

N. A. Shallik (✉)
Department of Clinical Anesthesiology, Weill Cornell Medical College in Qatar (WCMQ), Doha, Qatar

Department of Anesthesiology, ICU and Perioperative Medicine, Hamad Medical Corporation, Doha, Qatar

Department of Anesthesiology and Surgical Intensive Care, Faculty of Medicine, Tanta University, Tanta, Egypt
e-mail: Nshallik@hamad.qa

A. H. Moustafa
Department of Clinical Radiology & Medical Imaging, Hamad Medical Corporation, Doha, Qatar

Department of Diagnostic Radiology and Medical Imaging, El Minia University, Minia, Egypt

Y. Hammad
Department of Clinical Anesthesiology, Weill Cornell Medical College in Qatar (WCMQ), Doha, Qatar

Department of Anesthesiology, ICU and Perioperative Medicine, Hamad Medical Corporation, Doha, Qatar

© Springer Nature Switzerland AG 2019
N. A. Shallik et al. (eds.), *Virtual Endoscopy and 3D Reconstruction in the Airways*,
https://doi.org/10.1007/978-3-030-23253-5_4

face-to-face doctor–patient orientation. This is in contrast to bronchoscopy, in which the bronchoscopist is usually positioned behind the patient, having the same right–left orientation. Labeling the CT virtual endoscopic images may be necessary for clarification; however, the key guide usually present on the right corner of the reconstructed image is the cornerstone for orientation and overcomes any misinterpretation regarding the site. Postprocessing requires approximately 10 additional minutes per examination; however, continuous training on the workstation and familiarity with the software as well as the 3-D imagination will ultimately and significantly reduce the time needed for 3-D reconstructions [3].

4.2 Techniques (for More Details Please Refer to Chap. 3)

4.2.1 Modified Valsalva Maneuver

This is a simple trick of asking the patient to do a "modified Valsalva maneuver" by asking him/her to have a very deep inspiration, hold it inside, and to get it exhaled slowly through a slit-like orifice from the lips with buffed cheeks. This will help in increasing intrathoracic pressure to as much as 80 mmHg and subsequently result in full distension of the potentially collapsed airway fully and open the potentially under-filled different segments with air (Fig. 4.1).

4.2.2 Extension of Neck

A considerable neck extension is mandatory during the patient's intubation, and subsequently, special attention should be given to the patients with severe polytrauma for proper assessment of their cervical spine integrity as well as the cervico-cranial junction.

It is important to evaluate the cervical spine integrity, alignment, presence or absence of fractures or subluxations/displacement, and any pathology to give the anesthesiologist comprehensive data prior to the anesthesia procedure.

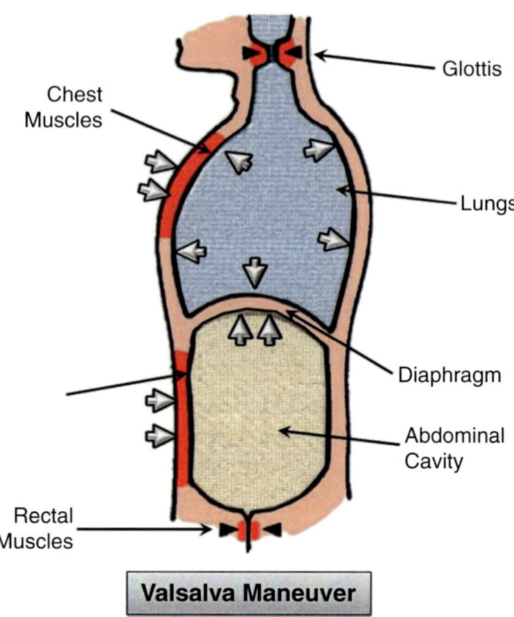

Fig. 4.1 Valsalva maneuver and increased pressure inside different body cavities (hand-drawn by the author)

4.3 Normal Finding of VE

Please refer to (Movies 4.1, 4.2, and 4.3) from nose to carina.

4.3.1 Nasal Cavity and Variant

Virtual endoscopic evaluation through the nasal orifice can demonstrate the collumella, nasal orifices, nasal cavities, inferior and middle turbinates, meatus, osteomeatal complex orifice, nasal septum, and vomer (Fig. 4.2).

VE can evaluate the posterior nares (choana), inferior turbinates, vomer, and Eustachian tube orifices (Figs. 4.3 and 4.10).

4.3.2 Nasopharynx and Posterior Nares

CT virtual endoscopy of the normal nasopharynx from a posterior viewpoint provides a look at the Eustachian tube orifices in reference to the choanae and nasopharyngeal walls, an area difficult to appreciate with conventional endoscopy.

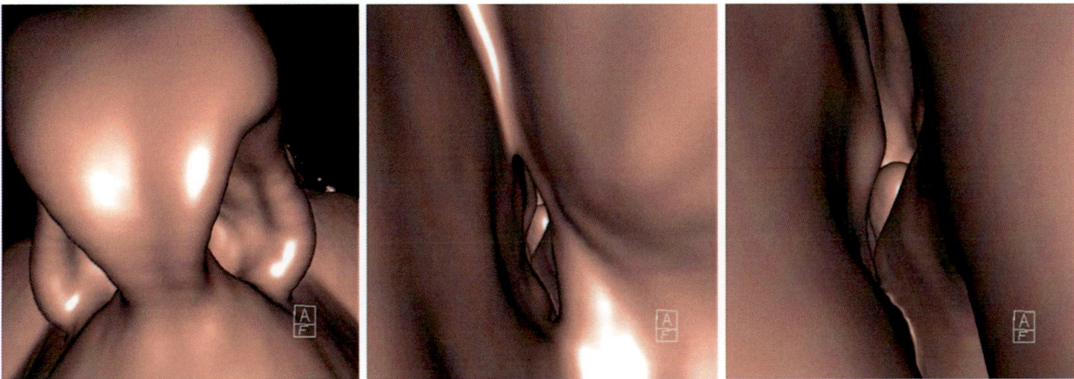

Fig. 4.2 Virtual endoscopy of nasal cavity

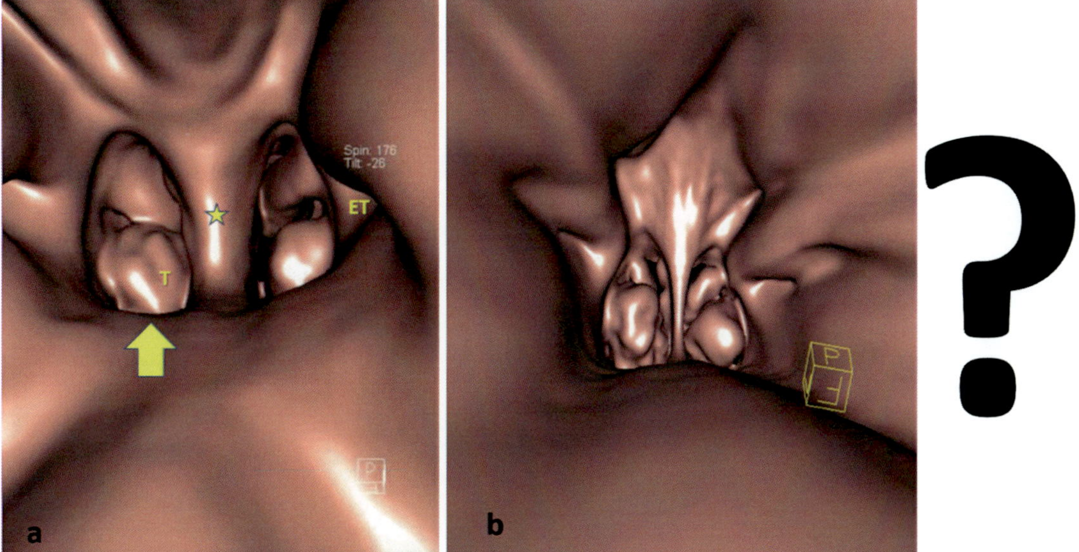

Fig. 4.3 (**a**) Unique view by virtual endoscopy showing the posterior vomer (∗), Turbinates (T), posterior nares (solid arrow), and the Eustachian tube orifice (ET). (**b**) Far View (?) image that cannot be physically duplicated

Posterior choanal projection is an image that cannot be physically duplicated except by the VE. Posterior nares (choana), vomer/posterior nasal septum, and Eustachian tube orifices are clearly visualized. Furthermore, evaluation and exclusion of the choanal atresia can be easily done.

4.3.3 Oropharynx Airway

4.3.3.1 Base of the Tongue, Vallecula, and Pyriform Sinuses

Aryepiglottic folds, pyriform sinuses, and vocal cords are seen (Figs. 4.4 and 4.5).

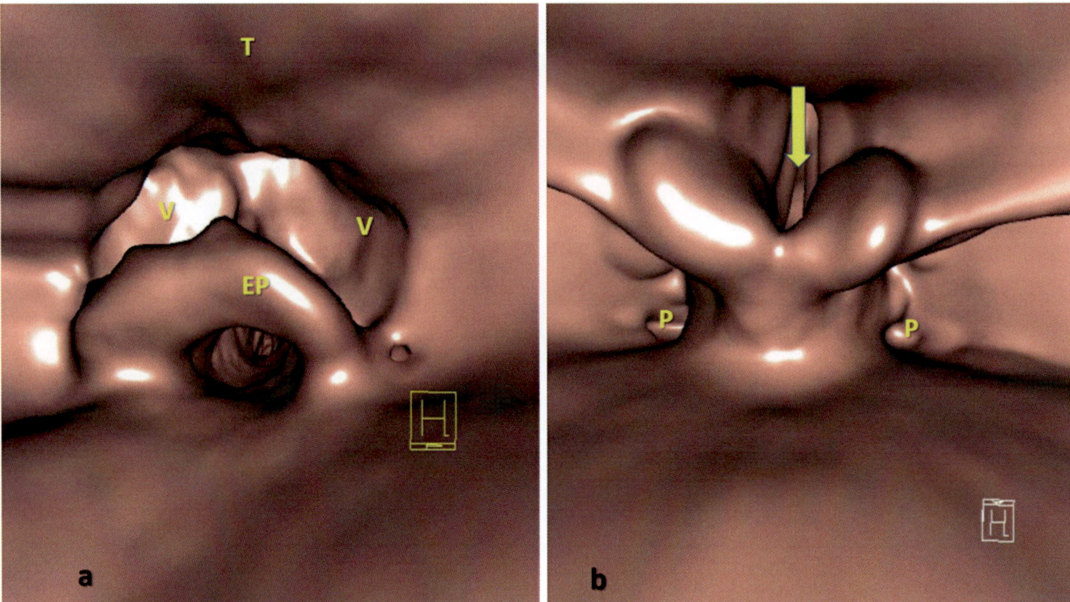

Fig. 4.4 (**a**): View showing (T) base of the tongue, (EP) epiglottis, and (V) Valecula. (**b**) View showing vocal cord (arrow) and (P) pyriform sinuses

4.3.4 Vocal Cord Proper (Ventricle and False Vocal Cord) (Figs. 4.5 and 4.6)

4.3.5 Trachea

Radiologists should be able to recognize the normal tracheal architecture and anatomic variants. In particular, normal structures such as the transverse aorta can indent the large airways and need not be confused with extrinsic lesions when viewed endoscopically (Figs. 4.7 and 4.8).

The trachea is usually 9–15 cm long in an adult and begins at approximately the sixth cervical vertebra, at the inferior border of the cricoid cartilage. The diameter of the trachea is typically 2–2.5 cm. The trachea has two sections. The cervical portion is superior to the thoracic inlet. The intrathoracic portion extends from the thoracic inlet to the bifurcation (carina). The trachea is supported anteriorly by 16–20 C-shaped rings of cartilage. In the posterior aspect, the trachea consists of the pars membranacea. This membrane is

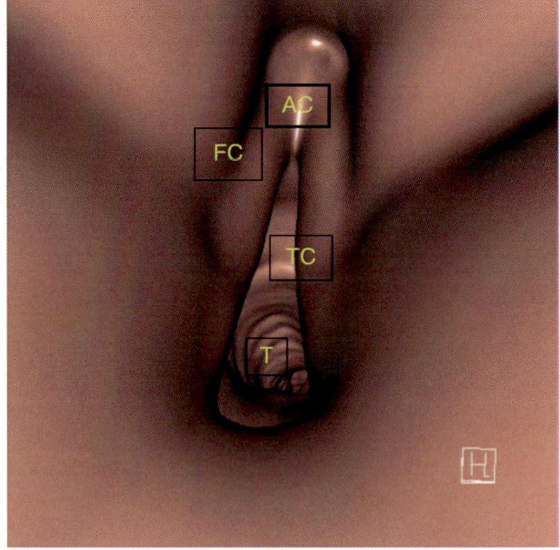

Fig. 4.5 Virtual endoscopy at the level of the vocal cord showing T, Trachea; AC, anterior commissure; TC, true cord; and FC, false cord

flexible, allowing the trachea to change in configuration during inspiration and expiration. The membrane normally bulges during expiration and coughing (Fig. 4.10).

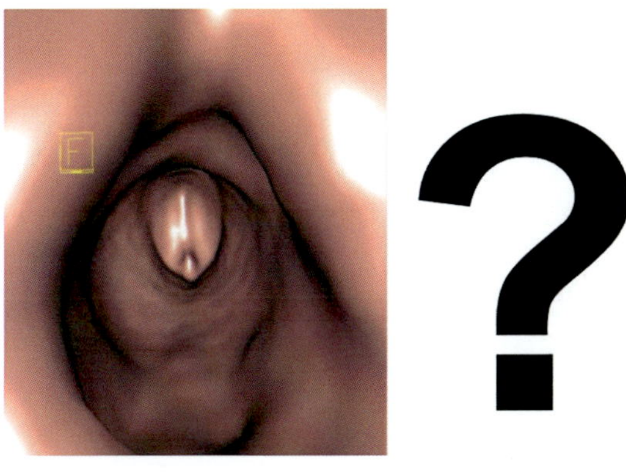

Fig. 4.6 Virtual endoscopy of the infraglottic region; the virtual endoscope is directed caudo-cephalic; image that cannot be physically duplicated by any other means including the real endoscope

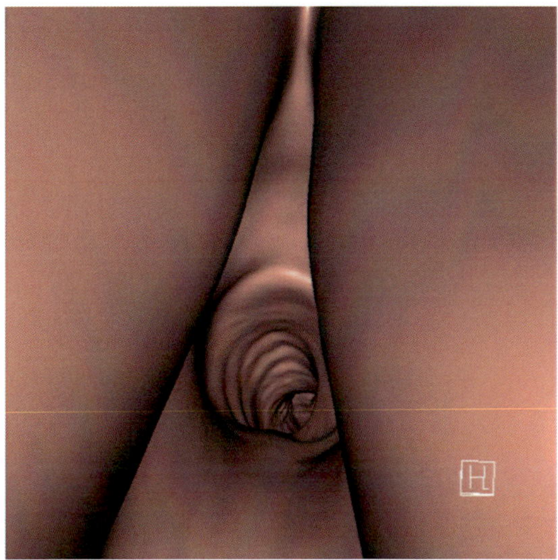

Fig. 4.7 View via the vocal cords showing the trachea in depth

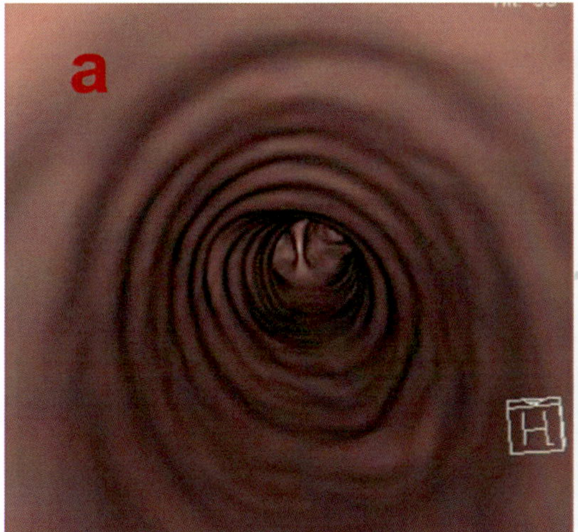

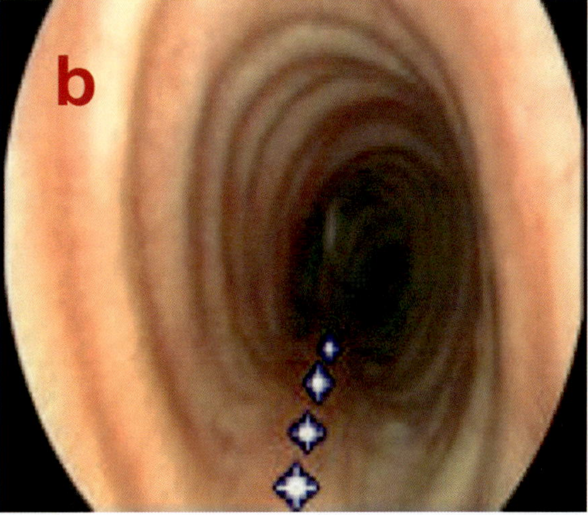

Fig. 4.8 (**a**) Virtual endoscopic evaluation inside the tracheal lumen showing anteriorly the c-shaped cartilage and posteriorly the membranous part which is indented by the effect of the esophagus. The virtual endoscopy is identical to the real one (**b**)

4.3.6 Carina

At the level of sternal angle (T4–T5), the trachea divides at the carina, a ridge formed by the downward and backward projection of the last tracheal ring, into the right and left main-stem bronchi (Figs. 4.9 and 4.10).

4.4   Technical Limitations

Asymmetry is a guide to pathology on endoscopy, but asymmetries on CT, particularly in the larynx, are most often caused by poor aeration [4, 5]. Because of this, virtual laryngoscopy has low specificity in evaluating mucosal lesions of the

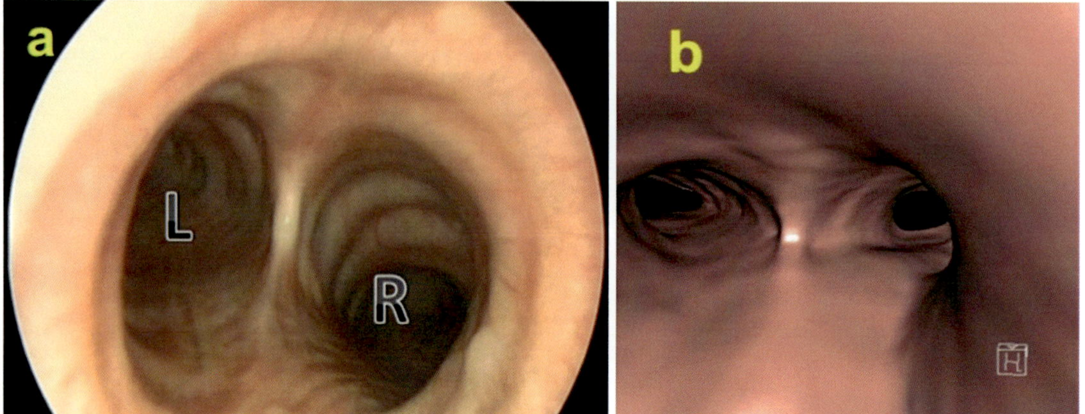

Fig. 4.9 Virtual endoscopy (VE) at the level of the carina showing the right and left main bronchi; kindly check the orientation index to have more right lower cube about the directions. (**a**) Normal video-endoscopic view and (**b**) Virtual endoscopic view

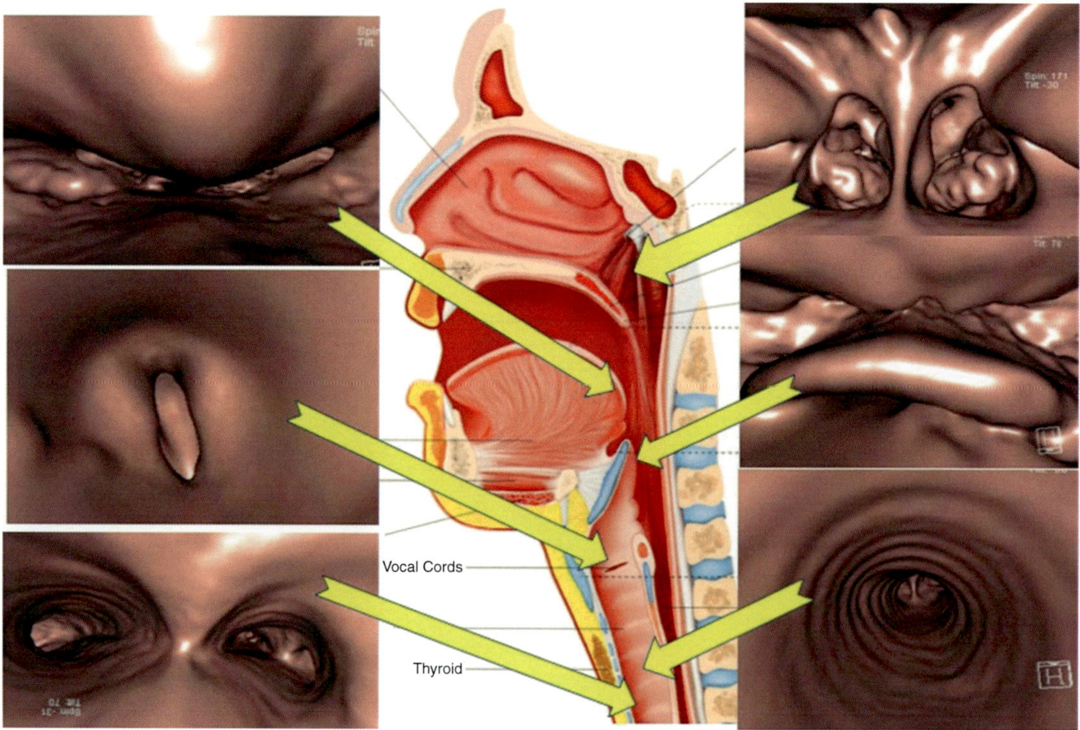

Fig. 4.10 Different levels of virtual endoscopic images with the referred arrows to their perspectives

valleculae, pyriform sinuses, and larynx. Therefore, findings on virtual laryngoscopy should always be evaluated in the context of the original CT data set. The extent of airway compromise may be overestimated on CT virtual endoscopy when the airway is significantly stenosed. The apparent degree of stenosis may vary with different tissue air threshold values. Lower threshold values increase the apparent stenosis, and higher thresholds can produce mucosal gaps.

This phenomenon is exemplified in the case of polypoid corditis, with different threshold values yielding different appearances of the pathology. The degree of glottic narrowing must be approximated with the source CT images. In this case, actual luminal compromise was estimated to be 85% by conventional endoscopy. Therefore, threshold values should be tailored to reflect relative lumen size. This can be performed easily at the workstation by using the mouse to appropriately "window" the threshold value of the 3-D image or by manually entering different values into the display options. This also applies to endoluminal lesions [4]. Note that mass lesion size is generally underestimated using CT virtual endoscopy, and measurements should instead be made from 2D source CT data. To reiterate, the CT virtual endoscopic images shown in this chapter were created retrospectively with no changes in routine departmental scanning protocols. However, in the evaluation of distal airway disease, advanced protocols such as cardiac gating and submillimeter collimation should be considered. Finally, we found no significant qualitative differences in CT virtual endoscopy images created from the 16-MDCT scanner versus those generated from the 64-MDCT scanner [5].

4.5 Normal Finding of TTP (Tissue Transparent/ Transition Projection)

Tissue Transparent Projection or tissue transition projection (TTP) is one of the applications available on most of the commercially avilable workstations that allow visualization of underlying objects/anatomical structures through a transpar-

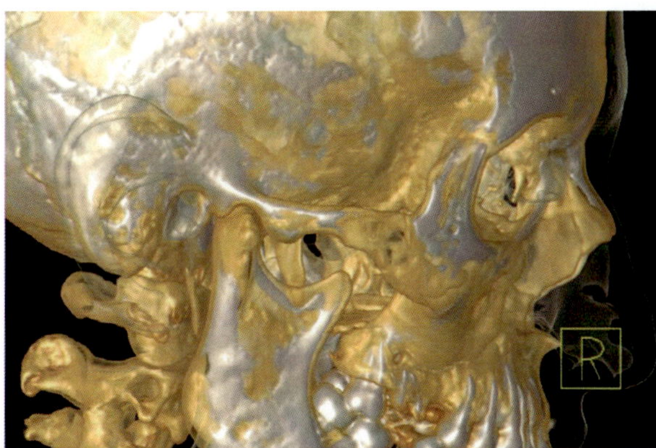
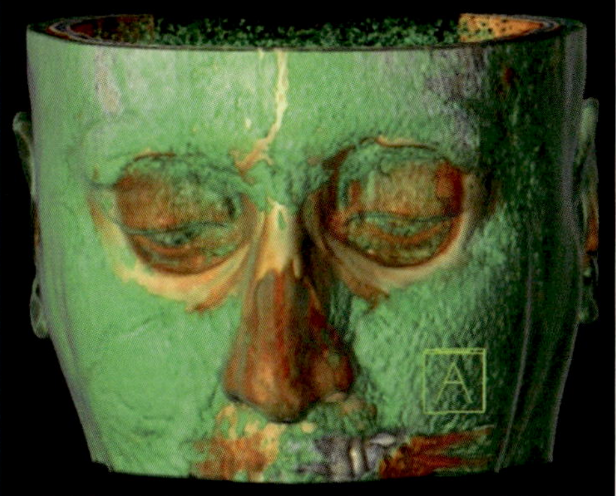

Fig. 4.11 Frontal and lateral projections of the generated 3D models using VRT with the overlying muscles and subcutaneous fat as well as the details of the nose including its bony and nasal cartilage components

Fig. 4.12 Surface-rendering VRT technique for the skin architecture of the patient to give a comprehensive idea about the facial features of the patient without encroachment upon the patient's privacy

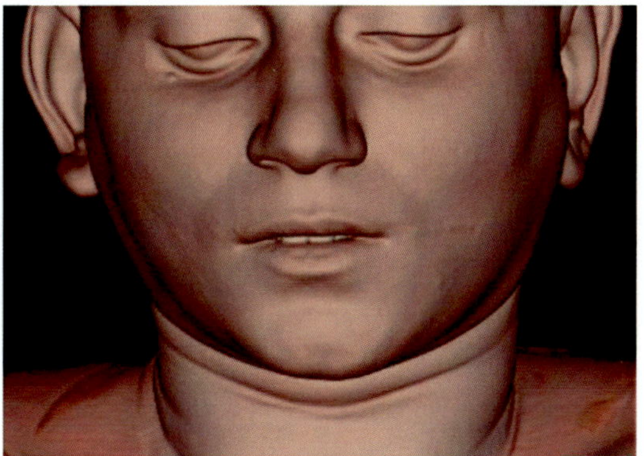

ent overlying tissues. We have two images: One AP and the other lateral

TTP reconstruction image of the skin contour as well as the cartilaginous framework of the nose is demonstrated clearly using the VRT model (Figs. 4.11 and 4.12) (Movie 4.4).

4.6 Conclusion

In summary, the airway being of inherent curved anatomical complex matrix makes the evaluation of its distensibility and the potential collapse a great obstacle and challenge for the proper assessment. Aero-digestive airway is unique regarding its anatomical and functional perspectives. So, 3-D reconstruction and VE volume rendering of CT images of the airway can provide anesthetists with an alternative view of the airway in patients with normal and difficult airway management. This way of assessing the airway in a complex group of patients allows us to better appreciate how the pathology may affect safe airway management and appears to influence us into formulating safer airway planning.

References

1. Burke AJ, Vining DJ, McGuirt WF, Postma G, Browne JD. Evaluation of airway obstruction using virtual endoscopy. Laryngoscope. 2000;110(1):23–9. https://doi.org/10.1097/00005537-200001000-00005.
2. Thomas BP, Strother MK, Donnelly EF, Worrell JA. AJR integrative imaging CT virtual endoscopy in the evaluation of large airway disease: review. AJR. 2009;19209(March):20–30. https://doi.org/10.2214/AJR.07.7077.
3. Thomas BP, Strother MK, Donnelly EF, Worrell JA. CT virtual endoscopy in the evaluation of large airway disease: review. Am J Roentgenol. 2009;192(Suppl. 3):20–30. https://doi.org/10.2214/AJR.07.7077.
4. Ferretti GR, Knoplioch J, Bricault I, Brambilla C, Coulomb M. Central airway stenoses: preliminary results of spiral-CT-generated virtual bronchoscopy simulations in 29 patients. Eur Radiol. 1997;7(6):854–9. https://doi.org/10.1007/s003300050218.
5. Horton KM, Horton MR, Fishman EK. Advanced visualization of airways with 64-MDCT: 3D mapping and virtual bronchoscopy. Am J Roentgenol. 2007;189(6):1387–96. https://doi.org/10.2214/AJR.07.2824.

Virtual Endoscopy and 3-D Reconstruction in Patients with Airway Pathology

5

Imran Ahmad, Britta Millhoff, Sarah Muldoon, and Kayathrie Jeyarajah

5.1 Introduction

The assessment and airway planning of patients with airway pathology can be challenging as the current bedside airway assessment tools are often inadequate due to their low sensitivity and specificity. Almost all of these patients would have had a multi-plane computerised tomography (CT) of the head and neck as part of the diagnostic process. In addition to this, many would also have had a flexible nasal endoscopy with an associated hand-drawing by the surgeon or a still image in the notes. With three-dimensional (3-D) reconstruction and virtual endoscopy (VE) performed by either the radiologist, the anaesthetist or the surgeon on an Apple Mac workstation with easily available software such as OsiriX® and HOROS, an inside simulated view of the airway or the pathology can be obtained. This can then be utilised to formulate an airway management plan. Three-dimensional reconstruction of the patient's head and neck anatomy gives a better understanding of how it is affected by pathology in and around the upper

Electronic Supplementary Material The online version of this chapter (https://doi.org/10.1007/978-3-030-23253-5_5) contains supplementary material, which is available to authorized users.

I. Ahmad (✉) · B. Millhoff · S. Muldoon · K. Jeyarajah
Guy's & St Thomas' NHS Foundation Trust,
London, UK

airway. This well-established tool has already shown its value in diagnosing intra-luminal lesions of the airway and bronchial tree, and there is now growing evidence demonstrating the benefits of this technology in visualising and mapping out an airway management plan in patients with head and neck pathology.

5.2 Assessment Tools for Airway Management

Predicting difficulty with mask ventilation, intubation or both is notoriously challenging for the anaesthetist, lacking as we are in tests of sufficient sensitivity and specificity to identify those patients at greatest risk.

These difficulties are more pronounced when attempting to plan appropriate airway management for patients with airway pathology, where the disease state, or indeed its treatment, can introduce further challenges.

The Fourth National Audit Project (NAP4) [1], published in the UK in 2011, demonstrated that patients with head and neck pathology accounted for 40% of patients suffering from serious morbidity and mortality during airway management, with key features being a failure to adequately assess the airway preoperatively, or to adapt the best anaesthetic technique to suit the patient's condition. In several cases, radiological imaging was available prior to theatre, which would have alerted the anaesthetist to the difficulty ahead if it had been reviewed appropriately. It was postulated that unfamiliarity with interpreting images such as CT scans may partly explain why this did not occur in some cases.

Many patients with airway pathology, for example neoplastic disease in the glottic region, are likely to need advanced airway management techniques such as videolaryngoscopy, awake tracheal intubation or even a primary tracheostomy. NAP 4 highlighted several cases where patients were exposed to harm due to suboptimal airway management when an awake tracheal bronchoscopic intubation or tracheostomy under local anaesthesia was indicated, but not performed first-line. An accurate judgement of which technique is most likely to result in the rapid, atraumatic and safe securement of the airway reduces the morbidity suffered by the patient, and the stress suffered by the anaesthetist.

Many organisations including the American Society of Anaesthesiologists (ASA) and World Health Organization (WHO) [2, 3] recommend a systematic airway assessment be performed prior to induction of anaesthesia, although consensus on what this should entail and the evidence that doing so improves outcomes, is lacking.

However, patients with head and neck pathology by their very nature should arouse suspicions of difficulty with the airway, and tend to have undergone several relevant diagnostic investigations prior to surgery, which are of benefit to the anaesthetist planning the airway management.

Virtual endoscopy offers particular advantages in such cases, utilising computer software to transform CT images of the head and neck into 3-D "fly-through videos" of the patient's airway anatomy in a format familiar to the anaesthetist who practices flexible bronchoscopic intubation. This allows the anaesthetist to determine preoperatively the degree of distortion and narrowing caused by any infective, inflammatory or neoplastic process and make a judgement as to whether ventilation and intubation can be performed in the asleep patient, or whether an awake technique utilising a flexible bronchoscope or tracheostomy is more appropriate. If flexible bronchoscopic intubation is

deemed the technique of choice, the anaesthetist can plan the best route to take and can anticipate at which level of the airway difficulty may be encountered.

5.2.1 Airway Assessment

The airway assessment of the patient with head and neck pathology begins as for any other patient undergoing anaesthesia, with a targeted history and simple bedside tests.

5.2.2 History

Important symptoms to illicit when taking a pre-anaesthetic history for a patient with pathology in the airway include dyspnoea—on exertion, at rest or worsened by the supine position; dysphagia, to solids and/or liquids, and is coughing provoked which may suggest aspiration; voice change, such as hoarseness or weakness of the voice, or the "hot potato" quality suggestive of base-of-tongue lesions; difficulty with mouth opening due to pain or true trismus. The time scale over which symptoms have developed, and whether they are static or progressive is important. A more rapid progression will of course be expected in acute, infective pathologies of the airway as compared to those of a malignant process. If a patient's dyspnoea or hoarseness has progressed since their last imaging or surgical review, one should be wary that this is likely to be accompanied by anatomical deterioration of the airway. A history of relevant treatment, such as previous head and neck surgery or radiotherapy, is also very pertinent.

5.2.3 External Examination

A general external examination may yield information about generic challenges for airway management, such as the presence of a beard or obesity. There may also be disease-specific signs, such as facial or neck swellings caused by infection, tumour or lymphadenopathy or a visible goitre. The classic woody texture and appearance of radiotherapy treatment may be apparent, along with the scars and tissue flaps from previous surgery. Patients with slowly progressive disease can appear deceptively lacking in symptoms, as their respiratory muscles adapt and compensate for the progressive narrowing of the airway; the severity of their airway obstruction may only reveal itself with the induction of anaesthesia and the resultant loss of skeletal muscle tone [4].

5.2.3.1 Mouth Opening, Inter-Incisor Gap and Mallampati

The ability to open the mouth is the most ubiquitous component of the airway assessment, allowing the anaesthetist to gauge the ease of access for airway instrumentation. The inter-incisor gap (IIG) is the most reproducible measure of mouth-opening, with a distance of less than 3 cm being suggestive of difficulty with direct laryngoscopy [5]. Some of the more streamlined videolaryngoscope blades can be inserted with an IIG of 2 cm [6], and successful insertion of supraglottic airway devices has been reported with an IIG below this [7].

With the mouth open and the tongue protruded maximally, the modified Mallampati score can be assessed. This compares the relative size of the tongue to that of the oral cavity, and a grading of 1–4 assigned depending on the structures visible to the assessor sitting opposite to the patient.

A Class 1 Mallampati view means that the soft palate and entirety of the uvula are visible, while a Class 4 view means that only the hard palate is visible to the observer. In Mallampati's original paper [8], 80% of those with a Mallampati Class 1 view had a Grade 1 view of the glottis at laryngoscopy, with the remainder a grade 2 view, with higher Mallampati classes showing increasingly higher rates of poorer glottic visualisation. However, if used in isolation, the Mallampati test has been shown to be an unreliable predictor of the difficult airway with varied inter-observer reproducibility [9].

Performing a Mallampati assessment can be of value in patients with head and neck disease, as looking into the oral cavity can reveal the presence of an abscess, tumour or other soft tissue swelling. An inability to protrude the tongue can suggest disease process in the tongue base or submandibular space, which is a red flag for difficult laryngoscopy.

5.2.3.2 Jaw Protrusion and Upper Lip Bite Test

Difficult laryngoscopy is more likely in patients with retrognathic mandibles or prominent maxillary incisors. An assessment of the patient's ability to prognath the jaw will highlight either of these deficiencies and also assess the temporomandibular joint. Jaw protrusion is defined as Grade A when the incisors of the mandible protrude beyond those of the maxilla, Grade B when the incisors meet and Grade C when the maxillary incisors protrude beyond the mandible. An alternative is to ask the patient to bite their upper lip and assess whether they are able to get above the vermillion border of the upper lip with the lower incisors. This test has shown variable sensitivity and specificity for predicting difficult laryngoscopy when compared to the Mallampati assessment [10, 11].

5.2.3.3 Thyromental and Sternomental Distance

The thyromental distance (TMD) is the distance from the cephalad border of the thyroid cartilage to the mental protuberance of the mandible, with the head held in extension. The sternomental distance is that between the sternal notch and the mental protuberance. Distances of less than 6.5 cm and 12.5 cm, respectively, are associated with difficult direct laryngoscopy. The World Health Organization advocates the combination of Mallampati with TMD as the most useful way of identifying patients at risk of difficult intubation [3]. A modification of the TMD by working out its ratio to the patient's height has been shown to be more accurate than the TMD itself at predicting difficult laryngoscopy [12, 13].

5.2.3.4 Neck Movements

Assessing whether a patient can adequately flex the cervical spine and extend at the atlanto-axial joint indicates their ability to adopt the optimal position for mask ventilation and direct laryngoscopy. It also allows an opportunity to assess the landmarks for cricothyroidotomy, and the ability to position the patient with full cervical spine extension should front of neck access be required electively or in an emergency. Previous radiotherapy to the neck can have a detrimental effect on the ability to flex the neck and palpate the necessary cartilaginous landmarks.

5.2.3.5 Multivariate Scoring Systems

As each of the tests outlined above has limited specificity and sensitivity when used in isolation, various attempts have been made to combine these components together to form a scoring system with a greater positive predictive value.

One of the first such scoring systems was the Wilson Score, which assesses the patient's weight, cervical spine flexibility, inter-incisor gap, retrognathism and prominent maxillary incisors [14]. The more unfavourable each component, the higher the score it attracts. A total score below 5 is reported to be reassuring for straightforward direct laryngoscopy, while a score greater than 7 warns of severe difficulty.

5.2.3.6 Simplified Airway Risk Index (SARI)

A more recently developed system is the Simplified Airway Risk Index (SARI) [15]. Again, this uses a weighted scoring system, and the factors assessed are mouth opening, thyromental distance, Mallampati score, neck movements, prognathic ability, weight and history of previous difficult intubation. However, a large, prospective Scandinavian trial detected no statistically significant change in the number of unanticipated or straightforward intubations when the SARI tool was compared with non-standardised airway assessment [16].

With the limitations that these simple bedside tests have in identifying the potentially difficult airway, the importance of imaging investigations in the planning of airway management for patients with head and neck pathology is emphasised.

5.3 Imaging of the Airway

Preoperative investigations can assist the anaesthetist by confirming the presence of any pathological abnormality detected during history and examination, and providing further information of the location and extent of disease. This allows us to make a more informed judgement as to how the airway pathology in question may impact on our ability to intubate, ventilate or both, and adjust our plan accordingly. The majority of airway investigations comprise some form of static radiological imaging, but some dynamic, real-time assessment can also be obtained by flexible nasendoscopy (Fig. 5.1) (Movie 5.1).

X-ray can provide useful information for airway assessment. Soft tissue views of the neck are informative in cases of suspected foreign body inhalation, as they may confirm the nature of the object and the level and extent of any resulting airway obstruction.

A chest radiograph may offer further information, such as distal airway obstruction or collapse and air trapping. A plain chest film may also reveal pathologies such as deviation or narrowing

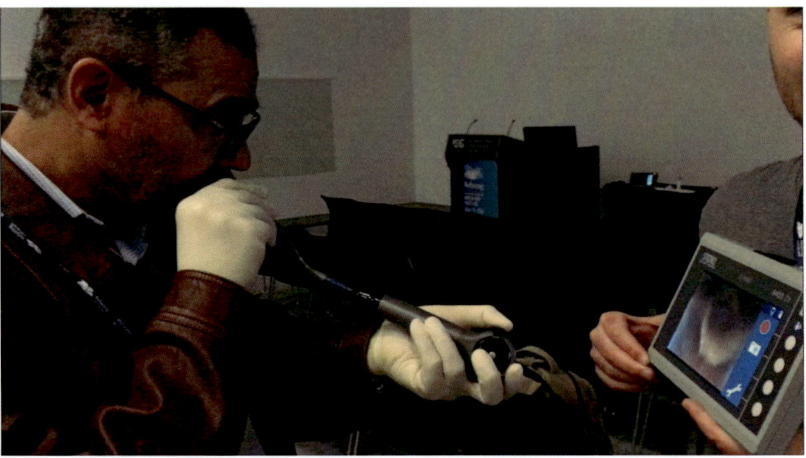

Fig. 5.1 Self demonstration of awake nasendoscopy

of the trachea, which may prompt further investigations such as nasoendoscopy or a CT scan.

A lateral c-spine radiograph, taken with the head in a neutral position, allows measurement of the distance between the C1 spinous process and the occiput. A distance less than 5 mm is suggestive of intubation difficulty [5].

Information can be gleaned from orthopantomograms (panoramic views) such as the presence of facial fractures. This can increase the likelihood of difficult mask ventilation and laryngoscopy due to the disruption of the anatomy and tissue swelling.

5.3.1 Ultrasound

The introduction of anatomical assessment with the help of ultrasound imaging in anaesthesia has been one of the more recent technological advances in this field. The increasing use of ultrasound has been accredited to its proven established clinical efficacy, cost-effectiveness and practicality as it allows anaesthetists to evaluate often complex and varied anatomy.

Ultrasound imaging can contribute to anatomical information that would otherwise not be evident on routine clinical screening tests for assessment of difficult laryngoscopy, e.g. thickness of anterior soft tissue on the neck, oedema and tumours. One of the primary uses of ultrasound is for the identification of the cricothyroid membrane. Additionally, it is employed for the discovery of midline vessels in gauging suitability for percutaneous tracheostomy. It also allows an assessment of vocal cord mobility.

Current literature suggests the novel use of ultrasound for predicting difficult intubation has been growing. Hui et al. describe a method of imaging oropharyngeal and laryngeal structures by performing sublingual ultrasound on the floor of the mouth [17, 18]. This produces sagittal views permitting visualisation of the base of tongue, hyoid bone and suprahyoid muscles. They postulate that failure to visualise the hyoid bone may indicate difficulty with intubation, as this suggests a more caudal placement of the hyoid which can be caused by a relatively short mandibular ramus or a more hypopharyngeal position of the tongue. Oesophageal intubation

can be easily determined by an ultrasound probe when placed 1 in. above the suprasternal notch, and the double trachea sign is easy to be seen and more diagnostic.

Ultrasound use has gained popularity; however, more extensive validation is required. Advantages of ultrasound imaging are as follows: it is safe; there is no use of ionising radiation or contrast agent; it is non-invasive, portable, widely available, painless and easily reproducible, and moreover gives real-time dynamic images. Although considered safer compared to other imaging modalities, exposure in terms of intensity and time should be limited as much as possible, as high-energy ultrasound can cause heating of the tissues. There is also a recognised learning curve for ultrasoud assessement of the airway, which requires training and practice to overcome.

5.3.2 Computed Tomography (CT)

Computed tomography scans have significantly enhanced the assessment of patients with complex airway pathology. Joint discussion between the head and neck/ENT surgeon and radiologist aids the interpretation of images with regard to the source of pathology, staging of neoplasms and severity of any stenosis, or any subglottic/retrosternal extension.

The CT scan, whilst providing extensive clinical information and aiding in diagnosis, to the extent of pathology, carries certain risks to patients, namely, exposure to ionising radiation, allergy to contrast and deterioration of renal function in patients with poor renal function when contrast is used.

5.3.3 Magnetic Resonance Imaging (MRI)

MRI is useful for delineating soft tissue pathology; however, the ability of many patients with multiple comorbidities to lie flat for prolonged periods can be a limiting factor for their use. The lack of radiation compared to CT scan is a huge advantage. Multi-planar reformations (MPR) in sagittal and coronal planes are more useful in indicating stenosis, as well as the degree of airway distortion, and in delineating airway anatomy than individual coronal slice images [3].

5.3.4 Nasendoscopy

Nasendoscopy is versatile in the fact that it is generally well tolerated and can be performed at pre-assessment clinic, in the ward setting and before induction of anaesthesia (Fig. 5.1). It is performed using a small-diameter flexible nasendoscope, and allows the operator to visualise the upper airway anatomy and identify any abnormalities. As the patient is awake and spontaneously breathing during the procedure and retains the ability to phonate various sounds, nasendoscopy allows a dynamic assessment of the position and movement of the vocal cords.

The procedure is commonly performed as part of the patient's assessment in the head and neck clinic, and the surgeons will usually document any pathology seen on a diagram in the patient's case notes so that other clinicians can refer to it, although still images or video recordings can also be taken and stored for reference. It is highly beneficial for the anaesthetist to perform or be present at the time of nasendoscopy rather than rely on these methods of documentation, as this allows a fuller assessment of the patient's upper airway anatomy and the ease with which a view of the glottis can be obtained with a flexible bronchoscope [19]. The procedure provides information on the bearing that a lesion will have on direct laryngoscopy, fibreoptic intubation, intubation and even direct tracheal access, and this information can be assimilated into the airway plan (Movie 5.1).

5.3.5 Radiographs

5.4 3-D Reconstruction and Virtual Endoscopy and Applications in Airway Pathology

In obstructing airway pathology, the assessment of the airway beyond what can be seen on examination is difficult, and therefore, advanced imaging can be helpful. Often nasendosopy is performed if tolerated and is a valuable tool in understanding the degree of airway compromise. In most cases, a CT scan of the head and neck will be performed; this provides extra information for the surgeon and the anaesthetist. Viewing of airway pathology on two-dimensional imaging such as CT slices and making an accurate identification of the size and location of the pathology can be a challenging task for the anaesthetist.

Modern post-processing software techniques such as 3-D volume rendering provide added diagnostic value to two-dimensional CT scans [20, 21]. Sharing the 3-D images enhances communication amongst clinicians and also improves procedural planning. The software tools are available to radiologists but often underutilised as they are slightly more time consuming and not all radiologists are familiar with them. Also the additional reconstruction is often not routinely requested. With newer software such as OsiriX® and Horos, the reconstruction has become easier and available to specialists outside radiology. The usefulness in the diagnostic process and airway management has been shown in the literature [22]. Virtual endoscopy and 3-D reconstruction also enhance communication amongst different specialities such as ENT and head and neck surgeons, radiologists, anaesthetists and also possibly the patient. It is important to understand that VE and 3-D reconstruction of the airway do not provide new information to the original CT scans but rather a complementary way of viewing the same data set. All the images and movies at our centre are created using the Osirix software (Osirix Viewer 9.5, Pixmeo Sarl, Bernex, Switzerland). Other software such as Horos (Horosproject.org, Nimble Co. LLC d/b/a Purview in Annapolis, MD, USA) and RadiAnt (Medixant 2009) used by the radiologists are equally accurate.

5.4.1 3-D Reconstruction

3-D reconstruction of the air–tissue interface is another application of post-processing software. This external 3-D rendering creates a 3-D model of the air-filled spaces that can be rotated in every direction and exported as an image (Fig. 5.2) or a

Fig. 5.2 3-D reconstruction of the air-filled spaces (**d**) from sagittal (**a**), axial (**b**) and coronal (**c**) views of the CT scans. Obstructing transglottic lesions show the severe narrowing of the trachea (**e**)

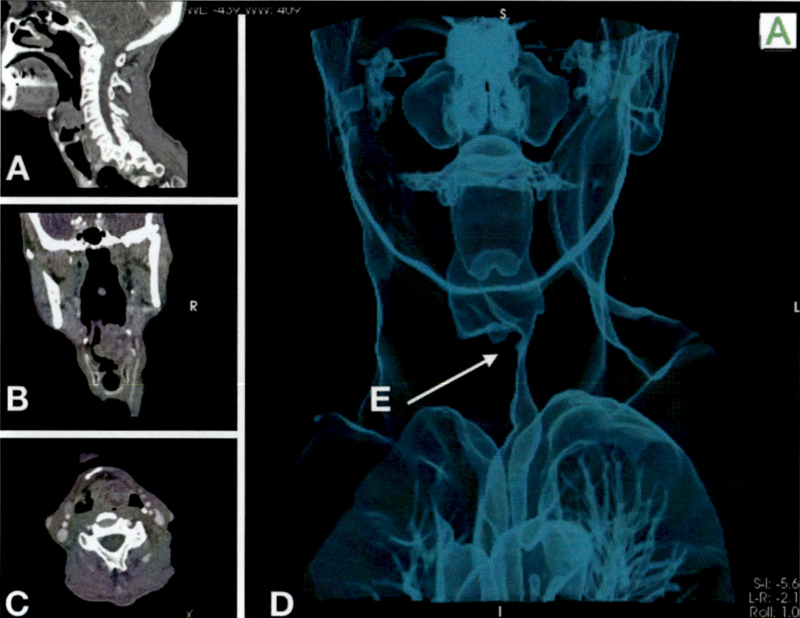

movie format (see Movie 5.2). Pathology within the airway or external lesions can be visualised by showing a narrowing of the air-filled spaces (Fig. 5.2).

With these techniques, subglottic lesions and abnormalities such as deviation of the trachea and long narrow stenosis can be appreciated better than those with a 2-D format or even virtual endoscopy.

5.4.1.1 Example

The three-dimensional aspect of an airway tumour can be better appreciated in the movie format. The extent of the obstruction of this adenoid cystic supraglottic tumour is shown in Movie 5.2 in the linked video files.

5.4.2 Virtual Endoscopy

Virtual endoscopy is another application of volume-rendering techniques whereby a virtual camera can be moved inside a hollow organ lumen. In airway assessment, this can be done in a similar way to moving a flexible bronchoscope through the patient's airway and down into the trachea. A focal point, which can be moved in every direction through the lumen, determines the pathway.

Several points are saved and computed to create a movie that can be viewed and shared. The advantage of VE in addition to conventional airway imaging is that it is non-invasive whereas flexible nasendoscopy is therefore not always tolerated by the patient. Also, VE does not require any additional radiation, as the CT scans are already part of the diagnostic process. By visualising the airway from the inside and thereby simulating an awake flexible bronchoscopic examination, the airway management can be planned in advance. Also, the virtual camera can move beyond the vocal cords and establish a retrograde view in a downward to upward direction.

5.4.2.1 Clinical Applications of VE

Virtual simulation training has good evidence as a tool to improve technical skills in the training of physicians [23, 24, 25].

NAP 4 has shown that patients with pathology of the head and neck have a higher proportion of complications during airway management as well as more severe complications than any other patient cohorts [1]. The evaluation and the subsequent airway management plan tend to be more challenging in patients with obstructing airway lesions [26]. As mentioned above, the usual methods of clinical airway assessment can be misleading or falsely reassuring or in fact be influenced by the airway pathology such as a dental abscess causing poor mouth opening.

Airway pathology can involve one or several parts of the supraglottic, glottic and subglottic larynx, and correctly pinpointing the location and extent of the lesion can be difficult for most anaesthetists [26, 27]. Advanced imaging of the airway such as helical CT scans or MRI can help to visualise the obstructing airway pathology (OAP). When available and performed close to the time of surgery, flexible nasendoscopy evaluation of the airway can change airway management [19]. Nasendoscopy is routinely done by the otolaryngologists if tolerated by the patient, but it is not always available to the anaesthetist. Also, the small calibre nasal endoscope can be passed after topicalisation of the nose to visualise structures down as far as the vocal cords and not beyond, and is not always available in theatre.

Other than nasal endoscopy, CT scans or MRI of the head and neck needs to be reviewed. Because of the two-dimensional aspect of these images and the way they need to be reviewed, it is not always easy to clearly identify the level of the obstructing airway pathology and quantify the impact onto the airway patency, especially by practitioners who have not been formally trained to do so. The endoscopic view of the airway is a view that anaesthetists are more familiar with as done during standard laryngoscopy, video-laryngoscopy or awake tracheal intubation using a flexible bronschoscope. Virtual endoscopy provides such a view of the airway from the patient's CT scans with no extra radiation as these images will have already been obtained during the diagnostic process. These virtual endoscopy views have been shown to accurately represent intraluminal lesions [28–37] and in fact are used in other specialities such as radiology and thoracic surgery to diagnose pathology in head and neck and the bronchial tree. More recent evidence shows that having virtual endoscopy views in addition to CT images improves the anaesthetist's diagnostic accuracy [22]. It has also been shown that they influence the airway plan. In the study by El-Boghdadly et al., the changes that were made to the airway management plan after

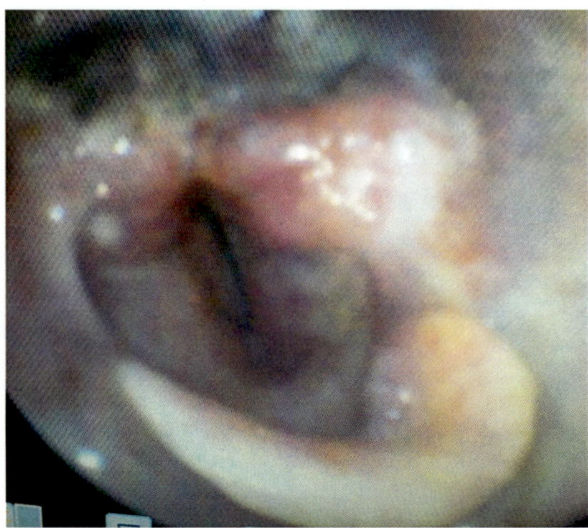

Fig. 5.3 Hypopharynx cancer involving the arytenoids as seen during awake tracheal intubation using a flexible bronchoscope

viewing the virtual endoscopy video were mostly to a more cautious approach and that was not dependent on the anaesthetist's level of experience with managing patients with OAP.

5.4.2.2 Example 1

This is an example of a glottic tumour involving the arytenoid cartilages. In Movie 5.3, the glottic tumour can be seen (Figs. 5.3 and 5.4).

5.4.2.3 Example 2

This is an example of a large supraglottic obstructing airway pathology arising from the right vallecula and pushing the epiglottis over to the left. The similar appearance of the large smooth-surfaced lesion wrapping around the epiglottis and obstructing the laryngeal inlet can be seen on the image taken from the flexible bronchoscopic airway assessment (Fig. 5.5) as well as from the virtual endoscopy (Fig. 5.6). In the VE video (Movie 5.4), a patent pathway can be seen beyond the lesion, which favours a possible awake tracheal intubation using a flexible bronschoscope.

5.4.2.4 Example 3

The following example is a patient with a base of tongue tumour and the abnormally shaped epiglottis can be seen on the movie (Movie 5.5) as well as on the images (Figs. 5.7 and 5.8).

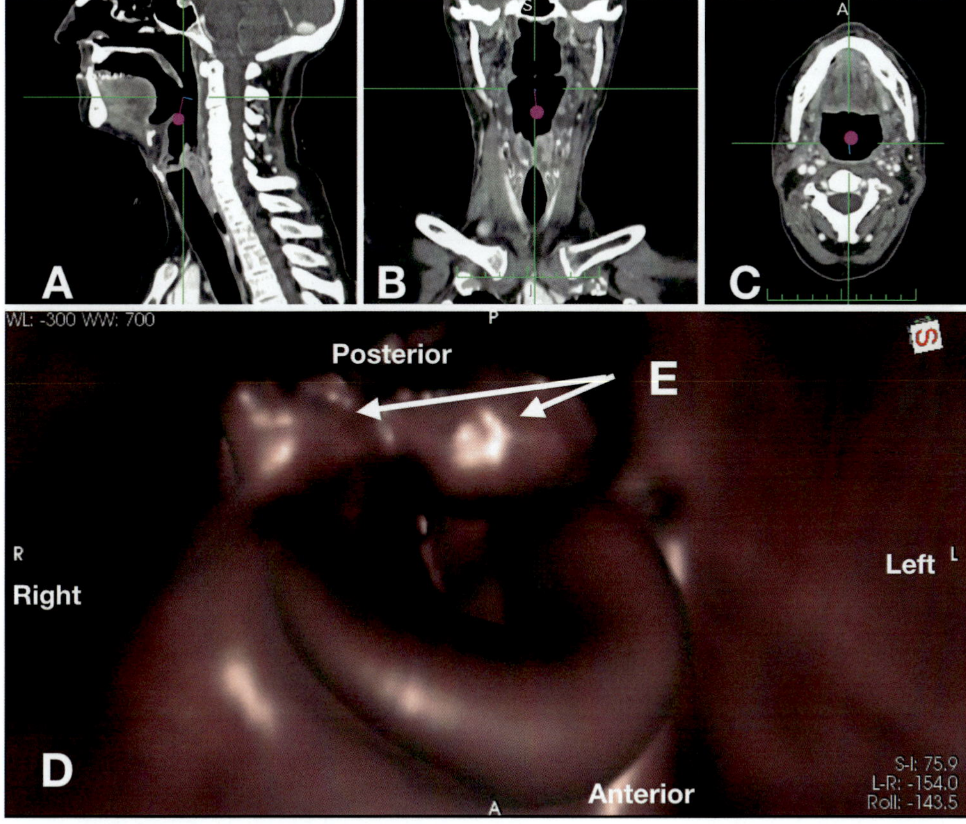

Fig. 5.4 Virtual endoscopy view 9 (**d**) of the epiglottis, vocal cords and arytenoid masses (**e**). The sagittal (**a**), coronal (**b**) and axial (**c**) views show the virtual camera position as a pink dot

5.4.3 Limitations of VE and 3-D Reconstruction

One of the limitations of VE and 3-D reconstruction is that it is based on static CT images in a supine position. In some cases, the supine position results in collapse of the airway and thus can give an appearance of the airway that is worser than it actually is. Also, it would be difficult to obtain a full VE run through down to the trachea if parts of the airway are collapsed, and there is no actual lumen for the virtual camera to go through. 3-D reconstruction of the air-filled spaces will still be possible but might give the impression of a more severe narrowing of the airway. This could be overcome by manoeuvres such as Valsalva or blowing through a straw during the CT scan, which is done in some institutions [38].

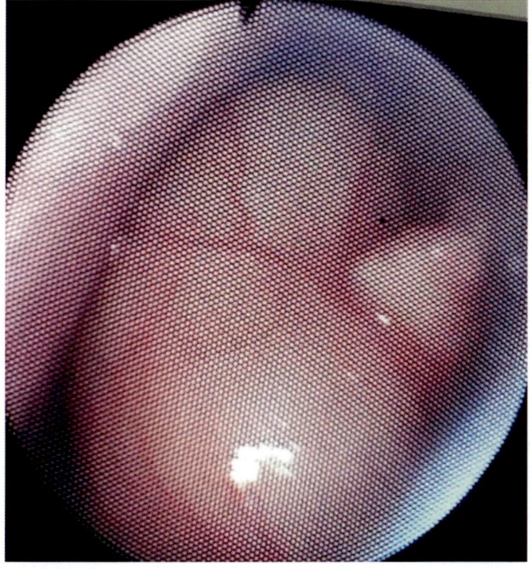

Fig. 5.5 Flexible bronchoscopic view of a large supraglottic mass lateral and posterior to the epiglottis. The epiglottis is seen on the right of the image

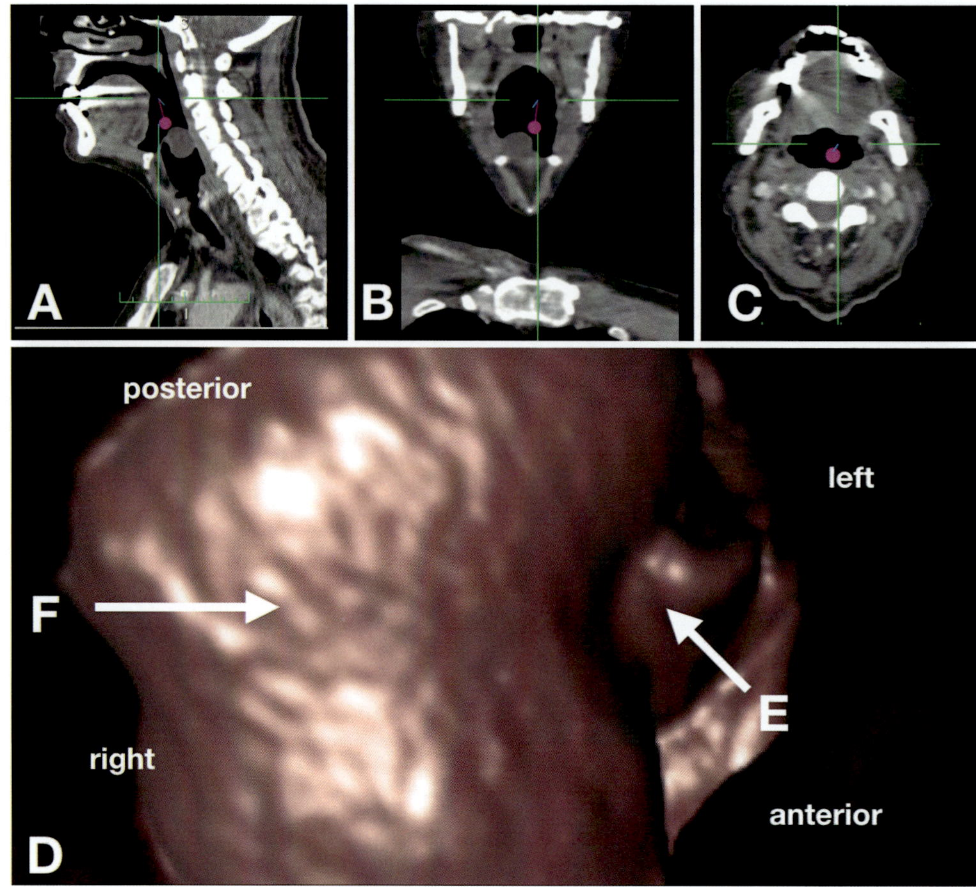

Fig. 5.6 Virtual endoscopic view (**d**) of a large exophytic lesion (**f**) arising from the right vallecula and pushing the epiglottis (**e**) over to the left. On the sagittal (**a**), coronal (**b**) and axial (**c**) views the virtual camera position can be seen as a pink dot

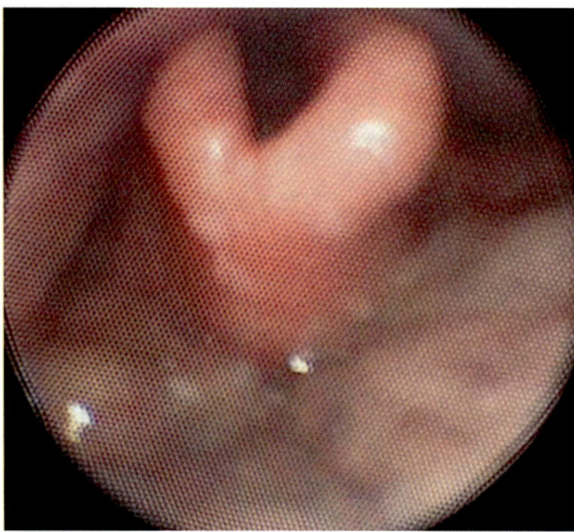

Fig. 5.7 Fibre-optic view of the epiglottis, which shows thickened edges, and some narrowing of the epiglottis is seen

The CT images are not always taken just prior to surgery and anaesthesia induction; therefore, caution should be taken in case the obstructing airway pathology has worsened or even improved.

Another limitation is the availability of the appropriate software and hardware as well as the CT scans. Radiologists can upon request reconstruct VE videos and a 3-D model of the air-filled spaces using the hospital's hardware and software and accessing the scans through the Patient Archive and Communication System (PACS). The downside of that is that radiologists do not always know what the anaesthetist is looking for to plan the airway, and some communication between specialities is required.

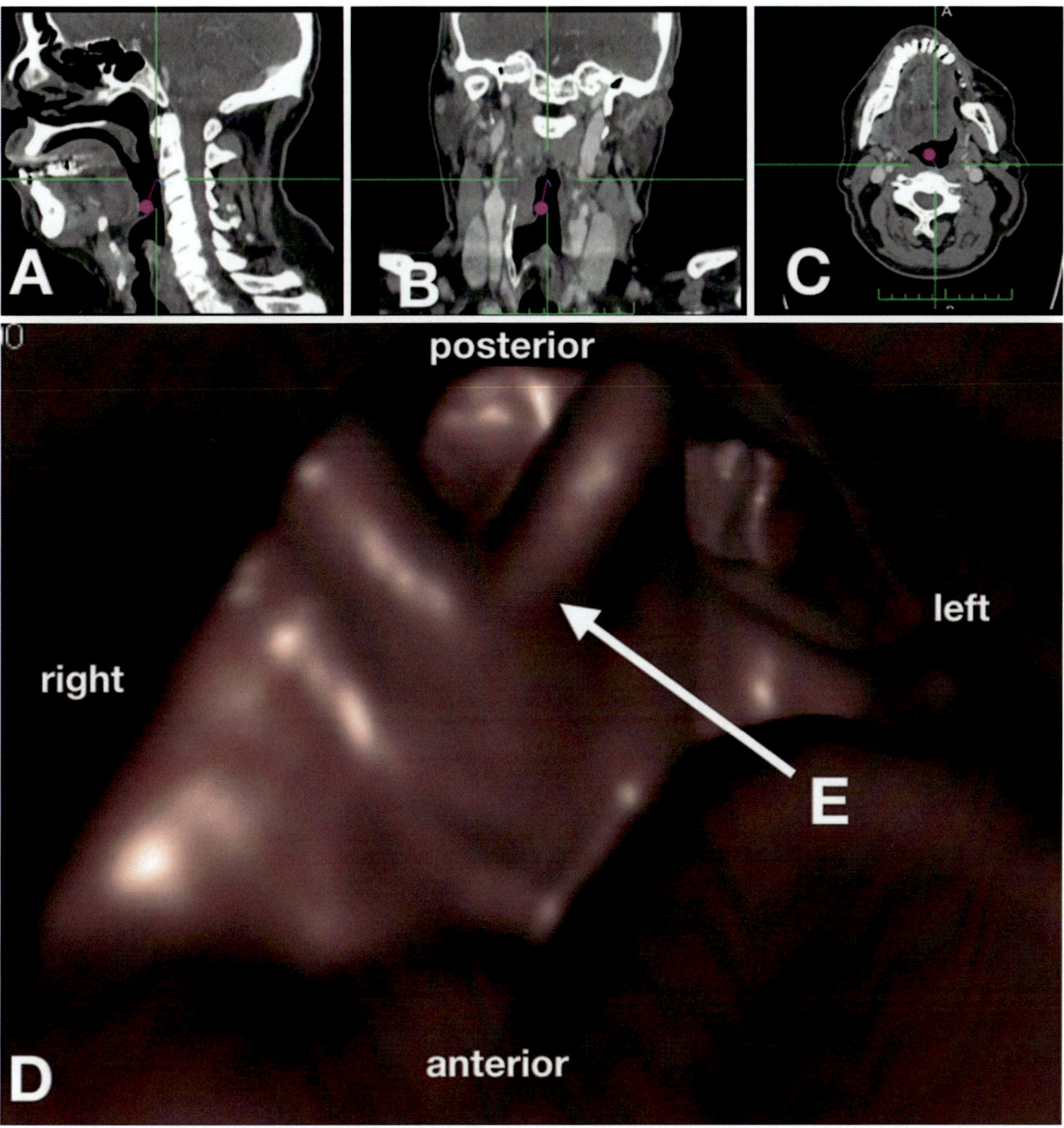

Fig. 5.8 Virtual endoscopy view (**d**) of epiglottis (**e**) reconstructed from the sagittal (**a**), coronal (**b**) and axial (**c**) views. The epiglottis is abnormally shaped and thickened edges in a patient with a supraglottic tumour

OsiriX® viewer and HOROS is a computer software program for Apple computer systems and that can be used to view Digital Imaging and Communications in Medicine DICOM data files as well as reconstruct VE and 3-D models of the airway in a user-friendly way. Most users without prior experience can create a video in 20 min whereas more experienced users are able to reconstruct VE in around 2 min.

5.5 3-D Printing in Airway Pathology

One must also consider the use of 3-D printed models, particularly of patients with airway pathology. These models, once printed from the patient's CT data, can not only be used in the assessment of the airway but also provide valuable anatomical information when they have been scoped by the anaesthetist pre-operatively. Manoeuvres of the flexible bronchoscope required to negotiate airway pathology can be practiced on the model without causing any airway trauma, with the added advantage that the operator will experience physical feedback, which is absent from VE. The creation of these models may also help in the teaching and training of fibre-optic intubation. There are, however, some areas of difficulty that need to be overcome such as cost and time required to produce each model, universal access to the software used to create the models and establishing the most appropriate materials to make the models.

5.6 Training Uses for Virtual Reality

Not only are 3-D reconstruction images useful for pre-emptive airway management planning, but the images are also of value for education and training. Both novice and expert airway anaesthetists can study the images, predict what aspects of airway management may be challenging and propose a strategy, which can be compared to how the case unfolded clinically.

There is precedent for the use of virtual reality in airway training, for example, the Operating Room Simulation (ORSIM)® System (Airway Simulation Limited, Auckland, New Zealand.) The ORSIM® comprises a replica bronchoscope associated with a sensor device, which communicates with a laptop configured with the ORSIM software package [25]. Users select a training package which displays on screen a high-fidelity, real-time run through a simulated patient's airway, and allows them to practice the endoscopy skills required to successfully navigate the airway. There are a variety of simulations to run, from normal airways through to complex airway pathology. The program will then give the operator feedback on the time taken for the procedure, whether hypoxia occurred during the procedure, and how often the simulated bronchoscope collided with soft tissues. The use of this system offers practitioners the opportunity to gain skills and experience in airway endoscopy in the safety of the virtual reality environment.

5.7 Summary

3-D reconstruction and VE volume rendering of CT images of the airway can provide anaesthetists with an alternative view of the airway in patients with head and neck pathology. This way of assessing the airway in a complex group of patients allows us to better appreciate how the pathology may affect safe airway management and appears to influence us into formulating safer airway planning.

References

1. Cook T, Woodall N, Frerk C. 4th National Audit Project (NAP 4) of the Royal College of Anaesthetists and The Difficult Airway Society, Major Complications of Airway Management in the United Kingdom, Report and Findings; 2011.
2. Apfelbaum JL, Hagberg CA, Caplan RA, et al. Practice guidelines for management of the difficult airway: an updated report by the American Society of Anesthesiologists Task Force on Management of the Difficult Airway. Anesthesiology. 2013;118:251–70. https://doi.org/10.1097/ALN.0b013e31827773b2.. Accessed 25 Mar 2018
3. Gawande A, Weiser T. Airway assessment. In: WHO Guidelines for Safe Surgery. Geneva: World Health Organisation; 2009. p. 29.. http://apps.who.int/iris/bitstream/handle/10665/44185/9789241598552_eng.pdf;jsessionid=170625B22-DD3F86FABAB55892724F269?sequence=1. Accessed 25 Mar 2018.
4. Ahmed-Nusrath A. Anaesthesia for head and neck cancer surgery. BJA Educ. 2017;17(12):383–9.
5. Crawley SM, Dalton AJ. Predicting the difficult airway. BJA Educ. 2015;15(5):253–7.
6. Karalapillai D, Darvall J, Mandeville J, Ellard L, Graham J, Weinberg L. A review of video laryngoscopes relevant to the intensive care unit. Indian J Crit Care Med. 2014;18(7):442–52.
7. Maltby JR, Loken RG, Beriault MT, Archer DE. Laryngeal mask airway with mouth opening less than 20 mm. Can J Anaesth. 1995;42(12):1140–2.
8. Mallampati SR, Gatt S, Gugino L, et al. A clinical sign to predict difficult tracheal intubation:a prospective study. Can Anaesth Soc J. 1985;32(4):29–34.
9. Lee A, Fan LT, Gin T, Karmakar MK, Ngan Kee WD. A systematic review (meta-analysis) of the accu-

racy of the mallampati tests to predict the difficult airway. Anesth Analg. 2006;102(6):1867–78.

10. Khan Z, Kashfi A, Ebrahimkhani E. A comparison of the upper lip bite test (a simple new technique) with modified mallampati classification in predicting difficulty in endotracheal intubation: a prospective blinded study. Anesth Analg. 2003;96(2): 595–9.

11. Hester C, Dietrich S, White S, Secrest J, Lindgren K, Smith T. A comparison of preoperative airway assessment techniques: the modified Mallampati and the upper lip bite test. AANA J. 2007;75(3):177–82.

12. Schmitt HJ, Kirmse M, Radespiel-Troger M. Ratio of patient's height to thyromental distance improves prediction of difficult laryngoscopy. Anaesth Intensive Care. 2002;30(6):763–5.

13. Krobbuaban B, Diregpoke S, Kumkeaw S, Tanomsat M. The predictive value of the height ratio and thyromental distance: four predictive tests for difficult laryngoscopy. Anesth Analg. 2005;101:1542–5.

14. Wilson ME, Spiegelhalter D, Robertson JA, Lesser P. Predicting difficult intubation. Br J Anaesth. 1988;61(2):211–6.

15. El-Ganzouri AR, McCarthy RJ, Tuman KJ, Tanck EN, Ivankovich AD. Preoperative airway assessment: predictive value of a multivariate risk index. Anesth Analg. 1996;82:1197–204.

16. Nørskov AK, Wetterslev J, Rosenstock CV, Afshari A, Astrup G, Jakobsen JC, et al. Effects of using the simplified airway risk index vs usual airway assessment on unanticipated difficult tracheal intubation - a cluster randomized trial with 64,273 participants. Br J Anaesth. 2016;116(5):680–9.

17. Hui CM, Tsui BC. Sublingual ultrasound as an assessment method for predicting difficult intubation: a pilot study. Anaesthesia. 2014;69:314–20.

18. Erzi T, Gewurtz G, Sessler DI, et al. Prediction of difficult laryngoscopy in obese patients by ultrasound quantification of anterior neck soft tissue. Anaesthesia. 2003;58:1111–4.

19. Rosenblatt W, Ianus AI, Sukhupragarn W, Fickenscher A, Sasaki C. Preoperative endoscopic airway examination (PEAE) provides superior airway information and may reduce the use of unnecessary awake intubation. Anesth Analg. 2011;112:602–7.

20. Rosset A, Spadola L, Ratib O. OsiriX: an open-source software for navigating in multidimensional DICOM images. J Digit Imaging. 2004;17:205–16.

21. Ahmad I, Millhoff B, John M, Andi K, Oakley R. Virtual endoscopy—a new assessment tool in difficult airway management. J Clin Anesth. 2015;27:508–13.

22. El-Boghdadly K, Onwochei DN, Millhoff B, Ahmad I. The effect of virtual endoscopy on diagnostic accuracy and airway management strategies in patients with head and neck pathology: a prospective cohort study. Can J Anaesth. 2017 Nov;64(11): 1101–10.

23. Boet S, Naik VN, Diemunsch PA. Virtual simulation training for fibreoptic intubation. Can J Anesth. 2009;56:87–8.

24. Boet S, Bould MD, Schaeffer R, et al. Learning fibreoptic intubation with a virtual computer program transfers to 'hands on' improvement. Eur J Anaesthesiol. 2010;27:31–5.

25. Baker PA, Weller JM, Baker MJ, et al. Evaluating the ORSIM_simulator for assessment of anaesthetists' skills in flexible bronchoscopy: aspects of validity and reliability. Br J Anaesth. 2016;117:i87–91.

26. Law JA, Morris IR, Malpas G. Obstructing pathology of the upper airway in a post-NAP4 world: time to wake up to its optimal management. Can J Anaesth. 2017;64(11):1087–97.   https://doi.org/10.1007/s12630-017-0928-7.

27. Norskov AK, Rosenstock CV, Wetterslev J, Astrup G, Afshari A, Lundstrom LH. Diagnostic accuracy of anaesthesiologists' prediction of difficult airway management in daily clinical practice: a cohort study of 188 064 patients registered in the Danish anaesthesia database. Anaesthesia. 2015;70:272–81.

28. Finkelstein SE, Schrump DS, Nguyen DM, Hewitt SM, Kunst TF, Summers RM. Comparative evaluation of super high-resolution CT scan and virtual bronchoscopy for the detection of tracheobronchial malignancies. Chest. 2003;124:1834–40.

29. Boiselle P, Reynolds KF, Ernst A. Multiplanar and threedimensional imaging of the central airways with multidetector CT. AJR Am J Roentgenol. 2002;179:301–8.

30. Men S, Ecevit MC, Topc̣u I, Kabakci N, Erdag TK, Sutay S. Diagnostic contribution of virtual endoscopy in diseases of the upper airways. J Digit Imaging. 2007;20:67–71.

31. Walshe P, Hamilton S, McShane D, McConn Walsh R, Walsh MA, Timon C. The potential of virtual laryngoscopy in the assessment of vocal cord lesions. Clin Otolaryngol Allied Sci. 2002;27:98–100.

32. Summers RM, Shaw DJ, Shelhamer JH. CT virtual bronchoscopy of simulated endobronchial lesions: effect of scanning, reconstruction, and display settings and potential pitfalls. AJR Am J Roentgenol. 1998;170:947–50.

33. Summers RM, Aggarwal NR, Sneller MC, et al. CT virtual bronchoscopy of the central airways in patients with Wegener's granulomatosis. Chest. 2002;121:242–50.

34. De Wever W, Vandecaveye V, Lanciotti S, Verschakelen JA. Multidetector CT-generated virtual bronchoscopy: an illustrated review of the potential clinical indications. Eur Respir J. 2004;23:776–82.

35. Bauer TL, Steiner KV. Virtual bronchoscopy: clinical applications and limitations. Surg Oncol Clin N Am. 2007;16:323–8.

36. Rogalla P, Nischwitz A, Gottschalk S, Huitema A, Kaschke O, Hamm B. Virtual endoscopy of the nose and paranasal sinuses. Eur Radiol. 1998;8:946–50.

37. Burke AJ, Vining DJ, McGuirt WF Jr, Postma G, Browne JD. Evaluation of airway obstruction using virtual endoscopy. Laryngoscope. 2000;110:23–9.

38. P H, Blum A, Toussaint B, Troufleau P, Stines J, Roland J. Dynamic maneuvers in local staging of head and neck malignancies with current imaging techniques: principles and clinical applications. Radiographics. 2003;23(5):1201–13.

Virtual Endoscopy and 3-D Reconstruction in the Nose, Paranasal Sinuses, and Skull Base Surgery: New Frontiers

Shanmugam Ganesan, Hamad Al Saey, Natarajan Saravanappa, Prathamesh Pai, Surjith Vattoth, and Michael Stewart

6

6.1 Introduction

Technological developments in the medical and surgical field have driven the diagnostic and surgical management to an advanced level over the past few decades. Introduction of computerized tomography (CT) and magnetic resonance imaging (MRI) has improved the diagnostic workup and understanding of anatomical structures in health and disease. Further digitalization of radiological procedures has helped obtain better preoperative evaluation. We can merge different radiological images (fusion of CT and MRI) to obtain accurate visualization of internal structures. These advances have helped improve patient care and surgical outcome. The anatomy of the head and neck is very complex. Endoscopic surgery has revolutionized the way we treat various nose and paranasal sinus lesions. The clarity of endoscopic images and advancement in radiological techniques have led to the extended application of endoscope to an advanced level in rhinology and neurosurgery. Extended endoscopic skull base procedures are performed in various institutions for complex cases where it would have been difficult to reach with conventional surgery.

The most recent advance with spiral CT processing is the use of a three-dimensional (3-D) virtual endoscopy (VE) to display hollow organs and anatomical cavities. It is a new and noninvasive imaging tool. The viewer can penetrate the

S. Ganesan (✉) · H. Al Saey
Otolaryngology-Head and Neck Surgery Division, Department of Surgery, Hamad Medical Corporation, Doha, Qatar

Department of Otolaryngology-Head and Neck Surgery, Weill Cornell Medicine-Qatar, Doha, Qatar
e-mail: sganesan@hamad.qa; halsaey@hamad.qa

N. Saravanappa
Department of Otorhinolaryngology-Head and Neck Surgery, University Hospitals of North Midlands, Stoke-on-Trent, UK

P. Pai
Tata Memorial Centre, Homi Bhabha National Institute, Mumbai, India

S. Vattoth
Department of Clinical Radiology and Medical Imaging, Hamad Medical Corporation, Doha, Qatar

Department of Clinical Radiology, Weill Cornell Medicine-Qatar, Doha, Qatar
e-mail: svattoth@hamad.qa

M. Stewart
Department of Otolaryngology-Head and Neck Surgery, Weill Cornell Medical College, New York-Presbyterian Hospital/Weill Cornell Medical Center, New York, NY, USA
e-mail: mgs2002@med.cornell.edu

© Springer Nature Switzerland AG 2019
N. A. Shallik et al. (eds.), *Virtual Endoscopy and 3D Reconstruction in the Airways*,
https://doi.org/10.1007/978-3-030-23253-5_6

walls and visualize the extent of disease within and beyond the wall. The technique has been used in other disciplines such as simulation bronchoscopy, angioscopy, cystoscopy, and colonoscopy [1, 2]. Recently, VE of the nasal cavity and paranasal sinuses has drawn attention of otolaryngologists. It provides simulated visualization of nasal, paranasal, and skull base images equivalent to those produced by the standard endoscopic procedures and sometimes even better images. (Fig. 6.1). VE can clearly demonstrate anatomical structures within the nasal cavity, septal deviation, middle meatal pathology, turbinate hypertrophy, and pathological masses larger than 3 mm in diameter [3] (Fig. 6.1). As we are in an era of computer-assisted surgery and simulation-based training, VE holds far-reaching potential in endoscopic sinus surgery (ESS), extended ESS and skull base surgery.

In this chapter, we describe VE techniques and their advantages and disadvantages. We also explore the applications of VE in diagnosis, preoperative planning, and opportunities for surgical training in various nasal, nasal airway, paranasal, and skull base conditions.

## 6.2	3-D and VE in Endoscopic Sinus Surgery (ESS)

Endoscopic sinus surgery (ESS) currently represents the most common and effective surgical treatment for nasal, paranasal sinus, and skull base pathology. ESS can be challenging for trainees and practicing otolaryngologists due to the complex and varying anatomy of the paranasal sinuses and skull base [1–4]. The risks of ESS, although rare, include a number of potentially serious complications such as orbital penetration, optic nerve injury, arterial bleeding and skull base injury [1, 2, 4–6]. Endoscopes facilitate superior illumination, higher magnification, and various angular views for surgery. Efficient use of endoscopes is associated with a steep learning curve, and it provides two-dimensional (2-D) views which demand the operating surgeon to mentally create a three-dimensional (3-D) view of the operating field during surgery [2, 7].

In the past two decades, various virtual reality (VR) surgical simulators have been introduced for ESS training which complement other established modes of training methods like endoscopic anatomy atlases, hands-on cadaver dissections, and VR simulation training [1, 5, 8–13]. The application of VR was first proposed by Satava et al. in 1993 to deliver reproducible, consistent models, which allow unlimited practice using standardized anatomy [11]. All the above-mentioned available methods of training aim to make trainees and practicing otolaryngologists familiarize with the complex anatomy of the paranasal sinuses and skull base in particular the vital structures such as orbit and its contents, optic nerve, skull base, and carotid artery.

Training in a 3-D virtual environment helps to achieve a greater breadth of simulated surgical

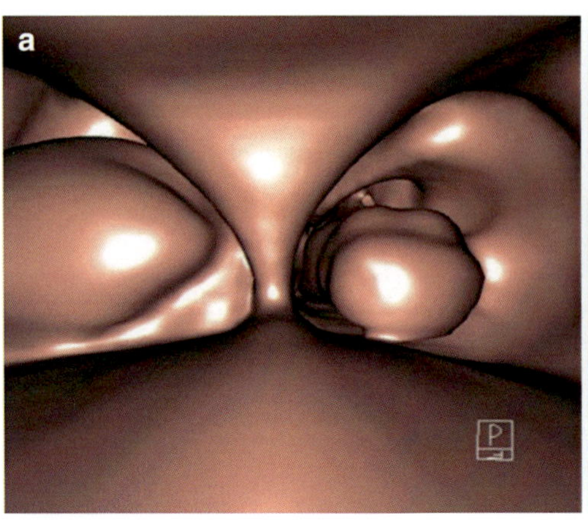
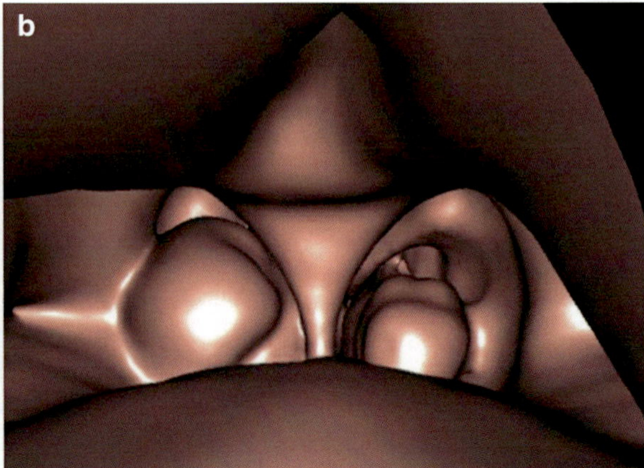

Fig. 6.1 Virtual endoscopic view from the posterior nares showing the vomer/posterior nasal septum, middle inferior turbinates, and partially the Eustachian tube orifices

scenarios resulting in acceleration of the learning curve. Surgical simulation allows the operating surgeon to develop a better preoperative planning and practice with the aim of providing better patient outcome facilitated by minimizing the complication rates [14].

6.3 Applications of VE and 3-D Reconstruction in Sinus and Skull Base Lesions

Virtual endoscopy (VE) provides a virtual three-dimensional view of intricate bony details of the sinus and skull base by computerized reconstruction of image data through a threshold process. It is possible to simulate three-dimensional visualization by virtual endoscopy and also possible to rotate the viewing position inside this virtual 3-D space. Merging the CT scan and MRI scan images enables us to produce 3-D images. This is helpful in better understanding of anatomical relations and the image of the lesions in hidden areas of the head and neck such as infratemporal fossa. Information technology now provides us with virtual endoscopy which is a valuable tool for visualizing the cavities and understanding the

anatomy to help in preoperative surgical planning and operative training [7]. Advancements in 3-D printing technology have enabled us to directly visualize intricate anatomical areas which help in surgical planning and to develop a tailored surgical approach to patients [15]. These technologies have also helped train future generations of surgeons and students. Furthermore, the extent of disease and the surgical procedure could be better explained to the patient who can understand the intricate details of their procedure, which in turn would improve the consenting process (Fig. 6.2). The 3-D printing is also expected to improve tissue engineering and provide further improvement in the management of biological tissue processing for prosthesis and reconstruction (for more details, refer to Chap. 11).

6.3.1 Benign Conditions of Nose and Sinuses

Endoscopic surgery of the nose, sinus, and skull base is widely practiced in rhinology and neurosurgery. Although CT scan and MRI scan allow for preoperative evaluation in these patients, virtual endoscopy has taken this step to another

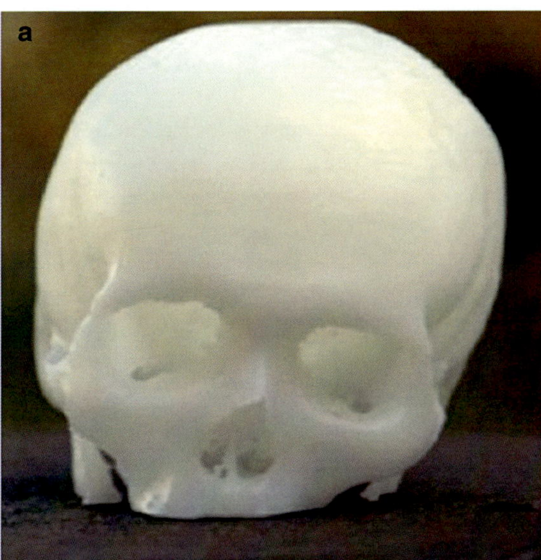
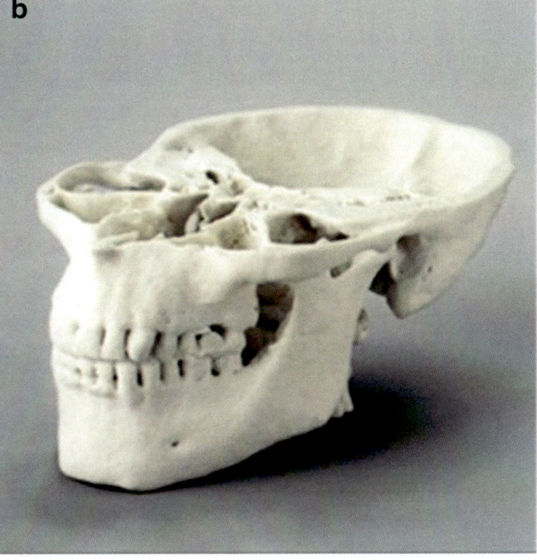

Fig. 6.2 Skull and mandible 3-D reconstruction printed model which is shuttered into two segments; A: including the bony calvarium, orbits, and nasal bone and part of the maxilla. B: 3-D printed model for the lower maxilla, mandible, skull base, and TMJ

level. Endoscopic approach to the frontal sinus is challenging even for an experienced rhinologist. Surgical trainees need to attend cadaver dissection courses to have a grasp of the anatomy and anatomical variations around the frontal sinus drainage pathway and anterior skull base. Comprehensive understanding of variations of frontal sinus cells and surrounding structures is of paramount importance for performing safe endoscopic frontal sinus surgery. Meticulous and careful presurgical planning is necessary by evaluating the CT scans to formalize a patient-specific surgery to avoid potential complications such as cerebrospinal fluid leak and intracranial injury. Three-dimensional reconstruction of paranasal sinus structure and anatomical variation obtained from CT scans of the human skull could be a valuable tool for trainee education [2]. Virtual endoscopy is an additional armamentarium which helps to study the structures around the frontal recess to aid the surgical planning [16–18].

6.3.2 Frontal Sinus Fractures

Management of frontal sinus fractures caused by major head injury can be a challenging task. Although CT scan provides two-dimensional imaging of fracture, visualization of fracture in relation to surrounding structures may be difficult. Virtual endoscopy and 3-D volume rendering can be very useful for delineating the fracture site in relation to surrounding structures and providing accurate information about the damage to the walls of the frontal sinus which would be useful for surgical planning and management of frontal sinus fractures [19]. Fujikura et al. reported the use of virtual endoscopy in endoscopic operations for mucocele and found that it is useful in sphenoid and ethmoid mucoceles avoiding injury to vital structures such as optic canal and lamina papyracea [20]. They also performed simulation based on virtual endoscopy images where it was possible to recognize the bone structure of the sinuses even if the endoscopic findings showed postoperative changes in the structure.

6.3.3 Pituitary Surgery and Skull Base Surgery

Endoscopic pituitary surgery has become a routine procedure and supra-sellar and para-sellar extensions can be reached safely via endoscopic procedures. Wolfsberger et al. compared the intraoperative endoscopic views during trans-sphenoidal pituitary surgery with the various anatomical structures identified on virtual endoscopy images and found that the images were comparable [21]. Virtual endoscopy was found to be useful in the preoperative understanding of nasal anatomy and sphenoid sinus septations for intraoperative orientation and in planning the opening of the sellar floor as it was possible to visualize the important structures related to the pituitary gland. Virtual endoscopy also provided a clear view of the choana, the ostium of the sphenoid sinus, bulging of the Sella, the clivus, tuberculum sellae, protuberances of the internal carotid artery, optic nerve and the optico-carotid recess, and the anterior clinoid process. Identification of these structures preoperatively would help in the preoperative planning of an individually tailored approach to patient management of sellar lesions. In their study, Wolfsberger et al. assessed the usefulness of virtual endoscopy in a series of 22 patients and observed that preoperative 3-D simulation of individual patient anatomy was feasible [21]. Virtual endoscopy could be used as a training tool for trainees to teach endoscopic pituitary surgery. Rotariu et al. reported the role of Osirix software (Osirix® Viewer 9.5, Pixmeo Sari, and Bernex, Switzerland) based visual endoscopy in endoscopic trans-sphenoidal surgery in 22 patients with pituitary adenomas [22]. While the Osirix-based visual endoscopy provided a good-quality image for preoperative planning, it was limited by the difficulty in obtaining information if the sphenoid sinus was not well aerated or filled by a tumor.

Three-dimensional printed skull base simulation could be used for trans-nasal endoscopic skull base surgery. In endoscopic pituitary surgery, the three-dimensional printed simulator could accurately reflect the spatial relationship between a tumor and internal carotid artery, and these simulators can be used for anatomical education and operative training. Although cadaver dissection is the gold standard for anatomical learning, combining the visual effect of virtual reality technology and the realistic tactile feedback of a 3-D printing simulator could complement surgical training [23] (Fig. 6.2).

Although the majority of studies discuss the use of virtual endoscopy in preoperative planning, surgical simulation, and training, virtual endoscopy has also been used intraoperatively to enhance the understanding of anatomical structures. Haerle et al. evaluated the intraoperative use of virtual endoscopy in skull base procedures [24]. In their study, the evaluation of virtual endoscopy image guidance systems and the usefulness of real-time visual/auditory alerts when the tracker drill approaches proximity zone positions were done on 16 patients whose pathology included pituitary adenoma, craniopharyngioma, and recurrent chordoma. They found that intraoperative virtual endoscopy image guidance system was a reliable and helpful technology in sinus and skull base surgery and suggested further studies to evaluate the impact on surgical workflow. In another study where virtual endoscopy was used intraoperatively in combination with image guidance, the authors found that visualizing the hidden anatomical structures behind the bony walls of sphenoid was most useful [18].

Intraoperative navigation is routinely used in various centers to guide surgeons in complex skull base procedures. Endoscopic skull base procedures can be technically challenging as the surgeon needs to operate in the surgical field surrounded by critical anatomical structures such as the carotid artery, optic nerve, and the brain. This becomes even more challenging as the disease process and the pathology might have destroyed the normal anatomical landmarks. Neuronavigation is another tool which helps surgeons identify various structures with the use of the navigational probe and advanced navigation protocols permitting continuous suction-tracked

navigation guidance that could be used for displaying fine paranasal sinus structures providing seamless integration of structures into the operating workflow during endoscopic transsphenoidal surgery [25]. In the future, virtual endoscopy images used for preoperative surgical planning could be integrated with the intraoperative image-guided navigation system to improve surgical precision for complex extended endoscopic skull base procedures including anterior skull base, pterygopalatine fossa, infratemporal fossa, and suprasellar lesions (Fig. 6.3).

6.3.4 Skull Base Tumors

Virtual endoscopy has been around for some time now, and its application in paranasal sinus and skull base tumors is well known. The image quality is still far from perfect, but it certainly gives an understanding of the pathway to the sinuses and skull base. The tumors involving the skull base are in the vicinity of the orbit, the dura, the internal carotid artery, and the cranial nerves—olfactory, optic, and trigeminal. The issues related to skull base tumors are defining the structures involved and the trajectory for access, which is currently decided based on the planar images provided by CT and MRI. Virtual endoscopy and its adjuncts could help in surgical planning by providing an opportunity to project the surgical access and to practice simulation.

6.3.5 Virtual Endoscopy in Surgical Access

Traditionally, open approaches were employed for accessing and excising the tumors. With the aid of virtual endoscopy and virtual reality or augmented reality, the tumor and its vicinity can be mapped with CT and MR along with angiography. This "mapping" can assist the surgeon to do preoperative planning and simulation or intraoperative real-time awareness. The possibilities are extensive.

Haerle and colleagues from Toronto, Canada, have reported on image-guided sur-

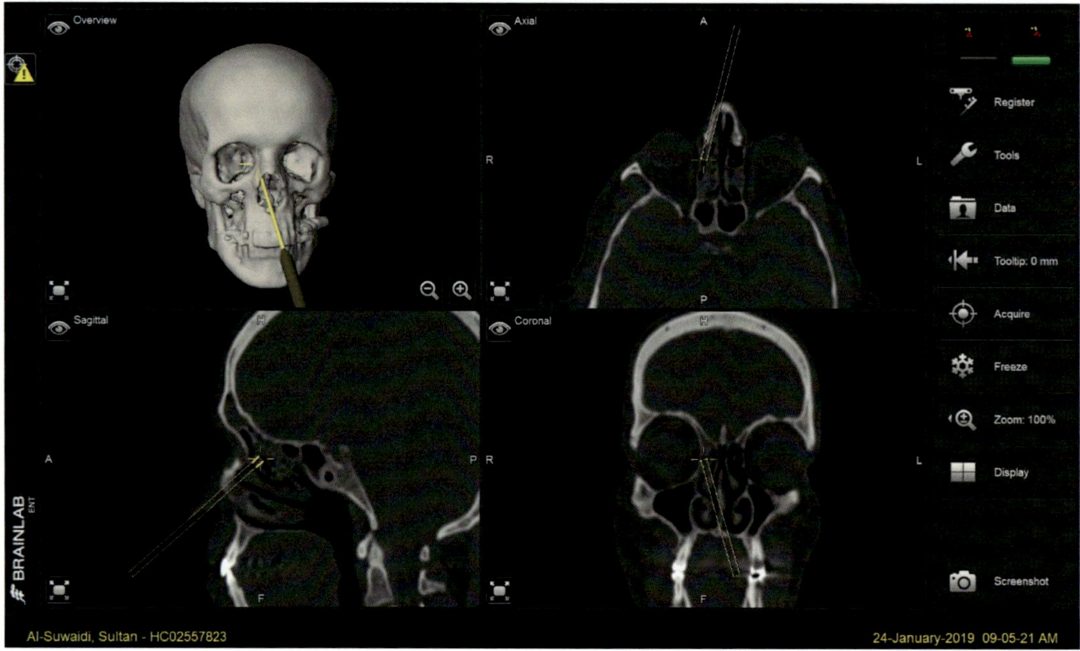

Fig. 6.3 Intraoperative image-guided navigation system using brain Lab

gery (IGS) navigation which is employed intermittently in the surgical procedure to confirm anatomical details [24]. They endeavored to provide a real-time feedback IGS system with high-resolution 3-D visualization. They used high-resolution MRI images to develop virtual endoscopy and augmented reality views and provide real-time visual and auditory alerts when encountered predetermined regions on the contoured images akin to radiation planning. They called it the "localized intraoperative virtual endoscopy," or LIVE-IGS (Fig. 6.4).

The study showed target registration error of 1 mm. They used a 3 mm alert zone for critical structures such as carotid arteries, optic nerves, and dura which reflected as the proximity of the drill to the carotid artery (1 mm) and optic nerve (0.5 mm).

The proximity of critical structures to the high-speed drill lends itself to the use of virtual and augmented reality views within intraoperative image-guided systems to be able to subjectively increase the surgeon's confidence.

6.3.6 Virtual Endoscopy in Simulation

Oishi and colleagues from Nigata and Tokyo, Japan, reported on the use of 3-D imaging techniques in neurosurgical planning and interactive virtual simulation (IVS) [26]. They acquired high-quality 3-D CG data from imaging (64 slice CT, CTA, and 3 T MR) and then developed CAD software with a haptic feedback device. Using IVS, they have simulated the best scenario for tumor removal and thereafter printed 3-D color models. They then performed IVS on the 3-D CG dataset simulating the surgical space, imitating craniotomy and retraction of the brain. Different approaches were simulated to determine the best surgical route, extent of the operative window, as well as tumor removal. They simulated brain tumors, vestibular and trigeminal schwannomas, and clival and para cavernous lesions. This was followed by 3-D printing of the model (Fig. 6.5).

The surgeons were then asked to perform the IVS and use the 3-D models for surgical simulation prior to surgery. Among the 25 cases, the

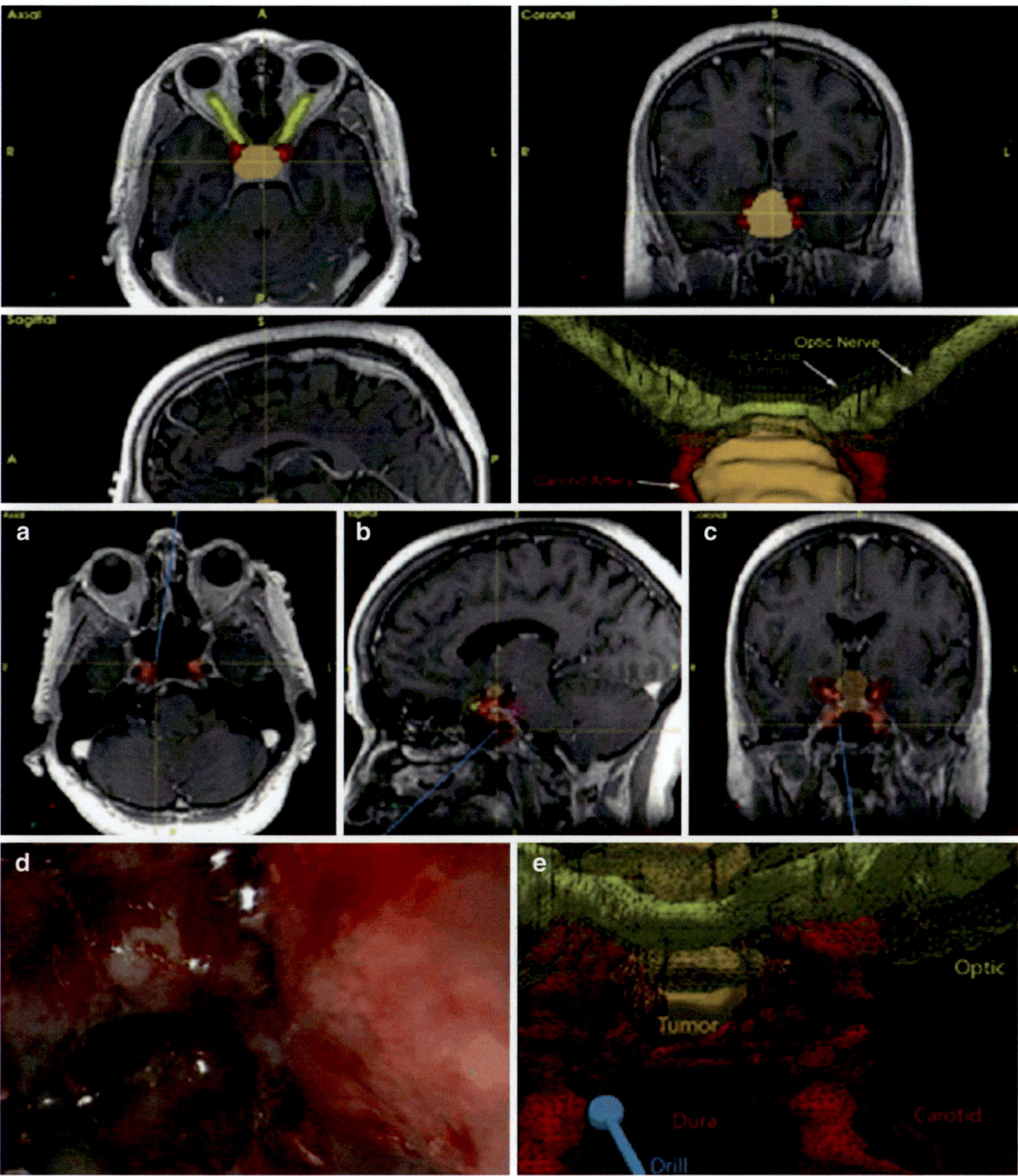

Fig. 6.4 (**a–c**) Views of drill in proximity to the carotid artery. (**d**) Endoscopic view. (**e**) Virtual view of the drill entering the "proximity zone" [26]

surgeons found benefit in 44% of cases. Some benefits included surgeons determining the most appropriate craniotomy to create a favorable working space, and also defining the complex bone work required in deep tumors, for example, the petrous apex with narrow surgical corridors. Identification of important deep veins around a tumor was made with confidence and strategies could also be determined in cases requiring staged operations ensuring appropriate planning for removal. The 3-D simulation with IVS and printed models has the potential for teaching and bridging the gap, reducing the learning curve in complex procedures by improving the microsurgical nuances and skills of trainees through repetition of surgical tasks (Fig.6.6).

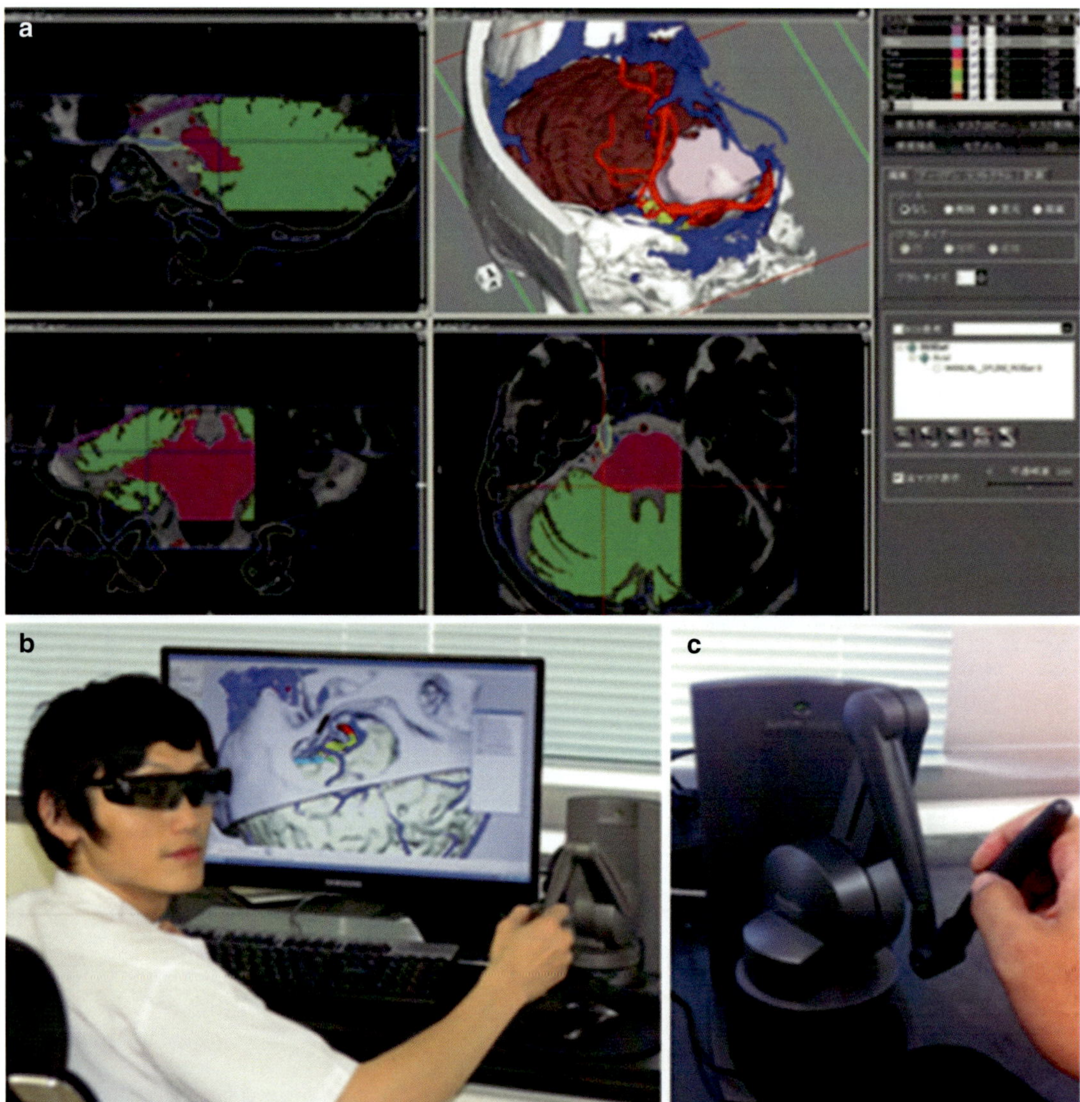

Fig. 6.5 (a) Operating window of the image analysis software (Zed-View, LEXI, Inc.) for data segmentation, fusion, and surface rendering of individual structures. (b, c) Interactive virtual simulation is performed using a Free Form Modeling system (SensAble Technologies, Inc.) characterized by unique 3-D computer-assisted designing software (b) with manipulation of a specific haptic device (c) [26]

6.3.7 Virtual Endoscopy and Diagnosis of Congenital Anomalies: Diagnosis of Choanal Atresia

Choanal atresia is a congenital condition which causes obstruction of one or both sides of posterior choanae. It is an uncommon condition with an estimated incidence of 1:7000 births. The obstruction can be bony (90%) or membranous or mixed. The atresia can be due to any of the bony components forming the borders of the posterior choana. The choanal atresia can be associated with other congenital anomalies including coloboma, heart defects, growth retardation, genital hypoplasia, and ear abnormalities (CHARGE syndrome). The clinical presen-

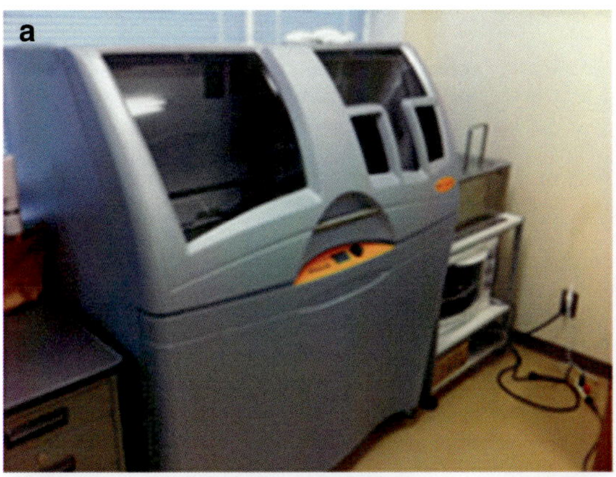

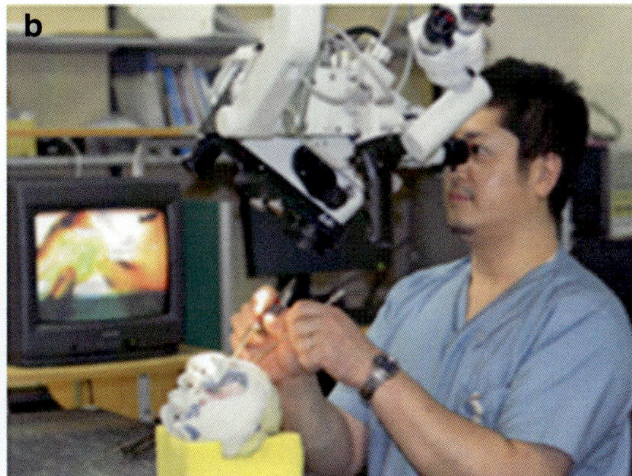

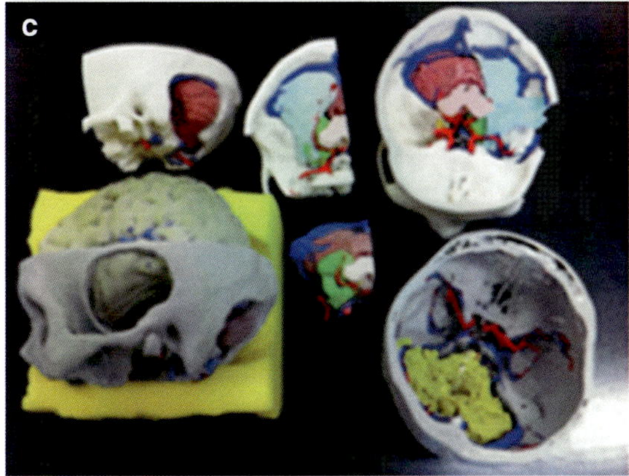

Fig. 6.6 The 3D color printer (Zprinter Z Corporation, Inc.); (**a**) the color-printed plaster models based on CG data modified through IVS (**b**). Realistic surgical sensa- tions can be experienced through microscopic observation of the models (**c**) [26]

tation varies from acute airway obstruction to recurrent sinus disease depending on whether the obstruction is unilateral or bilateral and presence of other congenital airway abnormalities.

The investigations for choanal atresia depend on the clinical presentation of the condition. Initial nasoendoscopy examination is a preferred method for making the diagnosis, as the point of obstruction can be directly visualized. Thin-section CT scan is a valuable tool in assessing the extent of obstruction and the bony involvement. In a recent study assessing the usefulness of helical 3-D reconstruction and virtual endoscopy, Yunus observed that CT and virtual endoscopy are valuable for defining the type and extent of the disease as CT virtual endoscopy of the nasopharynx from a posterior view can provide the view

of Eustachian tube opening with reference to bony borders of the nasopharynx [27]. Surgical management of choanal atresia can be difficult due to high re-stenosis, and the surgical approach includes transnasal, transseptal, transpalatal, and transmaxillary. Preoperative evaluation of the condition using CT scan and virtual endoscopy would be helpful in surgical planning. Intraoperative CT-guided navigation system can be used for endoscopic transnasal repair of choanal atresia in children with low birth weights and neonates with craniofacial abnormality where special anatomical considerations are needed [28] (Fig. 6.7). In the future, advances in virtual endoscopy techniques and 3 D printing may render useful information for preoperative planning. Further refinement of intraoperative navigation system, powered instrumentation,

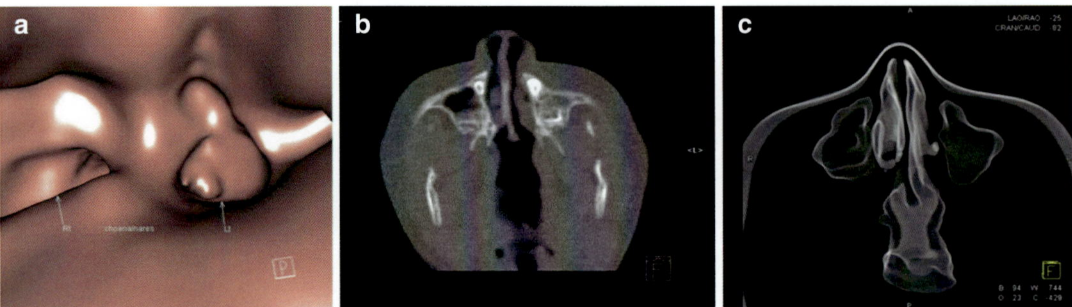

Fig. 6.7 Right-sided choanal atresia with significant bony narrowing at the level of the posterior nares (Choana) as well as membranous soft tissue component. (**a**) Virtual endoscopy projecting the posterior nares showing obliteration of the right nares, while the left nares are open. (**b**) Axial CT at the level of the posterior nares showing the mixed bony narrowing and soft tissue contribution for the right choana. (**c**) TTP showing nicely the airway continuation on the left side between the nasal cavity

and LASER-assisted surgery may be helpful in better surgical outcome of choanal atresia surgery in neonates and infants.

6.4 3-D Modeling in Skull Base Surgery

In recent years, advances in 3-D printing have enabled us to produce 3-D models useful for surgical planning of complex reconstruction of maxillofacial and skull base pathology. Advances in radiological techniques such as magnetic resonance imaging (MRI) and multi-detector computed tomography (MDCT) have provided surgeons with the necessary details for appropriate preoperative planning. However, accurate details may not be depictable as these techniques provide only two-dimensional images. Three-dimensional printing is used to address limitations in virtual image analysis and to provide physical models for surgical simulation and preoperative planning. The 3-D models are printed by converting 3-D digital models into physical models through the multi-layer fabrication process. This allows printing of patient-specific 3-D models which allows better visualization of the anatomy that can be useful for a better tactile understanding of the anatomical planes, preoperative planning, and surgical training and for explaining the procedure to the patient [29] (For more details about 3-D printing, please refer to Chap. 11).

6.4.1 3-D Printing Techniques

Three-dimensional printing is an umbrella term for creating 3-D printed models. 3-D printing is done by converting the digital images obtained by MRI and CT scanning into physical models. Multi-detector computed tomography is widely used for acquiring the image data. These images are processed using widely available CAD software packages to convert the data to Standard Tessellation Language (STL) format. The 3-D printing machine reads this data and converts the data into a physical 3-D model by layer-by-layer fabrication. This allows the production of patient-specific 3-D models, which can be used for surgical planning and training. Various methods can be used for converting the digital data into 3-D solid models, including rapid prototyping, material jetting printing, binder jetting printing, stereolithography (SLA), fused deposition modeling, laminated object manufacturing, and selective LASER sintering (SLS) [29, 30]. Of these, SLA and SLS techniques are typically used in the field of skull base surgery and maxillofacial trauma. The advantages of SLA and SLS techniques include the possibility of creating large models, high accuracy, and usefulness in device placement simulation. However, the main disadvantage of these techniques is the high production cost. Cost-effective and inexpensive methods of 3-D

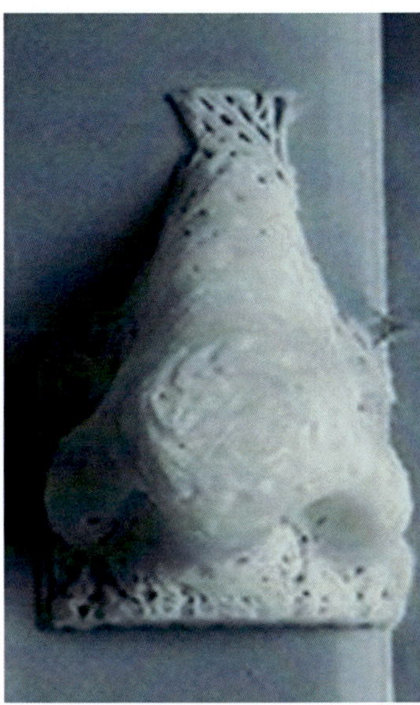

Fig. 6.8 3D printed nose for surgical planning, intraoperative guidance, and surgical simulation

models of the brain and skull using open-source desktop 3-D printers have been reported [31]. The 3-D printing of anatomical models can be used for patient discussion, informed consent, preoperative surgical planning, intraoperative guidance, and surgical simulation [30–40]. These models are useful for teaching and training of complex surgical procedures to surgical trainees. It is also possible to create complex anatomical models for prosthetics and implants for maxillofacial reconstruction (Fig. 6.8).

For more details about 3-D printing, please refer to Chap. 11.

6.4.2 Skull Base Procedures

The 3-D printed simulators are useful in endoscopic sinus and skull base surgery training and endo-nasal drilling practice providing accurate anatomical landmarks such as sphenoid, internal carotid artery, optic nerve, sella turcica, and upper clivus [32]. Various studies have looked at the application of 3-D printing technology for the management of skull base lesions, petroclival tumors, anterior skull base pathology, frontal

sinus models, various endoscopic skull base approaches, and surgical planning of resection of juvenile nasopharyngeal angiofibroma [29, 32]. Use of a 3-D printing model for preoperative planning of complex neurosurgical procedures and for the surgical management of multiple leak sites due to large skull base prolactinoma has also been reported [35]. Further, it is also possible to create models using 3-D printing to create patient-specific implants for rhinoplasty, complex nasal injuries, maxillofacial defects, and craniofacial reconstruction involving the skull base.

6.4.3 Cranio-Facial Trauma

Management of patients with severe cranio-facial trauma can be challenging due to the complexity and variations in the anatomy of the cranio-maxillofacial and skull base anatomy. 3-D printed models can be useful in such patients for appropriate surgical planning and precise reconstruction. A group of researchers reported the use of 3-D printing for presurgical planning and pre-shaping of the implant in cases of post-traumatic cranio-maxillofacial deformities [36]. 3-D printing can also be used for surgical planning and for precise modeling of titanium implants for the reconstruction of orbital floor fractures [37]. Stereolithographic printing models can be used in cases of post-traumatic skull base deformity, peri-orbital lesions, and for planning skull base, orbital, and nasoethmoidal osteotomies [26]. Three-dimensional printed implants can be used for the reconstruction of maxillofacial defects and facial injury including midface post-traumatic defects [36]. For more details about craino-maxillofacial 3-D printing, please refer to Chap. 7.

6.4.4 Rhinoplasty

Esthetic reconstructive surgery for complex nasal deformities may involve placement of an implant for an appropriate shaping of the nose. Although autologous cartilage is ideal, this can be limited by availability and the complications associated with acquiring the cartilage. Various alloplastic materials including silicone, hydroxyapatite, and high-density porous polyethylene have been used as implants. In a recent study, polycaprolactone has been used for nasal reconstruction, and the authors reported that polycaprolactone implants could be produced using 3-D printing which was useful in the craniofacial reconstruction [38]. They further concluded that 3-D printed models of polycaprolactone implants can be useful for nasal tip augmentation in rhinoplasty surgery. A group of researchers reported the use of patient-specific implant fabrication system (3-D carving system) where surgical planning was done with patient's participation resulting in designing of a 3-D printed patient-specific implant [39]. A cost-effective and affordable method has been described which allows printing of sterilizable, scaled, patient-specific, 3-D printed models for rhinoplasty, and the authors reported that such model can be useful for evaluating the extent of a dorsal hump reduction, assessing the alar shape, and reconstructing the nasal tip [40]. Three-dimensional printed patient-specific models can be used for intraoperative tissue contouring during surgery for an extensive osseous tumor as a result of fibrous dysplasia [41]. 3-D printed models can also be used for surgical training of septoplasty [42] and for the production of prosthesis for septal perforation [30].

6.4.5 Patient Education and Medical/Surgical Training

3-D printing has also provided models to communicate with patients to discuss the anatomy, surgical planning, disease state, and treatment options which further enhance the informed consent process. The patient can visualize the anatomy and pathology which enables a better understanding of the intricacy, risks, and complications of operative procedures which further helps in the informed consenting process [29]. 3-D printed models can also be used for teaching medical students where pathological conditions can be incorporated into the anatomical models. However, the time and cost spent on the generation of 3-D models might limit their widespread usage at present [29]. Three-dimensional printed models can pro-

vide patient-specific anatomical and pathological models that can be used for patient information, preoperative planning, and surgical training in neurosurgery [43]. However, the advantages and benefits of 3-D model printing have not yet been completely validated, and future studies are necessary for comparing 3-D models and the currently available surgical simulation training tools to evaluate the impact and use of 3-D models for surgical training and surgical outcome [44].

6.4.6 Future Directions in 3-D Printing

In the future, bio-printing might allow us to integrate tissue engineering and materials to create functional implants to repair, for example, nasal turbinate tissue or trachea. Zhong and Zhao suggested that further studies should be carried out to create 3-D printing models impregnated with airway epithelial cells or stem cells which could be used for functional disorders of nasal cavity such as empty nose syndrome and atrophic rhinitis [33]. Furthermore, three-dimensional printing opens up another exciting possibility of patient-specific customized instrumentation. Incorporating 3-D printing models to mimic anterior skull base pathologies could be used for surgical training allowing trainees to practice drilling via endonasal approach. Based on current research, Zhong and Zhao predicted that it might be possible to develop bio-printed nerve grafts to repair nerves in the future [33]. The use of 3-D printing to form soft structures has not been fully explored. Ganguli et al. believed that future developments in 3-D printed materials would provide additional realism in the surgical simulation which might result in increased success rates in surgical operations [29].

6.5 Conclusion

Thus, virtual endoscopy and its adjuncts—virtual and augmented reality surgery—seem to be the future of improvements in surgical training, which should reduce the learning curve, improve surgical planning, improve accuracy, reduce morbidity, and reduce surgical time. Intraoperatively, they can provide early warnings for vital structures, and also allow the opportunity to teach via remote observation and guidance by an expert surgical team. The current limitations are cost and availability.

The future seems bright, however, with more institutions and companies working on these technologies. We anticipate more applications for training involving sensory and haptic feedback systems and anticipate the use of available computing power for achieving these goals.

References

1. Anand SM, Frenkiel S, Le BQH, Glikstein R. Virtual endoscopy: our next major investigative modality? J Otolaryngol Head Neck Surg. 2009;38(6):642–5.
2. Han P, Pirsig W, Ilgen F, Görich J, Sokiranski R. Virtual endoscopy of the nasal cavity in comparison with fiberoptic endoscopy. Eur Arch Otorhinolaryngol. 2000;257(10):578–83.
3. Kettenbach J, Birkfellner W, Rogalla P. Virtual endoscopy of the paranasal sinuses. In: Image processing in radiology. Berlin, Heidelberg: Springer; 2008. p. 151–71.. (Medical Radiology). https://link.springer.com/chapter/10.1007/978-3-540-49830-8_11.
4. Parikh SS, Chan S, Agrawal SK, Hwang PH, Salisbury CM, Rafii BY, et al. Integration of patient-specific paranasal sinus computed tomographic data into a virtual surgical environment. Am J Rhinol Allergy. 2009;23(4):442–7.
5. Farneti P, Riboldi A, Sciarretta V, Piccin O, Tarchini P, Pasquini E. Usefulness of three-dimensional computed tomographic anatomy in endoscopic frontal recess surgery. Surg Radiol Anat. 2017;39(2):161–8.
6. Patel NS, Dearking AC, O'Brien EK, Pallanch JF. Virtual mapping of the frontal recess: guiding safe and efficient frontal sinus surgery. Otolaryngol Head Neck Surg. 2017;156(5):946–51.
7. Nakasato T, Katoh K, Ehara S, Tamakawa Y, Hayakawa Y, Chiba H, et al. Virtual CT endoscopy in determining safe surgical entrance points for paranasal mucoceles. J Comput Assist Tomogr. 2000;24(3):486–92.
8. Glaser AY, Hall CB, Uribe SJI, Fried MP. Medical students' attitudes toward the use of an endoscopic sinus surgery simulator as a training tool. Am J Rhinol. 2006;20(2):177–9.
9. Anand S, Frenkiel RV. Virtual endoscopy of the nasal cavity and the paranasal sinuses. Adv Endosc Surg. 2011. https://www.intechopen.com/books/advances-in-endoscopic-surgery/virtual-endoscopy-of-the-nasal-cavity-and-the-paranasal-sinus
10. Solyar A, Cuellar H, Sadoughi B, Olson TR, Fried MP. Endoscopic sinus surgery simulator as a teaching tool for anatomy education. Am J Surg. 2008;196(1):120–4.
11. Seymour NE, Gallagher AG, Roman SA, O'Brien MK, Bansal VK, Andersen DK, et al. Virtual reality training improves operating room performance: results of a randomized, double-blinded study. Ann Surg. 2002;236(4):458–63; discussion 463-464
12. Kapakin S. The paranasal sinuses: three-dimensional reconstruction, photo-realistic imaging, and virtual endoscopy. Folia Morphol (Warsz). 2016;75(3):326–33.
13. Arora A, Lau LYM, Awad Z, Darzi A, Singh A, Tolley N. Virtual reality simulation training in otolaryngology. Int J Surg Lond Engl. 2014;12(2):87–94.
14. Edmond CV. Impact of the endoscopic sinus surgical simulator on operating room performance. Laryngoscope. 2002;112(7 Pt 1):1148–58.
15. Andolfi C, Plana A, Kania P, Banerjee PP, Small S. Usefulness of three-dimensional modeling in surgical planning, resident training, and patient education. J Laparoendosc Adv Surg Tech A. 2017;27(5):512–5.
16. Agbetoba A, Luong A, Siow JK, Senior B, Callejas C, Szczygielski K, et al. Educational utility of advanced three-dimensional virtual imaging in evaluating the anatomical configuration of the frontal recess. Int Forum Allergy Rhinol. 2017;7(2):143–8.
17. Thomas L, Pallanch JF. Three-dimensional CT reconstruction and virtual endoscopic study of the ostial orientations of the frontal recess. Am J Rhinol Allergy. 2010;24(5):378–84.
18. Dearking AC, Pallanch JF. Mapping the frontal sinus ostia using virtual endoscopy. Laryngoscope. 2012;122(10):2143–7.
19. Belina S, Cuk V, Klapan I. Virtual endoscopy and 3-D volume rendering in the management of frontal sinus fractures. Coll Antropol. 2009;33(Suppl 2):43–51.
20. Fujikura T, Tanaka N, Sugiura E, Ide N, Miyajima K. Clinical application of virtual endoscopy as a support system for endoscopic sinus surgery. Acta Otolaryngol. 2009;129(6):674–80.
21. Wolfsberger S, Forster M-T, Donat M, Neubauer A, Bühler K, Wegenkittl R, et al. Virtual endoscopy is a useful device for training and preoperative planning of transsphenoidal endoscopic pituitary surgery. Minim Invasive Neurosurg. 2004;47(4):214–20.
22. Rotariu DI, Ziyad F, Budu A, Poeata I. The role of osiriX based virtual endoscopy in planning endoscopic transsphenoidal surgery for pituitary adenoma. Turk Neurosurg. 2017;27(3):339–45.
23. Zheng J-P, Li C-Z, Chen G-Q, Song G-D, Zhang Y-Z. Three-dimensional printed skull base simulation for transnasal endoscopic surgical training. World Neurosurg. 2018;111:e773–82.
24. Haerle SK, Daly MJ, Chan H, Vescan A, Witterick I, Gentili F, et al. Localized intraoperative virtual endoscopy (LIVE) for surgical guidance in 16 skull base patients. Otolaryngol Head Neck Surg. 2015;152(1):165–71.
25. Mert A, Micko A, Donat M, Maringer M, Buehler K, Sutherland GR, et al. An advanced navigation pro-

tocol for endoscopic transsphenoidal surgery. World Neurosurg. 2014;82(6 Suppl):S95–105.

26. Oishi M, Fukuda M, Yajima N, Yoshida K, Takahashi M, Hiraishi T, et al. Interactive presurgical simulation applying advanced 3D imaging and modeling techniques for skull base and deep tumors. J Neurosurg. 2013;119(1):94–105.

27. Yunus M. Helical CT scan with 2D and 3D reconstructions and virtual endoscopy versus conventional endoscopy in the assessment of airway disease in neonates, infants and children. J Pak Med Assoc. 2012;62(11):1154–60.

28. Kwong KM. Current updates on choanal atresia. Front Pediatr. 2015;3:52.

29. Ganguli A, Pagan-Diaz GJ, Grant L, Cvetkovic C, Bramlet M, Vozenilek J, et al. 3D printing for preoperative planning and surgical training: a review. Biomed Microdevices. 2018;20(3):65.

30. Crafts TD, Ellsperman SE, Wannemuehler TJ, Bellicchi TD, Shipchandler TZ, Mantravadi AV. Three-dimensional printing and its applications in otorhinolaryngology-head and neck Surgery. Otolaryngol Head Neck Surg. 2017;156(6):999–1010.

31. Naftulin JS, Kimchi EY, Cash SS. Streamlined, inexpensive 3D printing of the brain and skull. PLoS ONE. 2015;10(8):e0136198.

32. Rengier F, Mehndiratta A, von Tengg-Kobligk H, Zechmann CM, Unterhinninghofen R, Kauczor H-U, et al. 3D printing based on imaging data: review of medical applications. Int J Comput Assist Radiol Surg. 2010;5(4):335–41.

33. Zhong N, Zhao X. 3D printing for clinical application in otorhinolaryngology. Eur Arch Otorhinolaryngol. 2017;274(12):4079–89.

34. Muelleman TJ, Peterson J, Chowdhury NI, Gorup J, Camarata P, Lin J. Individualized surgical approach planning for petroclival tumors using a 3D printer. J Neurol Surg B Skull Base. 2016;77(3):243–8.

35. Grau S, Kellermann S, Faust M, Perrech M, Beutner D, Drzezga A, et al. Repair of cerebrospinal fluid leakage using a transfrontal, radial adipofascial flap: an individual approach supported by three-dimensional printing for surgical planning. World Neurosurg. 2018;110:315–8.

36. Cui J, Chen L, Guan X, Ye L, Wang H, Liu L. Surgical planning, three-dimensional model surgery and pre-shaped implants in treatment of bilateral craniomaxillofacial post-traumatic deformities. J Oral Maxillofac Surg. 2014;72(6):1138.e1–14.

37. Mustafa SF, Evans PL, Bocca A, Patton DW, Sugar AW, Baxter PW. Customized titanium reconstruction of post-traumatic orbital wall defects: a review of 22 cases. Int J Oral Maxillofac Surg. 2011;40(12):1357–62.

38. Park SH, Yun BG, Won JY, Yun WS, Shim JH, Lim MH, et al. New application of three-dimensional printing biomaterial in nasal reconstruction. Laryngoscope. 2017;127(5):1036–43.

39. Choi YD, Kim Y, Park E. Patient-specific augmentation rhinoplasty using a three-dimensional simulation program and three-dimensional printing. Aesthet Surg J. 2017;37(9):988–98.

40. Bekisz JM, Liss HA, Maliha SG, Witek L, Coelho PG, Flores RL. In-house manufacture of sterilizable, scaled, patient-specific 3D-printed models for rhinoplasty. Aesthet Surg J. 2018;39(3):254–63.

41. Darwood A, Collier J, Joshi N, Grant WE, Sauret-Jackson V, Richards R, et al. Re-thinking 3D printing: a novel approach to guided facial contouring. J Craniomaxillofac Surg. 2015;43(7):1256–60.

42. AlReefi MA, Nguyen LH, Mongeau LG, Bu H, Boyanapalli S, Hafeez N, et al. Development and validation of a septoplasty training model using 3-dimensional printing technology. Int Forum Allergy Rhinol. 2017;7(4):399–404.

43. Ploch CC, Mansi CSSA, Jayamohan J, Kuhl E. using 3d printing to create personalized brain models for neurosurgical training and preoperative planning. World Neurosurg. 2016;90:668–74.

44. Vakharia VN, Vakharia NN, Hill CS. Review of 3-dimensional printing on cranial neurosurgery simulation training. World Neurosurg. 2016;88:188–98.

Computer-Assisted 3D Reconstruction in Oral and Maxillofacial Surgery

Mathias Martinez Coronel, Ismail Farag, and Nabil A. Shallik

7.1 Introduction

Cranio-maxillofacial surgery (CMF) represents a broad range of sub-specialties, such as maxillofacial oncological surgery (resection of tumors and reconstruction of the site with different types of grafts), craniofacial corrective surgery of malformative syndromes (i.e., craniosynostoses, or cleft lip palate), orthognathic surgery and distraction osteogenesis (to correct craniofacial deformities), cranio-maxillofacial trauma surgery and associated reconstructive maxillofacial surgery, and implantology. Surgical engineering in CMF surgery is present at all levels of the CMF clinical workflow, from diagnostic tools to preoperative planning, intraoperative guidance, and transfer of preoperative planning to the operative theater [1].

Virtual endoscopy (VE) and 3-D reconstruction can generate 3-D printed models from craniomaxillofacial structures (soft and hard tissues) that can be used for preoperative planning, intraoperative navigation, and postoperative control. Surgery can be planned with these models with highly valuable information as the soft and hard tissue can be measured using the mirrored data set of the unaffected side; size and location of the graft can be chosen virtually. Intraoperatively, contours of transplanted tissues can be navigated to the preoperatively simulated reconstructive result. Preoperatively outlined safety margins could be exactly controlled during tumor resection. Reconstructions of oncologic and trauma patients can be designed and performed precisely as virtually planned. Image-guided treatment improves preoperative planning by visualization of the individual anatomy, intended reconstructive outcome, and objectivation of the effect of adjuvant therapy. Intraoperative navigation makes tumor and reconstructive surgery more predict-

Electronic Supplementary Material The online version of this chapter (https://doi.org/10.1007/978-3-030-23253-5_7) contains supplementary material, which is available to authorized users.

M. Martinez Coronel (✉)
Craniomaxillofacial Department, Hamad Medical Corporation, Doha, Qatar

Universidad de Carabobo, School of Dentistry, Valencia, Venezuela
e-mail: mcoronel@hamad.qa

I. Farag
Craniomaxillofacial Department, Hamad Medical Corporation, Doha, Qatar

N. A. Shallik
Department of Clinical Anesthesiology, Weill Cornell Medical College in Qatar (WCMQ), Doha, Qatar

Department of Anesthesiology, ICU and Perioperative Medicine, Hamad Medical Corporation, Doha, Qatar

Department of Anesthesia and Surgical Intensive Care, Faculty of Medicine, Tanta University, Tanta, Egypt
e-mail: Nshallik@hamad.qa

N. A. Shallik et al. (eds.), *Virtual Endoscopy and 3D Reconstruction in the Airways*, https://doi.org/10.1007/978-3-030-23253-5_7

able by showing the safety margins, locating vital structures, leading reconstruction to preplanned objectives, as well as operating room time-saving as a custom-made adaptation of osteosynthesis material can be done previously [2].

7.2 Computer-Assisted Treatment

Computer-assisted technology was initially developed to provide neurosurgeons with accurate guidance during surgical procedures. Stereotactic procedures were introduced to neurosurgery in the early 1980s, and currently systems with and without robotic navigation are in use for specific medical indications. For oral and maxillofacial surgery nowadays, mechanical, electromagnetic, and optic systems are available to perform navigational surgery by frameless stereotaxy.

Clinical application of computer-assisted treatment is performed in three steps. The first step is the analysis of the problem, planning of treatment, and simulation of surgical procedures. The second step is the navigational surgery performed as frameless stereotaxy. The third step consists of post-therapeutic control.

Indications in traumatology are primary and secondary reconstruction of the orbit and the decompression of the optic nerve. Using frameless stereotaxy, the decompression of the optic nerve in trauma or tumor cases becomes a safe and predictable, as well as a minimally invasive procedure [3].

7.3 Frameless Stereotaxy

Optic navigation system includes an infrared light located on the tip of a surgical tool which allows correlation of anatomic situation and patient's spiral CT or MRI data set. Defined reference points exposable in the anatomic situation and visible in the data set of the patient are needed for registration of the system.

Registration with anatomical landmarks or skin Fiducial markers lacks accuracy, registration with devices fixed within the oral cavity interferes with surgical procedures [4, 5], while Fiducial markers fixed to bone screws are invasive and limited to one surgical intervention a few days after data acquisition (Fig. 7.1).

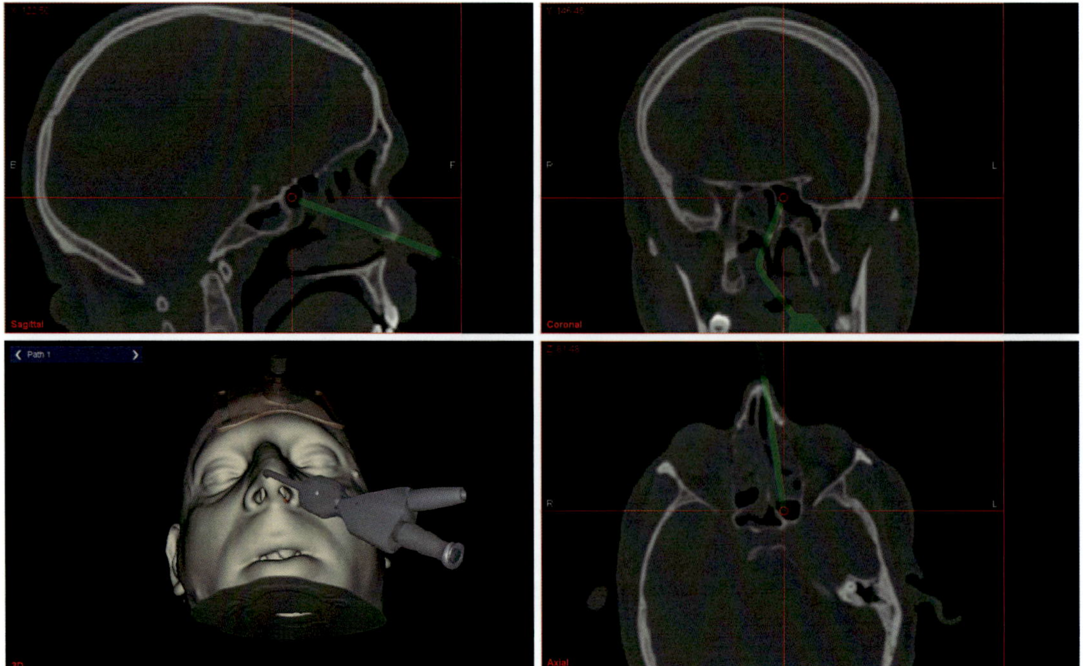

Fig. 7.1 Registration of Brain Lab Screen Shot

The head of the patient is normally fixed to a Mayfield clamp, which is tracked by a dynamic reference frame to allow changing of the position during operation. Noninvasive tracking can be achieved by fixing this dynamic reference frame to the occlusal splint. With this technique, navigational surgery of the mobile mandible can be performed. Frameless stereotaxy allows the surgeon to localize any desired anatomical structure with the pointer and lead the surgical intervention to the preplanned and simulated result; the surgeon is also able to guide the tip of any tracked surgical tool drill, fraise, chisel, or endoscope or to localize the focus of a surgical microscope [6].

7.4 Image-Guided Navigation

Image-guided navigation leads to improvement in surgical accuracy with the aid of software that uses images captured from CT or MRI and a tracking system for the surgical instruments [7]. The accuracy of image-guided navigation in CMF depends on the imaging modalities [8], patient-to-image registration procedures, the navigation system used [9], data acquisition [10], interaction of the surgeon with the system, technical errors [11], and instrument tracking [12, 13]. The technical accuracy and the navigation procedures seem to be of minor influence [14]. Image-guided navigation requires a means of registering anatomical points in the medical image (CT or MRI) and a software program to locate the surgical instruments [15–17]. Knowing the exact position of the instrument is the key to the success of the surgical intervention. CT/MRI images are used as a map to provide the surgeon with a real-time representation of the surgical instruments in relation to the images of the patient. This real-time representation allows for tracking the instrument position during the surgery and their visualization on the computer [9]. During the surgical phase, the surgeon is given interactive support with guidance in order to better control potential dangers and avoid complex anatomical regions [18]. Navigation is possible through a series of sensors attached to the rotator instruments, the surgical template, and a cap fixed on the patient's head, and the data are captured by different systems. The obtained data are transferred immediately to the computer and enable the surgeon to view the real situation [19].

Image-guided navigation is especially useful in tumor resection involving complex anatomy areas modified by tumor growth [19, 20] (such as the orbit), in proximity to cerebral structures, and when cranial nerves could be injured [21, 22]. Image-guided navigation allows for the immediate reconstruction of the unilateral resected area with an autologous graft designed and positioned under navigation with a preoperative plan based on the mirrored healthy side [23]. Computer-assisted surgery (CAS) navigation in CMF tumor resection can also be combined with new imaging modalities, such as positron emission tomography. In this combination, the surgeon is simultaneously provided with anatomical and functional (metabolic) details. The resulting fused images offer improved localization of malignant lesions and improve the targeting of the biopsy, especially for small lesions [24].

Intraoperative navigation has also been used in the resection of the ankylotic bone in temporomandibular joint (TMJ) gap arthroplasty and for TMJ arthroscopy using optoelectronic tracking technology [25–27].

7.5 Periorbital Reconstruction

In craniomaxillofacial surgery, advances in imaging techniques spiral-CT, 3-D imaging, and associated technologies (stereolithographic models and CAD/CAM) have led to improved preoperative planning within the past years. To assess asymmetry, proper measurement of distances between anatomic structures will help to determine the severity of a facial deformity. Within the orbit, transverse, cranio-caudal, and posterior-anterior measurements allow to determine areas of deficient bone and to evaluate how much grafted bone volume or reconfiguration of periorbital bone is necessary. By this procedure, the surgeon himself is not limited to a subjective clinical estimation of the asymmetry, but he gets familiar with the individual discrepancies in all three dimensions. The diagnostic value of the multiplanar assessment including the 3-D images is one of the most important features of the system.

Additionally, to measure functions, the volume rendering tool allows evaluation of affected and nonaffected orbital contents with individual cubic millimeter volume measures. By this method, the orbit can be directly compared to the other side. The majority of orbital deformities or traumatisms are unilateral, so that most of the cases can be approached by this side-to-side comparison. A further development of the idea to compare one side to the other is the mirroring tool. The surgeon has to define the individual level to which the data set shall be mirrored from the unaffected to the deformed side, and he has to set the range, within which the mirroring process shall be performed.

The software guides the surgeon step by step through this procedure. The optimal virtual reconstruction can be done and stored. During the operation, these new contours can be navigated and serve as a control of the ongoing orbital reconstruction [28].

7.6 Infection and Airway

Maxillofacial infections begin from the dentoalveolar area and then spread into the adjacent bone causing perforation of the bone cortex into the subperiosteal region. Fascial planes of the head and neck are virtual spaces, bounded by muscle attachments and bone. These anatomical structures will govern in which direction the infection spreads to the deeper soft tissues spaces (parapharyngeal and mediastinum) (Fig. 7.2).

Parapharyngeal abscess often has little clinical signs until the airway is compromised, as the swelling is located at the oropharyngeal or parapharyngeal region, so it is very important to make a complete anamnesis to get all the history of the illness [29].

Ludwig angina is an infection of the submandibular space, first described by Wilhelm Frederick Von Ludwig in 1836. It is an entity difficult to manage due to the rapid progression and difficulty in maintaining airway patency, resulting in asphyxiation and death in 8–10% of patients [30].

There are good predictors of sublingual involvement during head and neck infections; the patient usually cannot protrude the tongue, and we can find associated dysphagia and odynophagia.

During physical examination, stridor, difficulty managing secretions, anxiety, cyanosis, and sitting posture are late signs of impending airway obstructions, and they indicate the need for an immediate artificial airway (tracheotomy) [31].

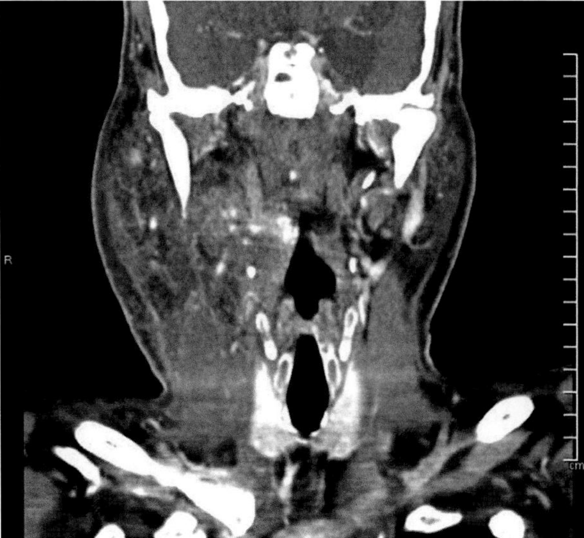
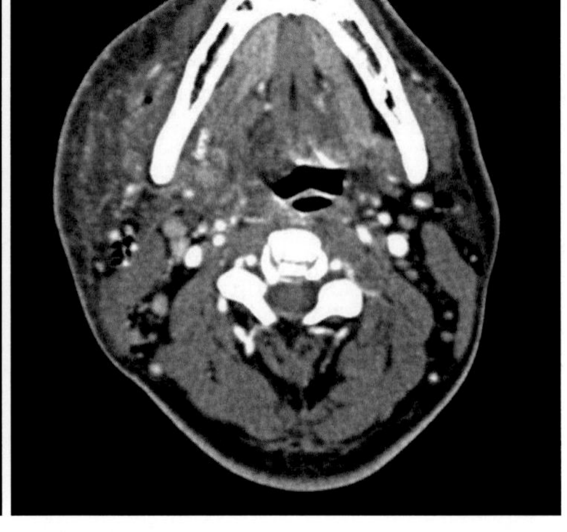

Fig. 7.2 CT scan coronal and axial view showing airway displaced in a maxillofacial infection case. Right-sided subcutaneous swelling edema and fat permeation is noted encroaching and violating deeply through the stylomandibular tunnel reaching to the oropharyngeal airway which is mildly compromised

Surgical tracheotomy in head and neck infections is often difficult and occasionally life threatening due to the involvement of the neck and pre-tracheal tissues. Incising through the pre-tracheal fascia and exposing the pre-vertebral tissues to pathogens risks the spread of infection into the mediastinum. Mediastinitis, despite modern healthcare, still carries significant mortality [32].

Sublingual hematoma, after traumatic injuries on the tongue or the floor of the mouth, is a rare but potentially fatal cause of upper airway obstruction. This condition has the potential for quick obstruction of the upper airway due to the tongue's vast vascularization. The increased lingual volume displaces it in a posterior and cephalic direction, thus blocking the airway; prompt evacuation will lead to avoid morbidity and mortality related to this complication [33].

3-D reconstruction and virtual endoscopy (VE) applied to these cases can give valuable information to the surgical and anesthesia team about airway displacements, relationship between collections (pus or blood), and vital structures and can also help with 3-D locations of multiple collections from infections or hematomas to proper evacuation during surgery.

7.7 Congenital and Developmental Abnormalities and Airway

Despite publishing after Shukowsky [34], Pierre Robin has been credited with describing a cluster of craniofacial anomalies with potential and specific physiologic sequelae. In the literature, this grouping is known as Pierre Robin syndrome [35], Pierre Robin sequence [36], Robin anomalad [37], or Robin complex [38], each justifying their own specific nomenclature. Pierre Robin sequence may manifest as micrognathia, cleft palate and glossoptosis with airway obstruction [39]. Infants with complications of Pierre Robin sequence are at increased risk of airway obstruction and resultant hypoxia, failure to thrive, and cerebral impairment [40]. The concept of "sequence" suggests that one anomaly causes subsequent anomalies, and micrognathia is believed to be inciting anomaly in patients with Pierre Robin sequence [41, 42]. Pierre Robin sequence can be life threatening during the neonatal period with the onset of airway obstruction, which can occur at any time right after birth. If left untreated, prolonged airway obstruction can lead to acute or chronic hypoxia, cyanosis, apnea episodes, aspiration, respiratory tract infection, feeding difficulties, malnutrition, and failure to thrive [43, 44].

There are numerous potential treatment options, and they range from conservative non-surgical interventions to surgical procedures including distraction osteogenesis (DO) [45]. The basic treatment of babies with suspected Pierre Robin sequence is to secure the pulmonary tract. Depending on the severity, tracheostomy is one of the options. In this decade, DO has been introduced for patients with the Pierre Robin sequence. DO makes a longer mandible and secures the upper pulmonary tract [46].

Mandibular distraction osteogenesis (DO) is currently the "gold standard" for the treatment of obstructive apnea secondary to micrognathia. It avoids the tracheotomy and/or other aggressive surgical procedures and treats the etiology of the disease, improving oxygen saturation and changes in feeding in a few days. For the surgical decision-making process, supplementary explorations are helpful, such as polysomnography, lateral cranial X-ray, and 2-D and 3-D CT scans. The horizontal or oblique distraction vector will be the vector of choice due to its positive effects on the sizes of the airway. It is a procedure whose results can be planned and reproduced, with minimum short-term complications [47].

Virtual technology can greatly improve the planning and execution of mandibular DO in Pierre Robin or syndromic patients [48]. The benefits of 3-D virtual planning in these cases fall into two categories:

1. Operative planning, the two key features of which are device and vector selection. Whether there is sufficient bone to place a device, and if so what would be the optimal angle and best location for the device. Virtual planning can help us to identify if the device

could be positioned appropriately. Once positioned on the virtual model, we could measure mandibular thickness at various holes and plan the appropriate screw length. Similarly, the inferior alveolar nerve and teeth buds could be viewed, identifying screw holes to avoid.

2. Surgical execution, the second major benefit, and the most novel aspect of this technique, is the ability to transfer the virtual plan to the operating room using operative guides and splints. Custom-designed cutting guides can be used in the virtual space and then provided as physical 3-D models. These will allow the device to fit in a proper position on the mandible during surgery, guide the osteotomy and the successful placement of the device to match our vector previously planned [49].

7.8 Temporomandibular Joint Ankylosis and Airway

Temporomandibular joint ankylosis (TMJA) is a disabling condition of the masticatory system that alters eating habits and speech ability. The features include hypomobility of the joint, micrognathia (TMJA is one of the most common causes for acquired mandibular hypoplasia), retrogenia, facial asymmetry, malocclusion, and airway compromise which in severe cases may manifest as sleep apnea/hypopnea syndrome [50] (Fig. 7.3) (Movie 7.1).

TMJA can be caused by bony or fibrous ankylosis of the TMJ as a sequel to trauma, infection, autoimmune disease, or failed surgery [51].

Posttraumatic ankylosis can be caused by different pathogenic mechanisms such as organization and ossification of hematoma, maltreated facial fractures, and systemic diseases such as ankylosing spondylitis, rheumatoid arthritis, psoriasis, and autoimmune disease that increase the effects of micro-trauma [52].

As observed in patients with micrognathia, the additional space occupied by tongue, soft palate, and redundant pharyngeal mucosa reduces the cross-sectional area of oropharyngeal airway by an average of 25%. Various cephalometric stud-

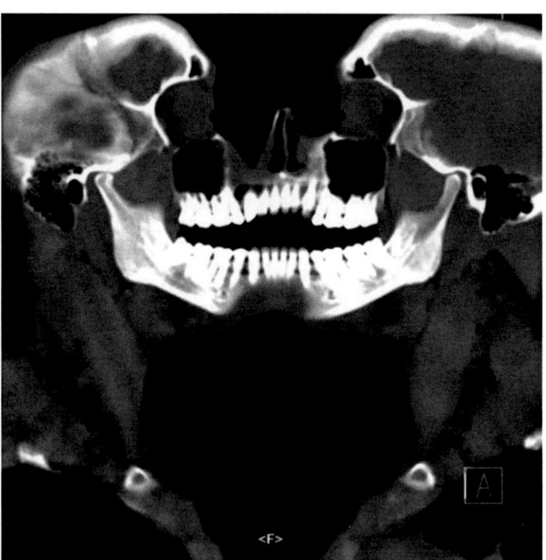

Fig. 7.3 Orthopantomogram-like reconstruction obtained from the volumetric study, and it is a post-processing technique which is called curved MPR C-MPR, the bony element and osseous framework of the mandible, maxilla, teeth, lamina dura, and TMJ can be instantaneously evaluated without extra radiation to the patient

ies have demonstrated the effectiveness of mandibular advancement procedures on the improvement in oropharyngeal dimensions. When TMJ ankylosis occurs during the growth of the mandible, varying degrees of facial deformities result. Since these children grow with facial asymmetry, the position of the larynx may be altered. Classically, bird-faced deformities with convex facial profiles have been described in chronic long-standing TMJ ankylosis characterized by micrognathic mandible with receding chin and steep occlusal plane [53].

Facial asymmetry, malocclusion, anemia, and malnutrition may be the consequences of TMJA. It also leads to increased airway obstruction, obstructive sleep apnea, and cor pulmonale. Airway obstruction is secondary to structural encroachment on oro-pharyngeal and hypopharyngeal lumen, subatmospheric intrapharyngeal pressure, and hypotonicity of oropharyngeal muscles. All these structural deformities lead to difficulty in ventilation, intubation, and extubation [54].

It has been reported that the three-dimensional (3-D) reconstruction models based on MRI can play an important role in TMD diagnosis by revealing morphological features of TMJ, thus being a powerful tool for characterizing different patterns of TMJ pathologies [55]. The use of 3-D models can help to classify the morphology of the articular eminence by correlating signs and symptoms of temporomandibular joint dysfunction to articular disc displacement on MRI images [56]. Understanding of the TMJ anatomy, biomechanics, and the imaging manifestations of diseases is important to accurately recognize and manage these various pathologies.

The application of virtual endoscopy (VE) and 3-D printed models in TMJA reconstruction enhances the clinical accuracy, and the following advantages can be described: First, the contour of the selected graft or alloplastic material could be guaranteed adequate matching with the lateral surface of ramus in shape, guiding precisely the implantation the grafts in an ideal position. Second, the better fixation position of the bone grafts could be determined preoperatively without the damage of the anatomical structures (e.g., inferior alveolar nerve). Third, the osteotomy orientation and bone trimming would be guided accurately intraoperatively. Moreover, the length of the titanium plate and each titanium screws also could be confirmed, with no need to measure during surgery (decrease in operation time) [57].

Therefore, 3-D printed models make the TMJ reconstruction more predictive and easier, and avoid the unplanned graft selection and the fixation of the bone graft. Custom-fitted implants for joint reconstruction also decreased the preoperative workup time of the design and the manufacture of the TMJ prosthesis and increased the accuracy of the model surgery [58] (refer to Chap. 11 for more details) (Fig. 7.4).

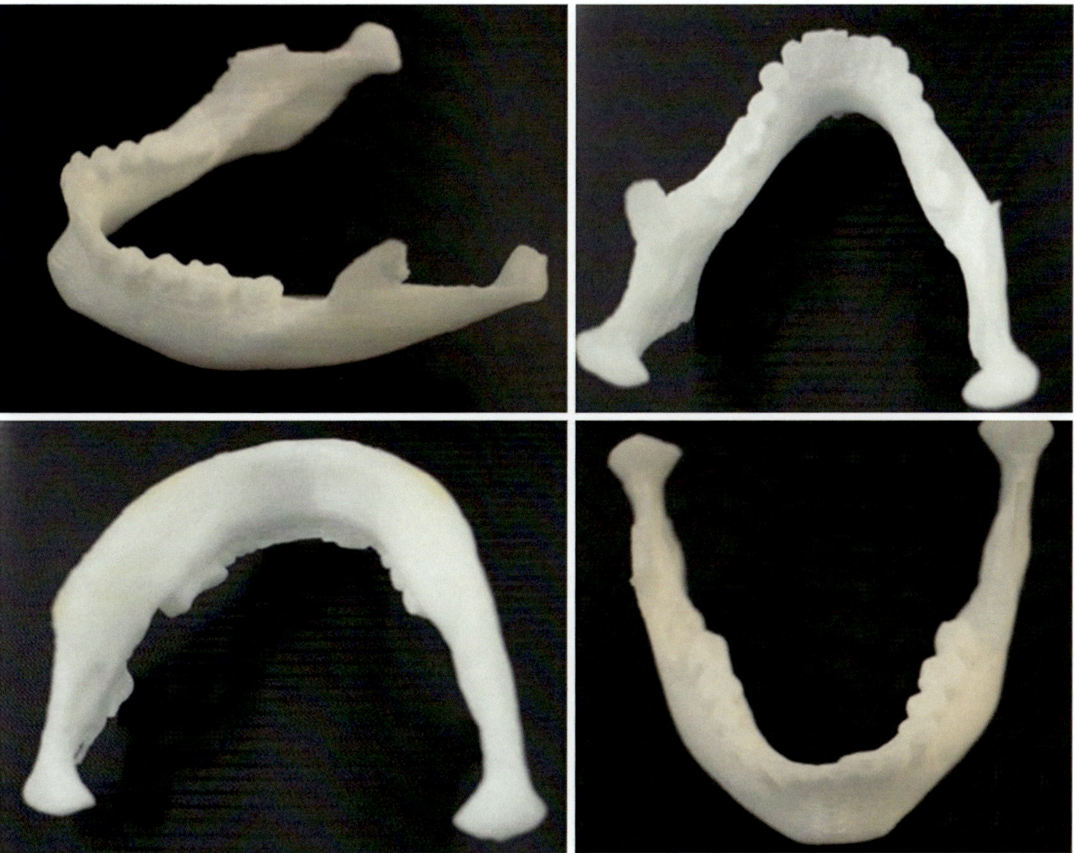

Fig. 7.4 Printed 3-D model for the mandible from different perspectives

7.9 Oral and Maxillofacial Tumor Surgery and Reconstruction

Oral cancer is the sixth most common cancer worldwide. The factors responsible for difficult airway during perioperative period in oral cancer patients are as follows: [58].

(a) Presence of cancer growth itself
(b) Anatomical changes and fibrosis due to prior surgery or radiotherapy
(c) Lengthy surgical procedure
(d) Bulky flap reconstruction
(e) Edema around the airway due to surgical manipulations
(f) Risk of bleeding, mainly because of surgical causes or multiple attempts of airway manipulation
(g) Risk of pulmonary aspiration.

Airway management in head and neck tumor patients undergoing major surgical procedures, including microvascular free tissue transfer, has often been routine tracheotomy. The necessity of this procedure has, however, been questioned [59]. Tracheotomy itself is not without complications, with rates as high as 4.1–8% in some series. Possible complications include hemorrhage, obstruction, cannula displacement, local infection, pneumonia, fistula, tracheal stenosis, and tumor recurrence due to tumor seeding [60]. Brickman et al. argued that maxillectomy and microvascular free tissue transfer do not negatively impact a patient's oropharyngeal airway, so elective tracheotomy should only be considered in patients with additional risk factors, such as cardiopulmonary diseases [61]. Recently, a tracheotomy scoring system to guide airway management after major head and neck surgery has been proposed, whereby tumor site, mandibulectomy, neck dissection, and reconstruction are scoring factors [62].

Tumor ablation leads to head and neck defects, which brings about significant esthetic and functional deficits. After tumor resection in the cranio-maxillofacial area, the patient needs reconstruction of hard and soft tissue defects with the use of soft tissue grafts, bone grafts, flaps, and surgical plates which have been exten-

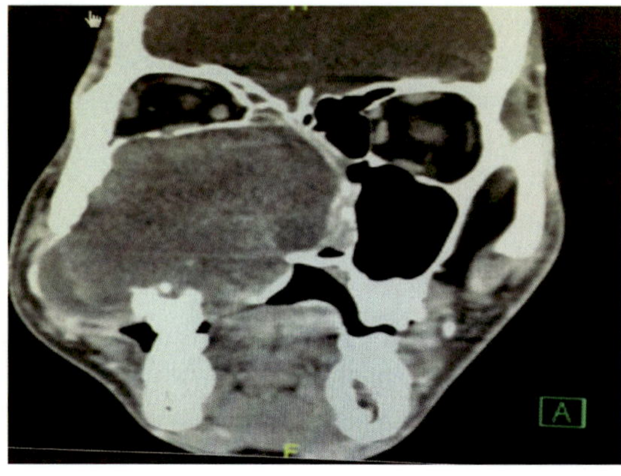

Fig. 7.5 Face CT scan coronal view showing soft tissue mass lesion epicentered over the right maxillary antrum causing its expansion violating and encroaching and partially obstructing the upper airway and ipsilateral nasal cavity

sively used in head and neck reconstruction to stabilize bone segments [63, 64] (Fig. 7.5).

The use of 3-D printed models facilitates the assessment of tumor extensions, the anatomical areas involved to plan the resections and visualize which structures will be involved in the resection's margins. These resections can be done on 3-D models previously and are valuable tools in order to plan contouring maxillofacial reconstruction preoperatively because the conventional surgical plates are mass-produced with universal configurations that should be manually bended to match the individual bone anatomy. The plate-bending procedure could be time- and energy-consuming, especially for inexperienced surgeons, so this technique also has a significant potential to shorten the length of operating room (OR) time for the surgical team and consequently reduce operative cost in the hospital [65]. The application of 3-D printed patient-specific surgical plates in head and neck reconstruction is feasible, safe, and precise [66] (refer to Chap. 11 for more details) (Fig. 7.6).

7.10 Maxillofacial Trauma

Patients with maxillofacial trauma present serious challenges for the physician because airway management in these patients can be complicated by their injury [67].

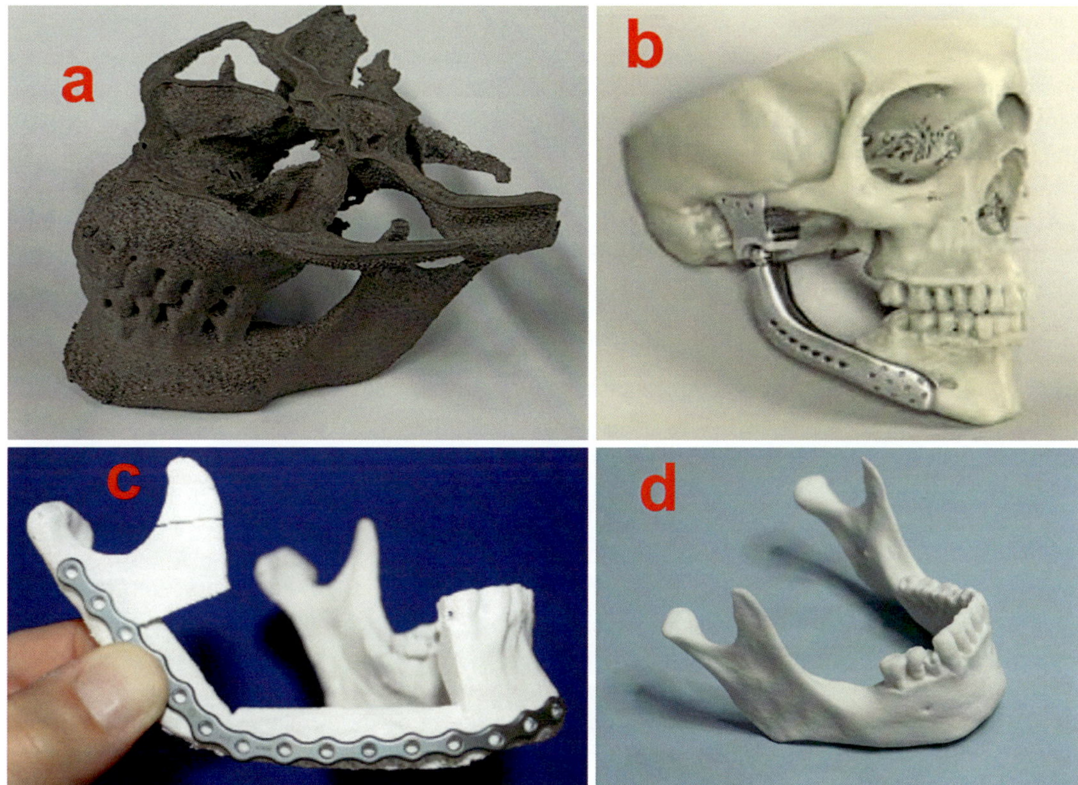

Fig. 7.6 3-D printed model for the mandible is of utmost benefit for planning for the reconstruction and plate and screws fixation in a step prior to the real surgical intervention. Rehearsal, measurement evaluation, and functional assessment will help the surgeons for better surgical outcome, and it is of high impact upon the teaching part for the junior staff colleagues

The first priority in assessing and managing the trauma patients is airway maintenance with cervical spine control. This is based on the Advanced Trauma Life Support (ATLS) concept for managing patients who sustained life-threatening injuries [68]. Immediate management of maxillofacial injuries is required mainly when impeding or existing upper airway compromise and/or profuse hemorrhage occurs [69].

Safe and optimal airway management of patients with maxillofacial trauma requires appreciation of the nature of the trauma. There are several maxillofacial injuries that result from critical care errors, with airway management being the most common [70].

A patient with a supraclavicular injury is considered to have a C-spine injury, until proven otherwise by imaging [71]. Since a complete C-spine clearance may take several hours and sometimes days to achieve, the patient must be fitted with a neck collar for cervical spine immobilization [72].

Using a video laryngoscope, or awake intubation techniques instead of a conventional laryngoscope with a Macintosh blade, may be beneficial for intubating patients whose neck position needs to be in a neutral position and their cervical spine requires immobilization [73, 74]. The surgical airway is considered to be the last option in airway management; however, inpatient with facial trauma sometimes it is the best solution [74]. To be prepared well, a qualified surgeon should stand onsite during conventional airway management in order to be immediately in-charge. Performing a cricothyroidotomy or tracheotomy under local anesthesia is a lifesaving procedure in selected patients in the "cannot intubate, cannot ventilate" situation.

Surgical creation of an airway is a safe method for securing the airway when the procedure is done by an experienced surgeon. However, this approach has its drawbacks: it carries some of complications such as hemorrhage or pneumothorax, in an elective scenario [75].

According to Hutchison et al., there are six specific situations associated with maxillofacial trauma, which can adversely affect the airway [69, 76].

1. Posteroinferior displacement of a fractured maxilla parallel to the inclined plane of the base of the skull may block the nasopharyngeal airway.
2. A bilateral fracture of the anterior mandible may cause the fracture symphysis and the tongue to slide posteriorly and block the oropharynx in the supine patient.
3. Fractured or exfoliated teeth, bone fragments, vomitus, blood, and secretions, as well as foreign bodies, such as dentures, debris, and shrapnel, may block the airway anywhere along the oropharynx and larynx (Figs. 7.6 and 7.7).

4. Hemorrhage from distinct vessels in open wounds or severe nasal bleeding from complex blood supply of the nose may also contribute to airway obstruction.
5. Soft tissue swelling and edema, which result from trauma of the head and neck, may cause delayed airway compromise (Figs. 7.8 and 7.9).
6. Trauma of the larynx and trachea may cause swelling and displacement of structures, such as laryngeal fracture, tracheal laceration, or complete transection of epiglottis or arytenoid cartilages injury or vocal cord trauma, and thereby increasing the risk of airway obstruction.

The maxillofacial surgery is done after stabilization of the patient; the radiographic tests are performed (VE and 3-D reconstruction of upper airway), and all the injuries are identified. In some patients, the surgery is performed at the same time as the surgery on other injured organs. The surgeon has to perform fracture reduction and internal fixation with plates and screws, repair soft tissue injuries, and restore the occlusion. In selected patients, naso-endotracheal intubation can be used for airway control during surgery [77].

Submental oro-tracheal intubation was developed in order to avoid the need for tracheotomy and to permit unfettered access to the oral region. This type of intubation is done (a) in patients with comminuted fracture of the midface or the nose, where nasal intubation is contraindicated, (b) inpatients who require restoration of the occlusion, and (c) patients whose condition permits extubation at the end of surgery [78]. The neck pathology and normal anatomy can be easily diagnosed using 3-D reconstruction of this submental region to prevent complication of submental intubation.

The patient with a difficult airway is also at high risk for postoperative complications. Following surgery, the mucous membranes are edematous, the soft tissues are swollen, and the airway may be compressed. Neck expandability is relatively low, and even a small hemorrhage in the region could result in airway compromise [79] (Figs. 7.10 and 7.11).

In intubated patients with maxillofacial trauma, extubation should be deferred until the edema subsides. During extubation, the patient

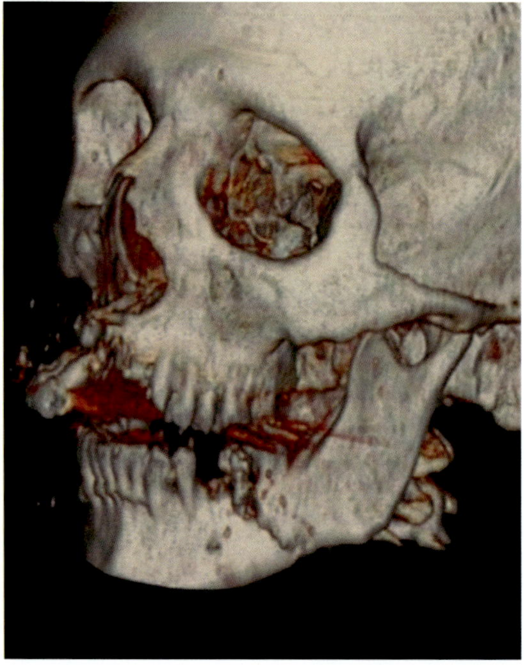

Fig. 7.7 3-D CT reconstruction showing loose teeth and bone that can cause obstruction of airway

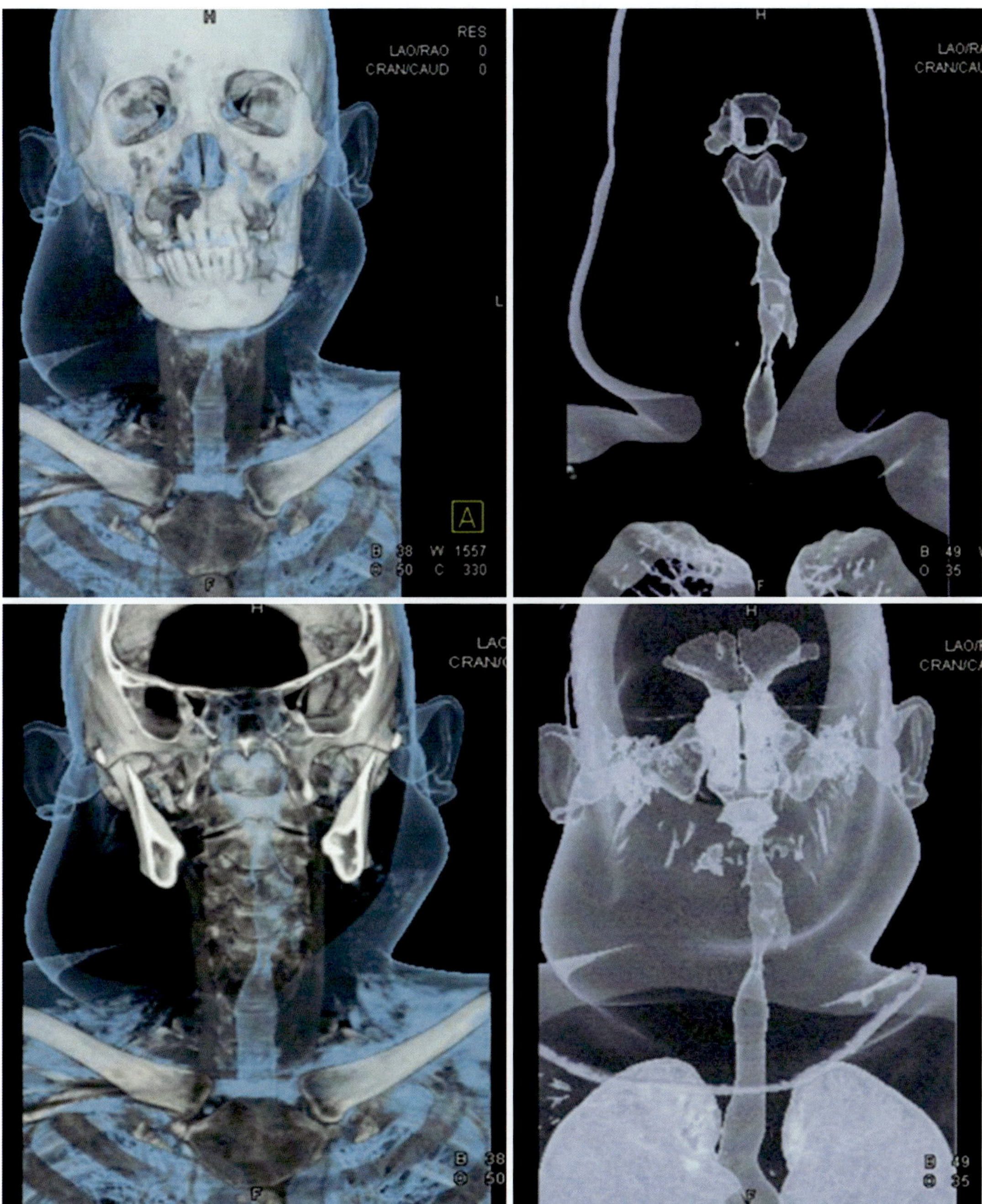

Fig. 7.8 A cancer maxilla patient with loose teeth on the right side. Lymph nodal sizable metastatic adenopathy, resulting in significant airway displacement to the left demonstrated clearly on the VRT models

should be monitored closely and the care providers should be prepared for the possibility of reintubation. It is important to prevent nausea and vomiting because of the risk of gastric content aspiration [80] (Figs. 7.10 and 7.11).

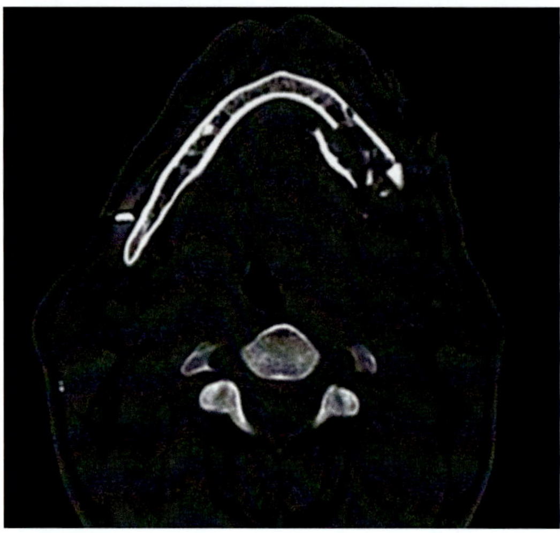

Fig. 7.9 Mandible CT scan axial view bone window settings with comminuted fracture of the left hemimandible with soft tissue surrounding edema and swelling resulting in partial obstruction and significant encroachment of the related airways

Pedicle screw fixation in the upper cervical spine is a difficult and high-risk procedure. The screw is difficult to place rapidly and accurately and can lead to serious injury of spinal cord or vertebral artery. The use of an individualized design 3-D printing navigation template for pedicle screw fixation in the upper cervical spine has been reported as a safe procedure, with a high success rate in the upper cervical spine surgery [81].

7.11 Virtual Surgical Planning (VSP)

Virtual surgical planning and 3-D printed models have been found to be more attractive and useful techniques recently. The usefulness and improvement of these models are beneficial tools that may be used to help the surgeon in the pre-surgical and intra-operative phase because it offers the surgeons the accuracy and precession of normal anatomical repair and reconstruction.

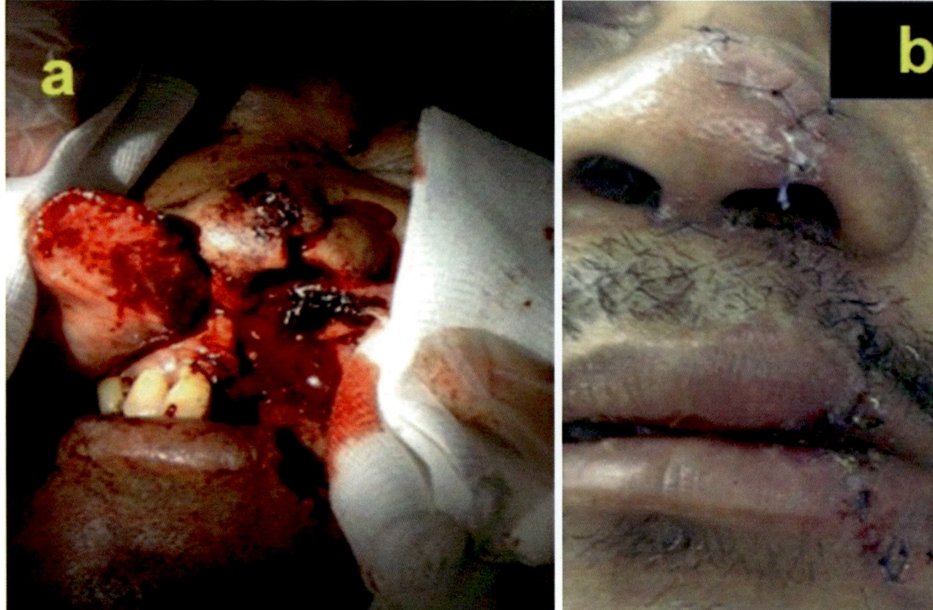

Fig. 7.10 (**a**) Upper lip and nose laceration preoperative. (**b**) Upper lip and nose laceration postoperative

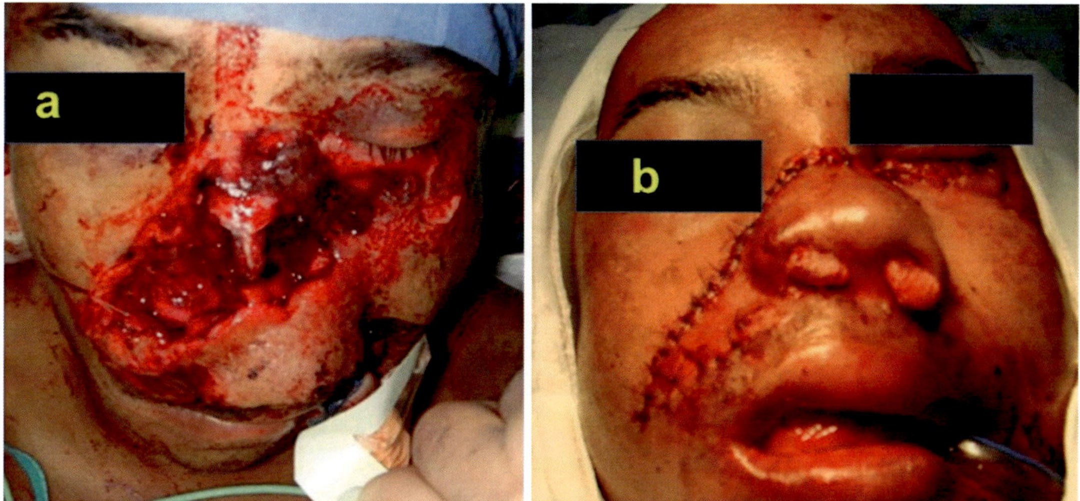

Fig. 7.11 (**a**) Facial laceration compromising the upper airway. (**b**) Facial laceration postoperative

7.11.1 Orbit and Sinus Surgery

Virtual surgical planning and 3-D printed models have been found to be especially useful for orbit and sinus surgery. The use of these models is beneficial that may be used to help the surgeon in the pre-surgical and intra-operative phases. This method can improve the precision and accuracy of the implant and hardware placement, preserving the neurovascular complex of the orbital area. Using virtual surgical planning in conjunction with 3-D, patient-specific implants can give surgeons an effective therapeutic solution in treating complex shape defects or secondary surgery for orbital reconstruction [82].

7.11.2 Maxillofacial Reconstruction

Virtual surgical planning (VSP) and 3-D printed models have proved to be very useful in complex maxillofacial reconstruction. In the area of mandibular reconstruction, this technique has been used in the shaping of free fibular flaps. With data obtained from high-resolution CT scans of the maxillofacial skeleton and lower extremity, stereolithographic models can be fabricated, whereas virtual surgery allows fabrication of mandible and fibular cutting guides

and a plate-bending template for shaping the fibula to best approximate the desired shape of the reconstructed mandible [83]. By using these planning methods, intraoperative time is decreased as bending and shaping of the plate and fibula can now be done with precision to match the dimensions of the defect, and not freehand as is the traditional technique. This is extremely valuable in decreasing ischemia time; the accuracy of the fibular osteotomies allows better shape and optimizes the position of the bones for eventual prosthetics rehabilitation [84, 85].

7.11.3 Mandibular Reconstruction

The use of 3-D printed models and VSP in mandibular reconstruction consists of a planning phase, modeling phase, and surgical phase [86]. High-resolution CT scans of the craniofacial skeleton and lower extremities are obtained. These images are forwarded to a company specializing in VSP. After an online meeting to discuss the case, a virtual resection of the mandible is performed. The 3-D image of the fibula is superimposed on the defect, and virtual osteotomies are performed. In the modeling phase, a stereolithographic model is fabricated (3-D model printed), as well as cutting guides for the mandible and fibula. Finally, in the surgical phase, the mandible cutting guides are used to guide resection of the lesion. A temporary external fixator may be placed to ensure that the remaining segments are kept in proper position. Otherwise, more commonly, a reconstruction plate and drilling of holes at appropriate locations on the remaining mandible are placed prior to performing the osteotomies. The reconstruction plate is removed and the cutting guides are placed in preparation for the osteotomies. The fibula is shaped using the fibular cutting guide, prior to or after division of the pedicle. The shaped fibula is used to reconstruct the mandible [87].

7.11.4 Midface Reconstruction

Virtual surgical planning with stereotactic navigation and 3-D printed models has been used for midface reconstruction with free fibular flaps [88]. Physical models are created using rapid prototyping techniques. Titanium plates are then bent to match the contours of the fibular flap and facial skeleton. In addition, custom-cutting guides are fabricated for the fibular osteotomies. Navigation is performed with fiducial markers on the patient's forehead, subsequently replaced by a navigation array fixed to the patient's calvaria at the time of surgery. Virtual surgical planning has also been used for complex reconstruction of the midface and mandible with two separate free fibular flaps [89]. In extensive defects, where the native anatomy of the face is distorted by trauma or irradiation, the amount of bone required for reconstruction can be underestimated. Virtual surgical planning and 3-D printed models obviate this problem by allowing the visualization of the pre-injury 3-D anatomy to aid planning of osteotomies preoperatively, saving valuable surgical time [90].

7.11.5 Total Replacement of the Temporomandibular Joint

Custom alloplastic total joint replacement implants of the temporomandibular joint (TMJ) have been used for the treatment of TMJ ankyloses in a single-stage surgery. Similar to the workflow for other applications in VSP, fine-cut CT scans of the TMJ and maxillomandibular complex are obtained, followed by the creation of 3-D models by a company experienced in VSP. Through an interactive online meeting, virtual surgery is performed, consisting of the resection of the ankylosed segment. The joint replacement is then designed, first with planning of the fossa component with a custom-made flange to fit the patient's zygomatic arch, followed by design of the mandibular ramus component. Accurate visualization of the 3-D anatomy of the mandible ensures that the prosthesis and fixation avoid the inferior alveolar nerve and tooth roots. Finally, a virtual 3-D prosthesis is designed. Screw holes can be placed away from vital structures such as the inferior alveolar nerve and maxillary artery and over the best bone thickness for fixation. In addition, measurement of screw depth is obtained to ensure that screw placement is bi-cortical for all holes [91].

7.12 Three-Dimensional Printing in Maxilla Facial and Oral Surgery

(Refer to Chap. 11 for more details.)

7.13 Future Plan

Virtual surgical planning has a clear role in facial transplantation where bone is a necessary component in the completion of the reconstruction [92]. If a Le fort III segment is planned, cutting guides and templates are fabricated for the recipient and for the donor at the appropriate times. Additionally, VSP can be used in surgical navigation. The use of VSP for this indication ensures a more accurate outcome while minimizing ischemia time when microvascular flaps are used for the reconstruction [93]. Also future perspectives are simulation of multiple osteotomies and moving various fragments to achieve virtual surgery for any kind of oral and cranio-maxillofacial surgery [94].

7.14 Conclusion

In conclusion, MDCT examination, as well as the post-processing techniques, has the following points to be addressed and thoroughly commented on dental assessment (panoramic-like view using curved MPR to create an orthopantomogram (OPG) for absent teeth or loosening or loss of the normal lamina dura. Denture artificial teeth or loose implant/prosthesis. Temporomandibular joint (TMJ) (ankyloses, dislocation, osteoarthrosis, osteomyelitis, or fractures).

Computer-assisted surgery (CAS) planning was implemented in CMF surgery so that the complex anatomy of the patient can be understood, and that the surgical task can be improved preoperatively. Orthognathic surgery represents an important part of CMF surgery and allows for correction of different dental and maxillofacial dysmorphoses, asymmetric faces, or craniofacial syndromes by cutting and moving the maxilla and/or the mandible according to a treatment plan.

Navigation system indications in craniomaxillofacial surgery, that is, navigational surgery, are a helpful tool for minimally invasive surgery, increasing radicality of tumor treatment, preventing damaging of vital structures, and leading the reconstruction to preplanned, defined results.

3-D printed models have been used in craniomaxillofacial surgery, bringing many benefits during planning and surgical phases with mainly advantages reported as improvement in precision and reduction of surgical time.

This technique can be used for planning mandibular distraction osteogenesis in a neonate with Pierre Robin syndrome, tumor resection, and reconstructions. Three-dimensional models are fabricated based on CT scan data of the craniofacial skeleton and distractors to ensure that the planned osteotomies would allow achievement of the planned distraction vector. One valuable advantage in DO is to allow preplanning of screw position and lengths to ensure bi-cortical screw placement, away from the inferior alveolar nerve, improving the efficiency and accuracy of placement of the distractors [90].

References

1. Olszewski R. Surgical engineering in craniomaxillofacial surgery: a literature review. J Healthcare Eng. 2012;3(1):53–86.
2. Schramm A, Schon R, Rucker M, Barth E-L, Zizelmann C, Gellrich N-C. Computer-assisted Oral and maxillofacial reconstruction. J Comput Inf Technol. 2006;14(1):71–6.
3. Schmelzeisen R, Schon R, Schramm A, Gellrich N-C. Computer-aided procedures in implantology, distraction and cranio-maxillofacial surgery. Ann R Australas Coll Dent Surg. 2003:46–9.
4. Ewers R, Schicho K, Wagner A, Undt G, Seemann R, Figl M, Truppe M. Seven years of clinical experience with teleconsultation in craniomaxillofacial surgery. J Oral Maxillofac Surg. 2005;10:1447–54.
5. Rubio Serrano M, Albalat Estela S, Peñarrocha Diago M, Peñarrocha DM. Software applied to oral implantology: update. Med Oral Patol Oral Cir Bucal. 2008;13(10):E661–5.. Review
6. Heiland M, Habermann CR, Schmelzle R. Indications and limitations of intraoperative navigation in maxillofacial surgery. J Oral Maxillofac Surg. 2004;62(9):1059–63.
7. Brief J, Edinger D, Hassfeld S, Eggers G. Accuracy of image-guided implantology. Clin Oral Implants Res. 2005;16(4):495–501.
8. Strong EB, Rafii A, Holhweg-Majert B, Fuller SC, Metzger MC. Comparison of 3 optical navigation systems for computer-aided maxillofacial surgery. Arch Otolaryngol Head Neck Surg. 2008;134(10):1080–4.
9. Hassfeld S, Mühling J. Computer assisted oral and maxillofacial surgery – a review and an assessment of technology. Int J Oral Maxillofac Surg. 2001;30(1):2–13.
10. Wagner A, Schicho K, Birkfellner W, Figl M, Seemann R, König F, Kainberger F, Ewers R. Quantitative analysis of factors affecting intraoperative precision and stability of optoelectronic and electromagnetic tracking systems. Med Phys. 2002;29(5):905–12.
11. Atuegwu NC, Galloway RL. Volumetric characterization of the Aurora magnetic tracker system for image-guided transorbital endoscopic procedures. Phys Med Biol. 2008;53(16):4355–68.
12. Widmann G, Stoffner R, Bale R. Errors and error management in image-guided craniomaxillofacial surgery. Oral Surg Oral Med Oral Pathol Oral Radiol Endod. 2009;107(5):701–15.. Review
13. Malthan D, Ehrlich G, Stallkamp J, Dammann F, Schwaderer E, Maassen MM. Automated registration of partially defective surfaces by local landmark identification. Comput Aided Surg. 2003;8(6):300–9.
14. Widmann G, Stoffner R, Schullian P, Widmann R, Keiler M, Zangerl A, Puelacher W, Bale RJ. Comparison of the accuracy of invasive and noninvasive registration methods for image-guided

oral implant surgery. Int J Oral Maxillofac Implants. 2010;25(3):491–8.

15. Luebbers HT, Messmer P, Obwegeser JA, Zwahlen RA, Kikinis R, Graetz KW, Matthews F. Comparison of different registration methods for surgical navigation in cranio-maxillofacial surgery. J Craniomaxillofac Surg. 2008;36(2):109–16.

16. Lee JD, Huang CH, Wang ST, Lin CW, Lee ST. Fast-MICP for frameless image-guided surgery. Med Phys. 2010;37(9):4551–9.

17. Ewers R, Schicho K, Truppe M, Seeman R, Reichwein A, Figl M, Wagner A. Computer-aided navigation in dental implantology: 7 years of clinical experience. J Oral Maxillofac Surg. 2004;62(3):329–34.

18. Nijmeh AD, Goodger NM, Hawkes D, Edwards PJ, McGurk M. Image-guided navigation in oral and maxillofacial surgery. Br J Oral Maxillofac Surg. 2005;43(4):294–302.

19. Bell RB. Computer planning and intraoperative navigation in cranio-maxillofacial surgery. Oral Maxillofac Surg Clin North Am. 2010;22(1):135–56.. Review

20. Casap N, Wexler A, Eliashar R. Computerized navigation for surgery of the lower jaw: comparison of 2 navigation systems. J Oral Maxillofac Surg. 2008;66(7):1467–75.

21. Voss PJ, Leow AM, Schulze D, Metzger MC, Liebehenschel N, Schmelzeisen R. Navigation-guided resection with immediate functional reconstruction for high-grade malignant parotid tumour at skull base. Int J Oral Maxillofac Surg. 2009;38(8):886–90.

22. Lübbers HT, Jacobsen C, Könü D, Matthews F, Grätz KW, Obwegeser JA. Surgical navigation in cranio-maxillofacial surgery: an evaluation on a child with a cranio-facio-orbital tumour. Br J Oral Maxillofac Surg. 2011;49(7):532–7.

23. Feichtinger M, Aigner RM, Santler G, Kärcher H. Case report: fusion of positron emission tomography (PET) and computed tomography (CT) images for image-guided endoscopic navigation in maxillofacial surgery: clinical application of a new technique. J Craniomaxillofac Surg. 2007;35(6–7):322–8.

24. Feichtinger M, Pau M, Zemann W, Aigner RM, Kärcher H. Intraoperative control of resection margins in advanced head and neck cancer using a 3-D-navigation system based on PET/CT image fusion. J Craniomaxillofac Surg. 2010;38(8):589–94.

25. Yu HB, Shen GF, Zhang SL, Wang XD, Wang CT, Lin YP. Navigation-guided gap arthroplasty in the treatment of temporomandibular joint ankylosis. Int J Oral Maxillofac Surg. 2009;38(10):1030–5.

26. Wagner A, Undt G, Watzinger F, Wanschitz F, Schicho K, Yerit K, Kermer C, Birkfellner W, Ewers R. Principles of computer-assisted arthroscopy of the temporomandibular joint with optoelectronic tracking technology. Oral Surg Oral Med Oral Pathol Oral Radiol Endod. 2001;92(1):30–7.

27. Belli E, Matteini C, D'Andrea GC, Mazzone N. Navigator system guided endoscopic intra-oral approach for remodelling of mandibular condyle in Garré syndrome. J Craniofac Surg. 2007;18(6):1410–5.

28. Schmelzeisen R, Gellrich N-C, Schon R, Gutwald R, Zizelmann C, Schramm A. Navigation-aided reconstruction of medial orbital wall and floor contour in cranio-maxillofacial reconstruction. Int J Oral Maxillofac Surg. 2004:753–7.

29. Marple BF. Ludwig angina. A review of current airway management. Arch Otolaryngol Head and Neck Surg. 1999;125:596–9.

30. Chow AW. Submandibular space infections (Ludwig's angina). Uptodate (serial on internet); 2013.

31. Saifeldeem K, Evans R. Ludwig angina. Emerg Med J. 2004;21:242–3.

32. Athanassiadi KA. Infections of the mediastinum. Thorac Surg Clin. 2009;19:37–45.

33. Kattan B, Snyder HS. Lingual artery hematoma resulting in upper airway obstruction. J Emerg Med. 1991;9(6):421–4.

34. Shukowsky WP. Zur atiologie des stridor inspiratorious congenitus. Jahrb Kinderheilk. 1911;73:459–74.

35. Oeconomopolous CT. The value of glossopexy in Pierre Robin syndrome. N Engl J Med. 1960;262:1267–8.

36. Carey JC, Fineman RM, Ziter FA. The robin sequence as consequence of malformation, dysplasia and neuromuscular syndromes. J Pediatr. 1982;101:858–64.

37. Parsons RW, Smith DJ. A modified tongue-lip adhesion for Pierre Robin anomalad. Cleft Palate J. 1980;17:144–7.

38. Cohen MM Jr. Robin sequences and complexes: causal heterogeneity and pathogenetic/phenotypic variability. Am J Med Genet. 1999;84:311–5.

39. Randall P. The Robin sequence: micrognatia and glossoptosis with airway obstruction. In: McCarthy JG, editor. Plastic surgery. Philadelphia: WB Saunders; 1990. p. 3123–34.

40. Tomaski SM, Howard GH, Aaal HM. Airway obstruction in the Pierre Robin sequence. Laryngoscope. 1995;105:111–4.

41. St-Hilaire H, Buchbinder D. Maxillofacial pathology and management of Pierre Robin sequence. Otolaryng Clin N Am. 2000;33:1241–56.

42. Dykes EH, Raine PAM, Arthur DS, Drainer IK, Young DG. Pierre Robin syndrome and pulmonary hypertension. J Pediatr Surg. 1985;20:49–52.

43. Benjamin B, Walker P. Management of airway obstruction in the Pierre Robin sequence. Int J Pediatr Otorhi. 1991;22:29–37.

44. Spranger JW, Benirschke K, Hall JG, et al. Errors in morphogenesis: concepts and terms. J Pediatr. 1982;100:160–5.

45. Berger JC, Clericuzio CL. Pierre Robin sequence associated with first trimester fetal tamoxifen exposure. Am J Med Genet A. 2008;146A:2141–4.

46. Abuzinada S, Alyamani A. Management of Pierre Robin sequence our experience and long-term follow-up. Int J Oral Maxillofac Surg. 2017;46(Supplement 1):252.

47. Miloro M. Mandibular distraction osteogenesis for pediatric airway management. J Oral Maxillofac Surg. 2010;68(7):1512–23.

48. Mofid MM, Manson PN, Robertson BC, Tufaro AP, Elias JJ, Vander CA, Kolk. Craniofacial distraction osteogenesis: a review of 3278 cases. Plast Reconstr Surg. 2001;108(5):1103–14.

49. Martínez A, Fernández R, Espana A, García B, Capitan L, Monsalve F. Changes in airway dimensions after mandibular distraction in patients with Pierre-Robin sequence associated with malformation syndromes. Revista Espanola de Cirugia Oral y Maxilofacial (English Edition). 2015;37(2):71–9.

50. Guven O. A clinical study on temporomandibular joint ankylosis. Auris Nasus Larynx. 2000;27:27–33.

51. Zhi K, Ren W, Zhou H, Gao L, Zhao L, Hou C, Zhang Y. Management of temporomandibular joint ankylosis: 11 years' clinical experience. Oral Surg Oral Med Oral Pathol Oral Radiol Endod. 2009;108:687–92.

52. Baykul T, Aydin MA, Nasir SN, Toptas O. Surgical treatment of posttraumatic ankylosis of the TMJ with different pathogenic mechanisms. Eur J Dent. 2012 Jul;6(3):318–23.

53. Neelima A. Ankylosis of temporomandibular joint and its management. Ch No.22. Text book of oral and maxilofacial surgery. 1st edn; 2002. pp. 207–219.

54. Soak I, et al. Nonsyndromal true congenital ankylosis of tempromandibular joint- a case report. West Indian Med J. 2006;55(6):444.

55. Falcão I, Carrazzone M, Da Silva L, Pereira S, Pichi L, Ferreira A. 3D morphology analysis of TMJ articular Eminence in magnetic resonance imaging. Int J Dentistry. 2017;

56. Hayakawa Y, Kober C, Otonari-Yamamoto M, Otonari T, Wakoh M, Sano T. An approach for three–dimensional visualization using high–resolution MRI of the temporomandibular joint. Dentomax Radiol. 2007;36(6):341–7.

57. Zheng J, Fan B, Zhong X, Qu P, Liu P, Guo K, Zhao H, Wang Y, Zhen J, Zhang S, Yang C. Application of computer-assisted surgical simulation for temporomandibular joint reconstruction with costochondral graft. Int J Clin Exp Med. 2016;9(9):17650–6.

58. Movahed R, Wolford LM. Protocol for concomitant temporomandibular joint custom-fitted total joint reconstruction and orthognathic surgery using computer-assisted surgical simu-lation. Oral Maxillofac Surg Clin North Am. 2015;27:37–45.

59. Benumof JL. Management of the difficult adult airway. Aneaesthesiology. 1991;75:1087–110.

60. Lin HS, Wang D, Fee WE, Goode RL, Terris DJ. Airway management after maxillectomy: routine tracheostomy is unnecessary. Laryngoscope. 2003;113(6):929–32.

61. Halfpenny W, McGurk M. Analysis of tracheotomy-associated morbidity after operations for head and neck cancer. Br J Oral Maxillofac Surg. 2000;38(5):509–19.

62. Brickman DS, Reh DD, Schneider DS, Bush B, Rosenthal EL, Wax MK. Airway management after maxillectomy with free flap reconstruction. Head Neck. 2013;35(8):1061–5.

63. Cameron M, Corner A, Diba A, Hankis M. Development of a tracheotomy scoring system to guide airway management after major head and neck surgery. Int J Oral Maxillofac Surg. 2009;38(8):846–9.

64. Supkis DE Jr, Dougherty TB, Nguyen DT, Cagle CK. Anesthestic management of the patient undergoing head and neck cancer surgery. Int Anesthesiol Clin. 1998;36:21–9.

65. Yanga W, Shan W, Yan Y, Curtina JP, Dub R, Zhang C, Chen X, Su Y. Three-dimensional printing of patient-specific surgical plates in head and neck reconstruction: a prospective pilot study. Oral Oncol. 2018;78:31–6.

66. Chan HH, Siewerdsen JH, Vescan A, Daly MJ, Prisman E, Irish JC. 3-D rapid prototyping for otolaryngology-head and neck surgery: applications in image-guidance, surgical simulation and patient-specific Modeling. PLoS One. 2015;10(9):e0136370.

67. Barak M, Bahouth H, Leiser Y, El-Naaj IA. Airway management of the patient with maxillofacial trauma: review of the literature and suggested a clinical approach. Biomed Res Int. 2015

68. Committee on Trauma American College of Surgeons. Advanced Trauma Life Support for Doctors ATLS. 8th edn, American College of Surgeons, Chicago, Ill; 2008.

69. Hutchison I, Lawlor M, Skinner D. ABC of major trauma. Major maxillofacial injuries. BMJ. 1990;301:595–9.

70. Garcia A. Critical care issues in the early management of severe trauma. Surg Clin N Am. 2006;86(6):1358–87.

71. Jamal BT, Diecidue R, Qutub A, Cohen M. The pattern of combined maxillofacial and cervical spine fractures. J Oral Maxillofac Surg. 2009;67(3):559–62.

72. Rahman SA, Chandrasala S. When to suspect head injury or cervical spine injury in maxillofacial trauma? Dental Res J. 2014;II(3):336–44.

73. Kill C, Risse J, Wallot P, Seidl P, Steinfeldt T, Wulf H. Videolaryngoscopy with glidescope reduces cervical spine movement in patients with unsecured cervical spine. J Emerg Med. 2013;44(4):750–6.

74. Bhardwaj N, Jain K, Rao M, Mandal AK. Assessment ofcervical spine movement during laryngoscopy with Macintoshand Truview laryngoscopes. J Anaesthesiol Clin Pharmacol. 2013;29(3):308–12.

75. Apfelbaum JL, Hagberg CA, Caplan RA. Practice guidelines for management of the difficult airway: an updated report by the American Society of Anesthesiologists Task Forceon Management of the difficult air way. Anesthesiology. 2013;118(2):251–70.

76. Hamaekers AE, Henderson JJ. Equipment and strategies for emergency tracheal access in the adult patient. Anaesthesia. 2011;66(2):65–80.

77. Kearney PA, Griffen MM, Ochoa JB, Boulanger BR, Tseui BJ, Mentzer RM Jr. A single-center-8-year experience with percutaneous dilational tracheostomy. Ann Surg. 2000;231(5):701–9.

78. Vezina M-C, Trepanier CA, Nicole PC, Lessard MR. Complications associated with the Esophageal-tracheal comb tube in the pre-hospital setting. Can J Anesth. 2007;54(2):124–8.

79. Peterson GN, Domino KB, Caplan RA, Posner KL, Lee LA, Cheney FW. Management of the difficult airway: a closed claims analysis. Anesthesiology. 2005;103(1):33–9.

80. Jahromi HE, Gholami M, Rezaei F. A randomized double-blinded placebo controlled study of four interventions for the prevention of postoperative nausea and vomiting in maxillofacial trauma surgery. J Craniofacial Surg. 2013;24(6)

81. Guo F, Dai J, Zhang J, Ma Y, Zhu G, Shen J, Niu G. Individualized 3-D printing navigation template for pedicle screw fixation in upper cervical spine. PLoS One. 2017;12(2)

82. Herford A, Miller M, Lauritano F, Cervino G, Signorino F, Maiorana C. Virtual surgical planning and navigation in the treatment of orbital trauma. Chin J Traumatol. 2017 Feb;20(1):9–13.

83. Efanov J, Roy A, Huang K, Borsuk D. Virtual surgical planning: the pearls and pitfalls. Plast Reconstr Surg Glob Open. 2018;6(1):e1443.

84. Antony AK, Chen WF, Kolokythas A, Weimer KA, Cohen MN. Use of virtual surgery and stereolithography-guided osteotomy for mandibular reconstruction with the free fibula. Plast Reconstr Surg. 2011;128(5):1080–4.

85. Roser SM, Ramachandra S, Blair H, et al. The accuracy of virtual surgical planning in free fibula mandibular reconstruction: comparison of planned and final results. J Oral Maxillofac Surg. 2010;68(11):2824–32.

86. Hirsch DL, Garfein ES, Christensen AM, Weimer KA, Saddeh PB, Levine JP. Use of computer-aided design and computer-aided manufacturing to produce orthognathically ideal surgical outcomes: a paradigm shift in head and neck reconstruction. J Oral Maxillofac Surg. 2009;67(10):2115–22.

87. Chim H, Wetjen N, Mardini S. Virtual surgical planning in craniofacial surgery Harvey. Semin Plast Surg. 2014 Aug;28(3):150–8.

88. Hanasono MM, Jacob RF, Bidaut L, Robb GL, Skoracki RJ. Midfacial reconstruction using virtual planning, rapid prototype modeling, and stereotactic navigation. Plast Reconstr Surg. 2010;126(6):2002–6.

89. Saad A, Winters R, Wise MW, Dupin CL, St Hilaire H. Virtual surgical planning in complex composite maxillofacial reconstruction. Plast Reconstr Surg. 2013;132(3):626–33.

90. Doscher ME, Garfein ES, Bent J, Tepper OM. Neonatal mandibular distraction osteogenesis: converting virtual surgical planning into an operative reality. Int J Pediatr Otorhinolaryngol. 2014;78(2):381–4.

91. Haq J, Patel N, Weimer K, Matthews NS. Single stage treatment of ankylosis of the temporomandibular joint using patient-specific total joint replacement and virtual surgical planning. Br J Oral Maxillofac Surg. 2014;52(4):350–5.

92. Chandran R, Keeler GD, Christensen AM, Weimer KA, Caloss R. Application of virtual surgical planning for total joint reconstruction with a stock alloplast system. J Oral Maxillofac Surg. 2011;69(1):285–94.

93. Chim H, Amer H, Mardini S, Moran SL. Vascularized composite allotransplantation in the realm of regenerative plastic surgery. Mayo Clin Proc. 2014;89(7):1009–20.

94. Eggers G, Mühling J, Marmulla R. Image-to-patient registration techniques in head surgery. Int J Oral Maxillofac Surg. 2006;35(12):1081–95.. Review

Virtual Endoscopy and 3-D Reconstruction/Prototyping in Head and Neck Surgeries

8

Hassan Mohammed, Hassan Haidar,
Nabil A. Shallik, Amr Elhakeem, Majid Al Abdulla,
and Zenyel Dogan

8.1 Introduction

The use and application of the three-dimensional (3-D) reconstructions generated from suitable files Digital Imaging and Communications in Medicine (DICOM) of computed tomography (CT) or magnetic resonance (MR) have been expanding recently. Such reconstructions allow physicians to observe anatomic cavities and structures within our body with an incredible amount of detail in addition to displaying the textures of variety of tissues [1–3]. The applications of such reconstructions have varied from simple illustrations in exams up to the help in the diagnosis and preoperative planning in several ENT proce-

dures. An example of such application is virtual upper airways endoscopies and laryngoscopies. Such application has been practically abandoned due to its complexity and need for computers with high power of graphic processing [4]. However, with the evolution of proper compute softwares for reading and reconstruction of the DICOM files, some applications of such 3-D reconstructions have been recovered for evaluation and preoperative planning in ENT, especially for head and neck surgeries and sinus surgery [5, 6]. Such 3-D reconstructions may offer potentially more usable information than those obtained with 2-D views in the axial, coronal, and sagittal planes. Two-dimensional images are of more difficult comprehension for surgeons [7]. We live in a three-dimensional world, and despite a large part of the endoscopes still do not allow the performance of 3-D stereoscopic surgeries, the images obtained in the traditional endoscopic surgeries allow us

Electronic Supplementary Material The online version of this chapter (https://doi.org/10.1007/978-3-030-23253-5_8) contains supplementary material, which is available to authorized users.

H. Mohammed · A. Elhakeem · M. Al Abdulla
ENT Department, Hamad Medical Corporation,
Doha, Qatar

H. Haidar (✉)
ENTDepartment, Hamad Medical Corporation,
Doha, Qatar

ENT Department, Weill Cornell Medical College in Qatar (WCMQ), Doha, Qatar
e-mail: hahmed2@hamad.qa

N. A. Shallik
Department of Clinical Anesthesiology, Weill Cornell Medical College in Qatar (WCMQ), Doha, Qatar

Department of Anesthesiology, ICU and Perioperative Medicine, Hamad Medical Corporation, Doha, Qatar

Department of Anesthesiology and Surgical Intensive Care, Faculty of Medicine, Tanta University, Tanta, Egypt
e-mail: Nshallik@hamad.qa

Z. Dogan
Head of Head and Neck Department at St. Anna Hospital Otolaryngology-Head and Neck Surgery, Teaching Hospital of University of Dusseldorf, Dusseldorf, Germany

the creation of 3-D relationships in our mind. These relationships may help in the performance of specific tasks, and the excellent preoperative preparation may sometimes prevent generally challenging complications [8]. Some researchers have studied the utility of the 3-D reconstruction tools for the surgeries of the ear, nose, and throat and of the recess and frontal sinus. Other possible applications include preoperative surgical planning, preoperative measurement for production of prostheses, air flow analysis, and proper teaching to resident doctors [5, 6, 8, 9, 10].

8.2 VE and 3-D in Head and Neck Surgery Planning

Surgical procedures in otolaryngology—head and neck surgery—can be so challenging even to the most experienced surgeons during resection of infiltrative diseases and reconstruction of anatomical structures. These challenges arise from performing excision of lesions within critical and anatomically complex areas in the head and neck region.

Head and neck anatomy is intricately unique in having compact condensation of neuromusculovascular structures. In addition, it is composed of multiple anatomical subsites which are essential for vital functions, namely, breathing, phonation, and swallowing. These structures have different embryological origins and give rise to various disease processes and pathologies. Esthetics is also a unique hallmark in the head and neck region for social acceptance and self-esteem.

Staging workup of head and neck cancers is important for prognosis assesment and for choosing the most appropriate treatment modality. Although there have been advances in nonsurgical treatment options, that is, chemoradiation, adequate surgery is still the mainstay of treatment for many benign and malignant tumors in head and neck region. Performing complete excision while minimizing effects on breathing, phonation, swallowing, and esthetic appearance greatly improves loco-regional control and minimizes short- and long-term complications with improved quality of life scores. Surgical planning for excision and/or reconstruction requires not only surgical expertise but also detailed knowledge of the disease topography in relation to the normal structures surrounding it.

Currently, endoscopic examination in the clinic or operating theatre is a valuable tool for disease mapping and assessing its effects on the upper aerodigestive tract and anticipating the function loss from adequate tumor resections. However, endoscopy is an invasive examination; may cause discomfort, bleeding, and airway compromise; and may often require local or even general anesthesia. In addition, it may yield limited information due to limited views depending on tumor localization and depth of extension and on individual patient's anatomy variations, patient's compliance, body habitus, and comorbidities, which should be taken into consideration. Therefore, reliance on other modes of information gathering is becoming more essential in assessing different head and neck pathologies. The current common modalities utilized in head and neck imaging are US, CT, and MRI, which have their own advantages and limitations in assessing head and neck tumors.

Virtual endoscopy (VE) and 3-D reconstructions have become a more attractive imaging modality concept used in head and neck surgical planning. Virtual endoscopy is the processing of computerized tomography image data to create a virtual environment of the human body to allow diagnosis of disease processes. This technique combines latest imaging techniques with modern computer software to provide interactive reconstruction of the 3-D anatomy and pathology of the head and neck from 2-D images. This mental task usually takes less time of experience to master as a radiologist or a head and neck surgeon. This concept will also be a useful tool for systematic and standardized way to help trainees develop their knowledge in dealing with the complex 3-D anatomy of the head and neck. VE allows the surgeon the opportunity to interact with an image that is artificially generated by the computer that mimics reality.

8.3 Airway Management in Head and Neck Pathology

Managing the airway in head and neck surgery is a shared responsibility between the anesthetist and the surgeon. The surgeon needs to be knowledgeable about how to keep the airway patent.

Traditional approaches to the development of surgical competency and image-guidance technology involve the use of biological specimens in a pre-clinical setting. However, the use of cadaveric specimens requires considerations of resource availability and bio-safety factors. In contrast, animal studies raise ethical issues and may not provide a realistic representation of human anatomy. In both scenarios, there are costs associated with specimen transport and storage.

The development of realistic 3-D reconstruction images and virtual endoscopy for head and neck surgery has the potential to provide a threefold advantage: (1) from an educational perspective, it provides realistic and customizable environments for surgical trainees; (2) from a surgical perspective, it enables the creation of patient-specific models for surgical planning and procedure simulation before starting the actual surgery; and (3) from a research perspective, it facilitates technology development in an environment that mimics clinical practice [2].

8.4 Some Major Problems Solved by VE and 3-D Redemonstration

In this chapter, the current applications and implications/limitations of VE in head and neck surgery are discussed. And processes that create rapid prototype models for VE applications of head and neck surgery are also given.

8.4.1 VE and 3-D in Head and Neck Foreign Body Diagnosis

8.4.1.1 Deceiving Duck Bone Which Turned Out to be a Needle

Foreign body ingestion is a very common presentation in ENT practice and can have different sequelae. It can arrest anywhere in the pharynx, or it can continue further down either taking the airway tract to end up in the bronchus, or the digestive tract up to the intestines. A young female patient presented with possible ingestion of duck bone. CT imaging and 3-D reconstruction are shown in Figs. 8.1 and 8.2 (Movie 8.1). The characteristics of FB determined to be more of metallic in nature. The FB was traversing the sternocleidomastoid muscale and peircing the internal jugular vein; it was removed and it was actually an injection needle with a bore, and with a pinged proximal end suggestive of a break-off from its base. Although she didn't not know how she ingested the needle, she recalled a dental procedure where she received a local anesthetic. The bottom line is that 3-D reconstruction and VE were helpful in localizing the FB and in surgical planning as well.

8.4.1.2 Fish Bone as a Diagnostic Tool

VE and 3-D reconstruction play a very important role in the diagnosis of foreign body ingestion like fish bone, and to see how the diagnosis becomes easy and accurate please refer to Movies 8.2, 8.3 and 8.4.

Please refer to Chap. 12, Challenge case discussion.

8.4.2 3-D and VE in Tracheo-Esophageal (TEF)

Tracheo-esophageal fistula is an abnormal communication between the trachea and the esophagus. Causes of TEF are numerous and could be classified into congenital and acquired. The acquired could be further subclassified into being benign (commonest is iatrogenic causes) or malignant. Although benign acquired TEF is uncommon, the incidence seems to be rising due to increase in long term intubations and tracheos-

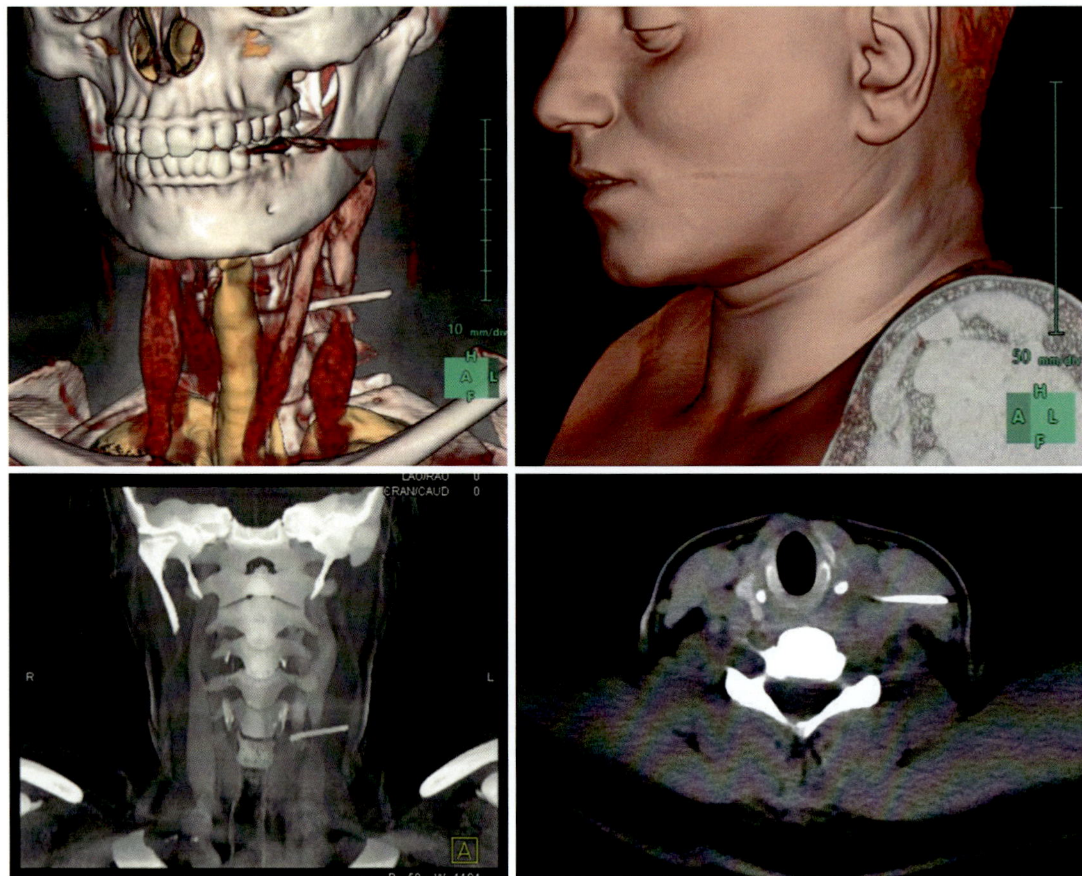

Fig. 8.1 FB needle transversely oriented with metallic density F.B. is noted as traversing and embedded within the left sternocleidomastoid muscle abutting the apparently intact left carotid sheath vessels with partial compression/effacement of the left IJV. The subcutaneous region showed subtle bulge which was the guide for easy surgical intervention (arrow).

tomies.) Patients typically present with cough after deglutition and/or recurrent chest infections/aspiration pneumonia. The latter is a reason for increased morbidity and mortality of TEF. Therefore, early detection and appropriate management is vital. Esophagoscopy and bronchoscopy are currently the gold standard for diagnosis. Radiological studies using VE and 3-D are important to plan surgical intervention. Size, location, and depth of the fistula are important factors to consider when planning the best approach for surgical closure or to plan the use of regional flaps (Fig. 8.3). Please refer to Chap. 12, Challenge case discussion.

Clinical scenario of one of our patient: a 60-year-old female patient who was intubated for 2 months with viral meningoencephalitis complained of recurrent cough while eating soon after extubation. Bronchoscopy and esophagoscopy aided to identify a small tracheoesophageal fistula in the cervical esophagus. The patient was initially managed conservatively with NPO and NG feeding. However, several months later, the fistula persisted and the patient presented to the ED with collapse due to septic shock secondary to aspiration pneumonia. Full recovery was made after 2-week course of intravenous (IV) total parenteral nutrition (TPN) feeding. VE was utilized in this frail patient to assess the size and location of the TEF and also the integrity of the posterior wall of the trachea/anterior wall of the esophagus. Please refer to Chap. 12, Challenge case discussion (Fig. 8.4).

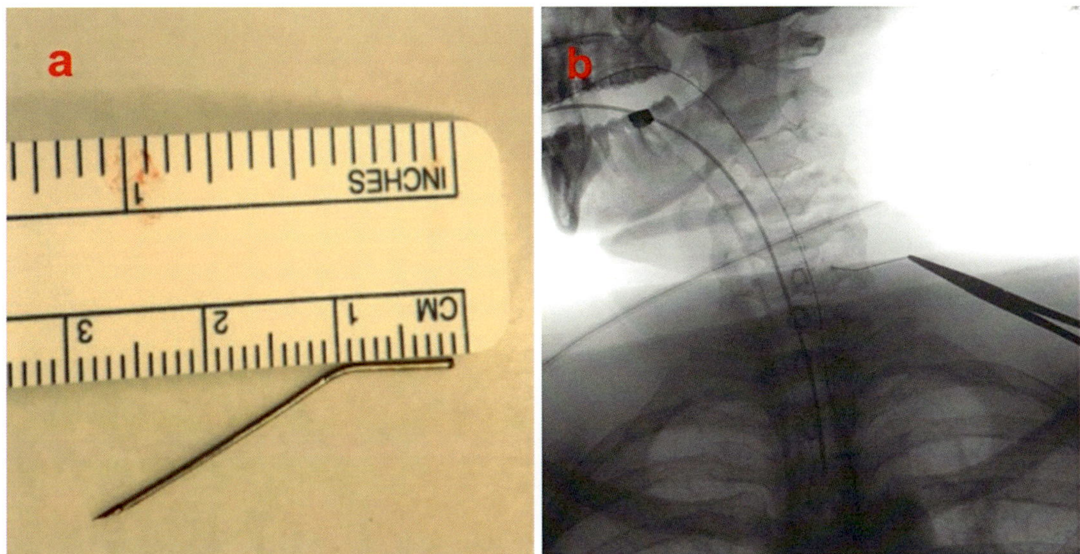

Fig. 8.2 (**a**) Curved metallic needle averaging about 3 cm in length with one beveled end. (**b**) The X-ray image showed the forceps caption of the needle during its extraction

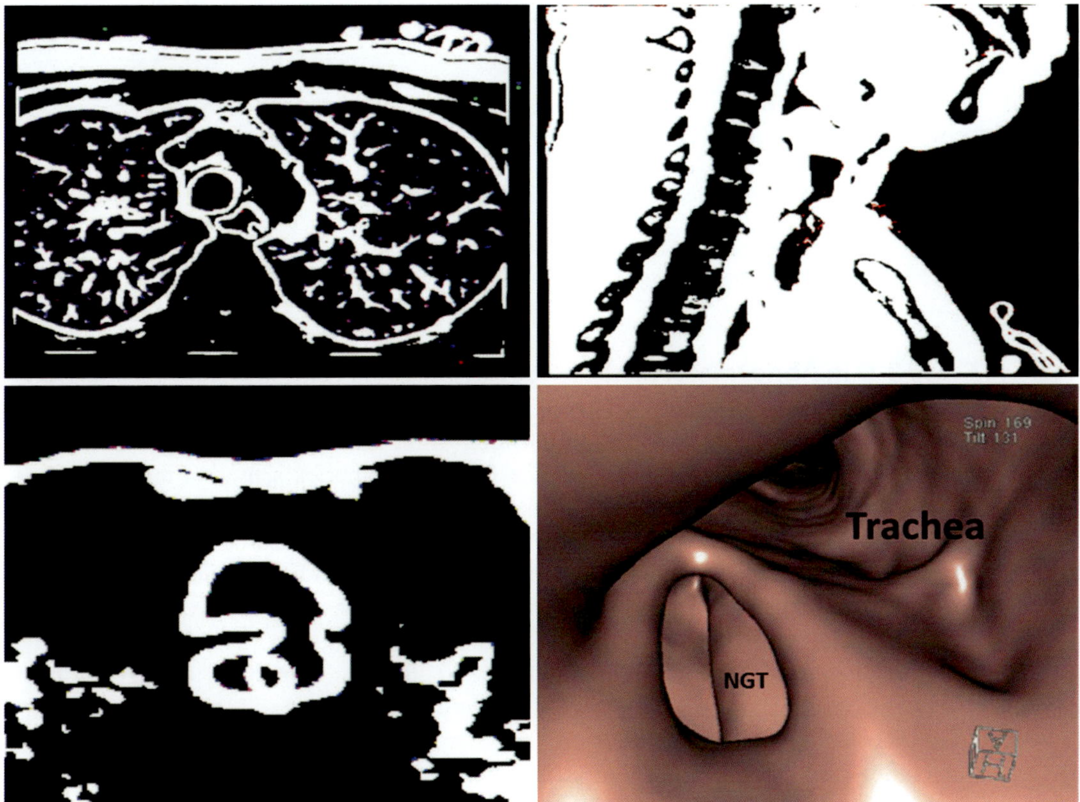

Fig. 8.3 Patient with TEF diagnosed after nondiagnostic several contrast studies; CT was carried out using modified Valsalva maneuver with nice demonstration of the fistula tract

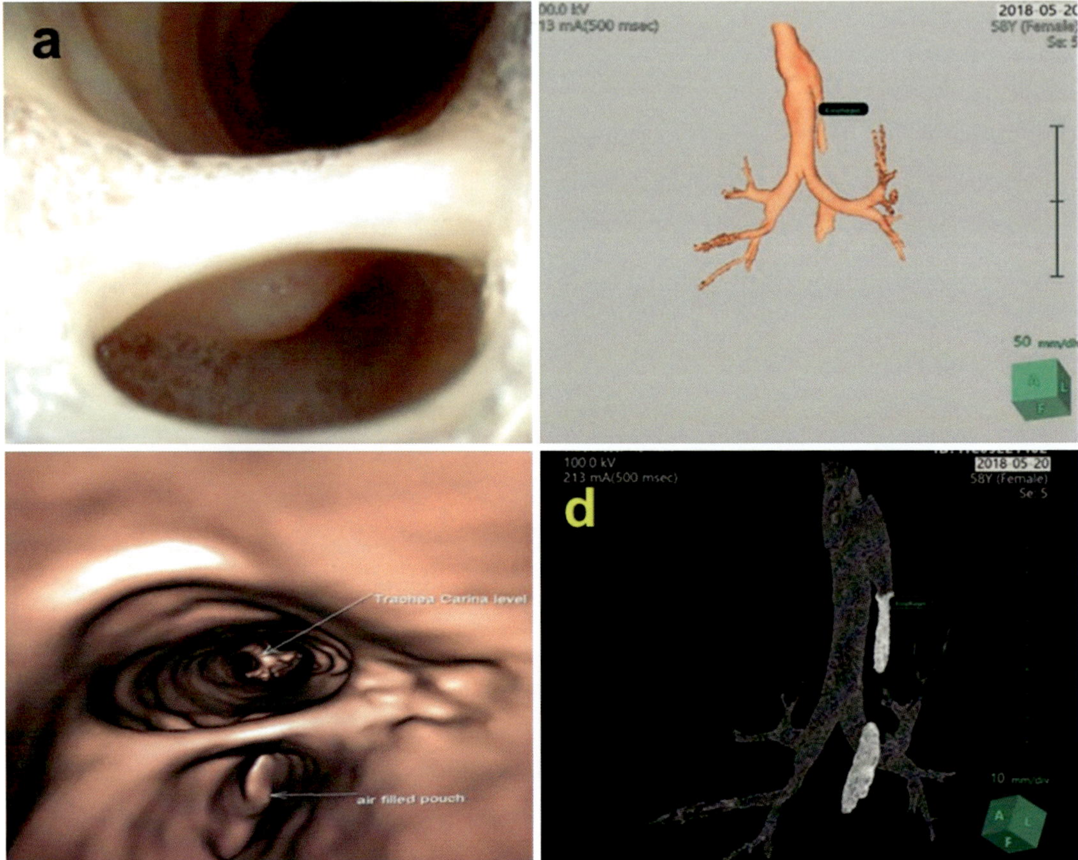

Fig. 8.4 TOF nicely demonstrated by virtual endoscopy and VRT and SSD techniques. The virtual endoscopy images and findings were identical and in accordance with the conventional endoscopy images, however, without the need for a local anesthetic and risk of aspiration, which is considered a breakthrough in safe patient management

8.4.3 VE and 3-D in Abnormal Hyoid Bone Diagnosis

8.4.3.1 Circular Hyoid Bone

Hyoid bone is a free-floating horseshoe-shaped, single bone located in the anterior neck. The hyoid bone consists of a central body and two horns (cornuas) on each side, a greater horn and a lesser horn. The hyoid bone is embryologically derived from the second (greater horns) and third (lesser horns) pharyngeal arches. Developmental abnormalities of the hyoid bone can be seen in clinical conditions such as Pierre Robin syndrome and cleft lip and palate. Only a few cases were reported on abnormal hyoid bone [11].

Circular hyoid bone with subsequent narrowing of airway in a 32-year-old male patient presenting to the clinic with dysphagia and having the feeling of pinprick sensation in the neck all the time for the past 1.5 years. Fiber optic examination revealed prominent corniculate cartilages and prominent hyoid bone horns protruding into the pharyngeal lumen.

CT imaging and 3-D reconstruction show abnormal thick and abnormal configuration of the hyoid bone causing mild oropharyngeal airway narrowing and indenting posterior upper hypopharyngeal wall. With the use of VE, the diameter of the airway was determined, and surgical, as well as anesthesia, planning was done accordingly. Microlaryngoscopy was done with a CO_2 laser and mucosa over the abnormal part of the bone and the abnormal part of the bone was exposed and removed. Please refer to Chap. 12, Challenge case discussion (Fig. 8.5), and kindly refer to Chap. 12, Movies 12.1 and 12.2.

8.4.3.2 Displaced Hyoid Bone

Our second patient presented earlier with a recent diagnosis of thyroid carcinoma for preoperative anesthesiology assessment for which clinical evaluation was carried out, and preoperative naso-endoscopic evaluation revealed the presence of abnormal mucosal lined drumstick-shaped structure of odd presentation, yet with no signs of malignancy or hyper-vascularity (Movie 8.5).

Its exact etiology origin was unclear till this point. Subsequently, 3-D reconstruction was carried out which solves this mystery as the etiology was due to displaced blade of the hypoid

bone, in which the thyroid mass lesion was clearly visualized. Please refer to Fig. 8.6 and Movie 8.6.

For more details, please refer to Chap. 12, Challenge case discussion.

8.4.4 Tracheal Stenosis (Please Do Referencing)

A 40-year-old lady presented with chief complaints of difficulty in breathing when she walks for 300 meters or more or during any form of exercise.

She had a past history of an acquired tracheal stenosis for which she was treated by balloon dilatation, after which she had improved.

Her presenting history is otherwise unremarkable.

Examinations are all within normal.

Laboratory workup including complete blood count, serum urea, and electrolytes is within normal limits.

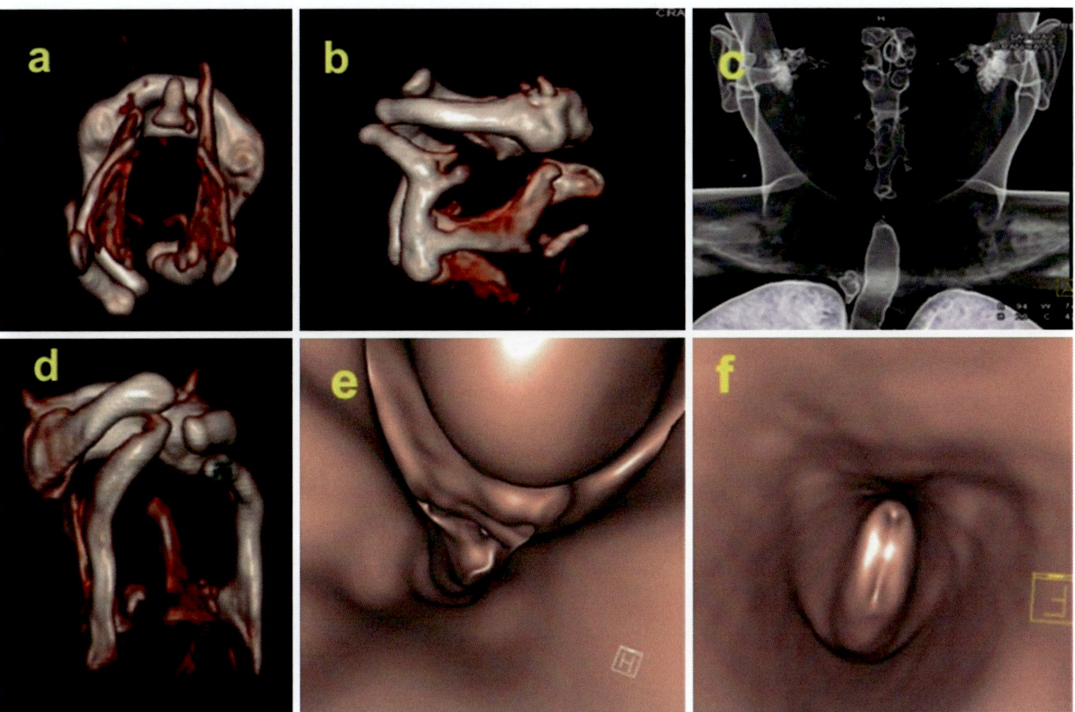

Fig. 8.5 Extremely rare anomaly (circular hyoid bone) with over-riding of its posterior aspect forming incomplete ring; the thyroid cartilages' superior conu share in the same process with subsequent signal encroachment on the related airway column. The 3-D images: (**a**) caudocranial, (**b**) right lateral, (**c**) TTP for the airway column with a narrow segment, (**d**) posterior aspect of the 3-D model, (**e**) VRT of the severely compromised airway, and (**f**) unique caudocranial view of the subglottic region

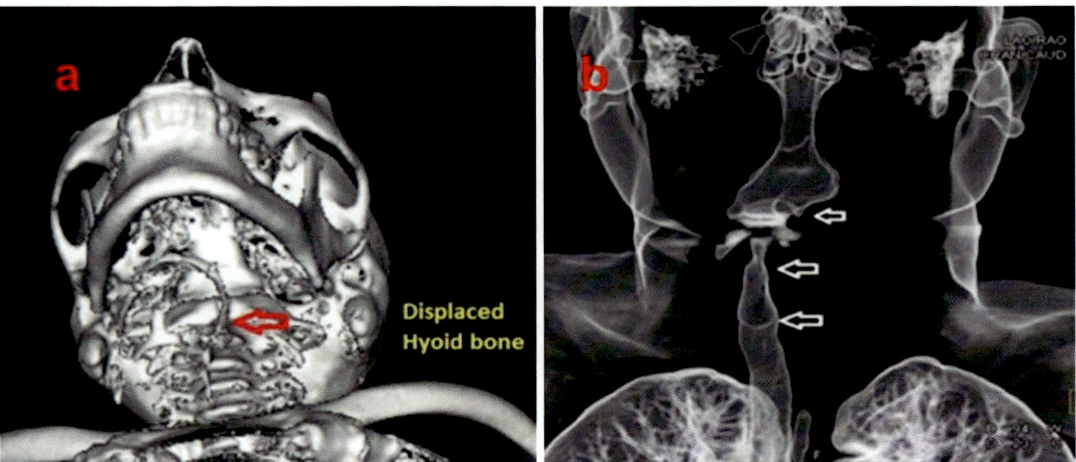

Fig. 8.6 Displaced and rotated hyoid bone (red arrow) with significant encroachment upon the airway, which is violated and replaced by a soft tissue mass lesion (white arrows)

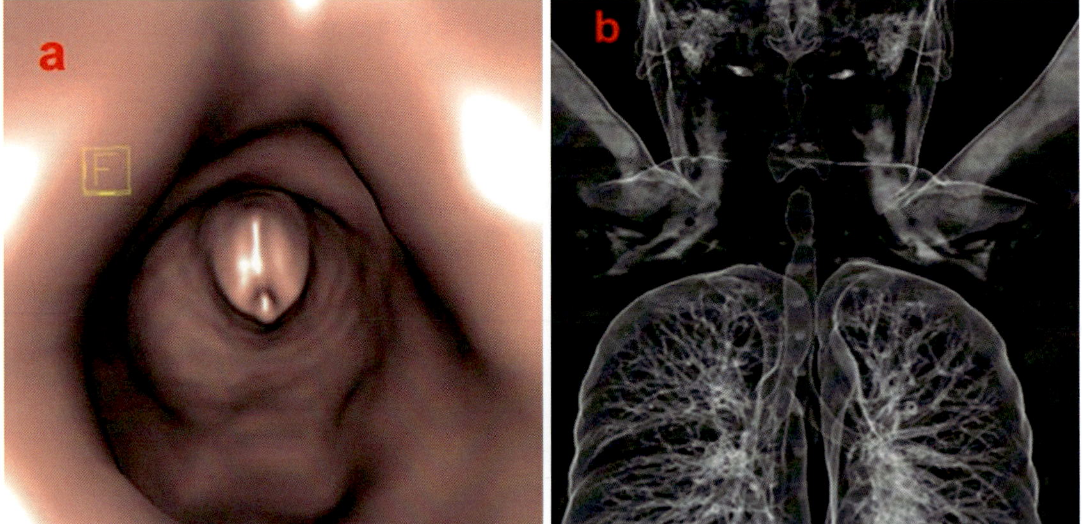

Fig. 8.7 Virtual endoscopy and TTP of the airway showing significant encroachment and subtotal occlusion, narrowing

CT of the neck and thorax was done (Fig. 8.7), which showed the severity and extent of stenosis:

A 1.5 cm short segment tracheal luminal narrowing of around 50% at the level of the thyroid gland and opposite to C5 vertebral body, corresponding to the previous tracheostomy site.

Diagnosis: Recurrent subglottic and tracheal stenosis.

Treatment planned: Microlaryngoscopy and balloon dilatation of the stenotic segment.

8.5 Traumatic Supraglottic Stenosis

This is the case of a patient with hoarsness of voice and exertional dyspnea. ENT clinical evaluation based on clinical and naso-endoscopy assessment revealed a web formation at the level of the glottis extending from the anterior commissure to the junction between the anterior two-thirds and posterior one-third of the vocal cord (glottic area) (Movie 8.3).

Virtual endoscopic evaluation was done which showed the web to be at a supraglottic region, 8 while the glottic region was clear) (Movies 8.7, 8.8, and 8.9).

The anesthesiologist's decision based on the VE findings was to give the patient light sedation in addition to topical surface spray airway anesthesia (Fig. 8.8).

8.6 Eagle Syndrome

Eagle syndrome is a rare disease due to elongation of the styloid process. Patients with this syndrome present with odynophagia, sensation of a foreign body in the throat, pain in the neck, and other non-specific symptoms such as otalgia and tinnitus. In most cases, elongation is an acquired condition, often occurring as a result of a traumatic incident, including tonsillectomy. Diagnosis is usually made through clinical symptoms, physical examination, and radiological findings (Fig. 8.9).

8.6.1 First Case

We describe the case of a 57-year-old man who experienced unremitting right neck pain for several years following an accidental fall. A multidisciplinary investigation identified an elongated

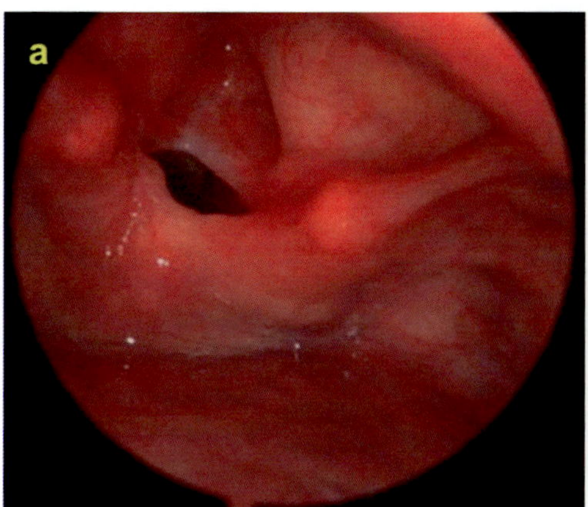
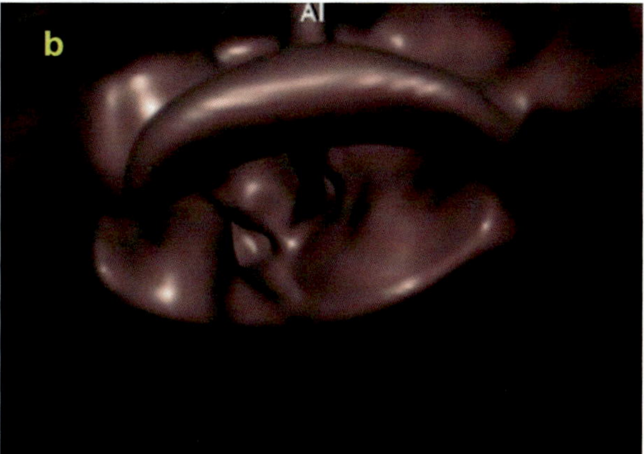

Fig. 8.8 Web formation at the level of the glottis extending from the anterior commissure to the junction between the anterior two-thirds and posterior one-third of the vocal cord (glottic area). The (**a**) image is for the conventional endoscopic evaluation, while the (**b**) image is the virtual endoscopy view [12]

Fig. 8.9 Cropped view of the VRT model nicely demonstrated the elongated styloid process with partial calcification and ossification of the stylohyoid ligament in a case of Eagle syndrome

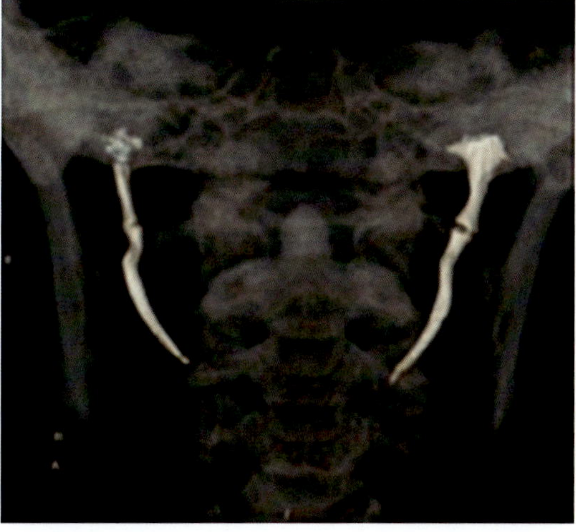

styloid process. Surgical shortening of the structure provided definitive relief of the patient's symptoms. We review the anatomy of the peristyloid structures and discuss the etiology, diagnosis, and treatment of Eagle syndrome.

8.6.2 Second Case

A 35-year-old male patient had tonsillectomy 5 years ago for chronic tonsillitis. One year later, he started to complain of pricking sensation in his throat upon swallowing along with severe pain during swallowing with significant weight loss because of fear of eating-related pain.

3-D reconstruction and virtual endoscopy were helpful in measuring the length and the relation with carotid artery because the plane of the styloid process is not pure in the coronal and sagittal planes.

8.7 Laryngocele

Laryngoceles are uncommon cystic lesions of the larynx, which may be internal type, external type, or combined. Laryngoceles are usually filled with air but could also be filled with mucus (laryngomucocele) or pus (laryngopyocele). They may be congenital or acquired mostly arising in the sixth decade of life. The association between acquired laryngoceles and squamous cell carcinoma is well established in the literature.

A 73-year-old had a 1-year history of anterior neck swelling which was slowly increasing in size, and 6-month history of dysphonia and dysphagia. Naso-pharyngo-laryngoscopic examination revealed a large left supraglottic cystic lesion with a normal overlying mucosa overhanging the glottic opening. CT showed a mixed fluid-filled laryngocele/laryngomucocele. VE reconstruction was helpful to navigate the upper airway to intubate the patient and avoid an upfront tracheostomy. Both components of the lesion were completely excised through a combined approach with airway reconstruction [13] (Fig. 8.10).

8.8 Blunt Neck Trauma

Blunt neck trauma is not common in children, but these injuries can be potentially life-threatening. The presentation could be vague and nonspecific. Voice change and stridor may not be evident early and could be life threatening when occurring late; imaging is very important for diagnosis and management.

We present a 6-year-old female child, previously healthy, presented with a history of falling down at the edge of the bed (wooden part); after that she had some little change in the voice. She also reported coughing a small amount of blood soon after trauma. With mild degree of odynophagia, no dysphagia, and no stridor, flexible fiberoptic laryngoscope revealed left aryepiglottic fold edema, a small hematoma above the posterior third of the left vocal cord, left vocal cord almost in the midline with sluggish movement, suspected thyroid cartilage fracture on the left side above the left vocal cord, mild to moderate airway compromise, no external injuries seen on the neck, she had mild to moderate tenderness on the neck at the level of thyroid cartilage. CT of the neck showed tiny air loculi at the level of the hyoid bone and thyroid cartilage on the left side and suspected upper airway injury with the help of 3-D reconstruction and VE; it was determined that we proceed with conservative management. The child did well and was discharged after full recovery and improvement in her voice and the above findings.

8.9 3-D Printing and Its Applications in Otorhinolaryngology and Head and Neck (for More Details Please Refer to Chap. 11)

8.9.1 Splints and Stents for Trachea

Recently, researchers and clinicians are investigating the use of 3-D printing for more delicate and critical implants such as tracheobronchial splint for pediatric patients, where the challenge

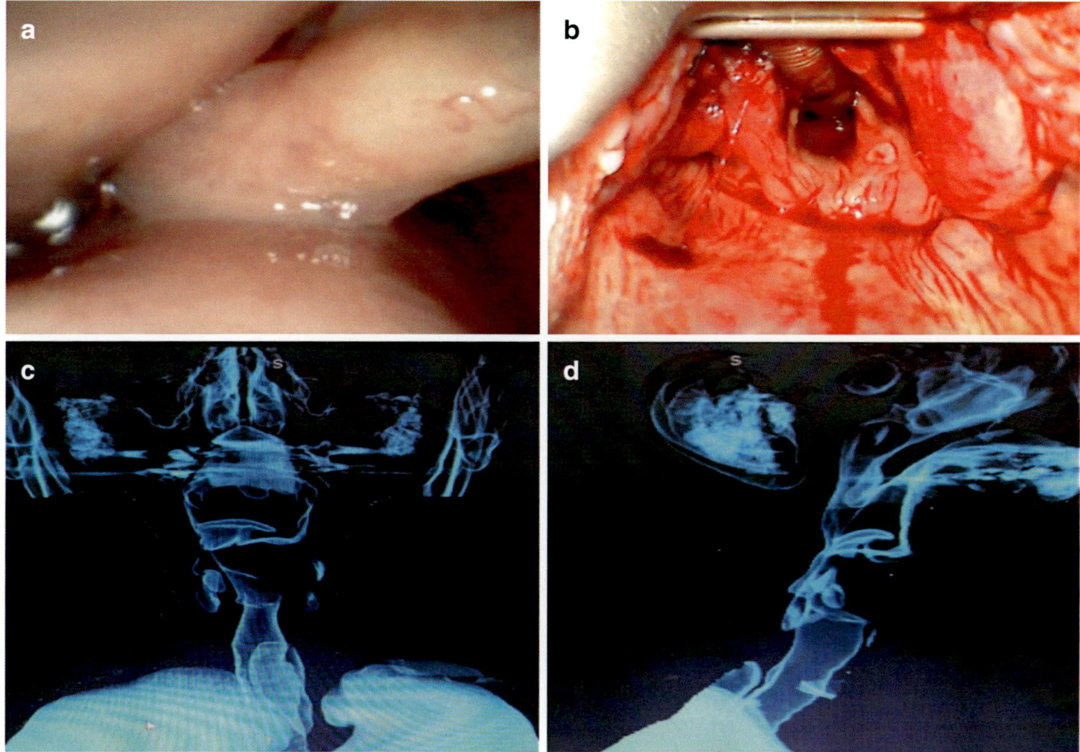

Fig. 8.10 A sizable combined internal and external laryngocele encroaching significantly upon the aerodigestive tract: (**a**) laryngoscopic view, (**b**). intraoperative photo, (**c**, **d**) airway reconstruction for the airway frontal and right lateral projections

is to create an external splint responsive to geometry changes. The case proves that 3-D printing can be useful to accommodate physiological behavior of the patients over time, in what many started to coin as four-dimensional (4-D) printing, in which materials with thermomechanical properties have shape-morphing behavior.

Surgeons succeeded in treating airway stenosis with customizable 3-D printed airway stent [14]. 3-D printing proved useful in this case due to the complexity of the geometry of the stenosis. In this case, the patient suffering from a complex case of a complete stenosis of the bronchus intermedius (BI) with partial dehiscence of the bronchial anastomosis after lung transplantation [15]. The complexity of the case excluded the use of conventional airway stents (Figs. 8.11 and 8.12).

By using computer-assisted segmentation and by conducting a virtual operation, the stenosis and dehiscence were treated and a 3-D stent was designed.

8.9.2 Bio-absorbable Polymer Vascular Stents in Head and Neck Area

Currently, most vascular stents, which are used as flow diverters or to treat stenosis, are manufactured using multi-step manufacturing processes that include, but not limited to, LASER precision micro sheet and tube machining and micro wire braiding. Essential post processing includes heat treatment to dispose internal stresses and manufacturing defects as well as surface electrochemical treatments. Materials used for stent manufacturing include nickel titanium (NiTi) and cobalt chromium (CoCr) [16]. 3-D printing seemed to be unsuccessful to present any added value to the clean room manufacturing of stents. However, many are investigating 3-D printing for direct digital manufacturing of stents that can better fit with complex geometries of critical vessels in head and neck, thus reducing the probability of failure. Furthermore, 3-D printed flexible, biodegradable polymer stents, which are customized to patient-specific geometries, can be coated with drugs that aim to reduce complications and expedite the healing process [16].

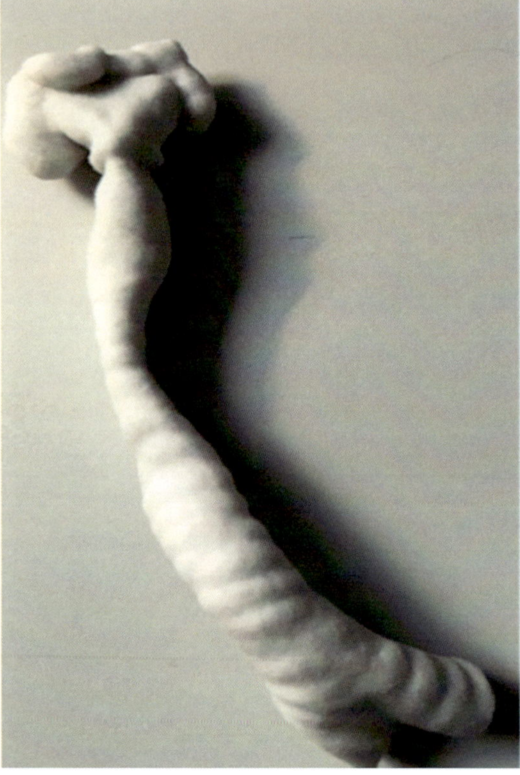

Fig. 8.11 3-D printed tracheal model shows mass effect on the wall of the trachea due to pressure from outside

8.9.3 3-D Printing for Design and Manufacture of Implantable Devices

Advances in 3-D printing now allow for the creation of biocompatible structures with impressive complexity. 3-D printed implantable models of auricle can be used for reconstruction of patients with microtia or arrhinia.

Researchers have begun exploring the feasibility of printing multi-material biomimetic tympanic membrane (TM) grafts that could be implanted into a patient.

The goal is to overcome the limitations of current graft materials to improve the outcomes following tympanoplasty. If we could design a graft material from the ground up and include optimized features, this would be a huge step forward. I think 3-D printing may now offer the means to produce such a graft.

Currently, physicians use materials such as temporalis fascia, perichondrium, and cartilage for TM grafts. The problem with these materials is that they do not possess similar structural features as those of the native TM, and this can leave the patient susceptible to chronic otitis media, a long-standing infection of the middle ear. 3-D printers can fabricate biomimetic TM grafts.

Using nonabsorbable materials, as well as biologics, such as collagen and fibrin, they have created tympanic membrane grafts with acoustic properties that can be tuned to correct the sound-induced motion patterns of the human TM.

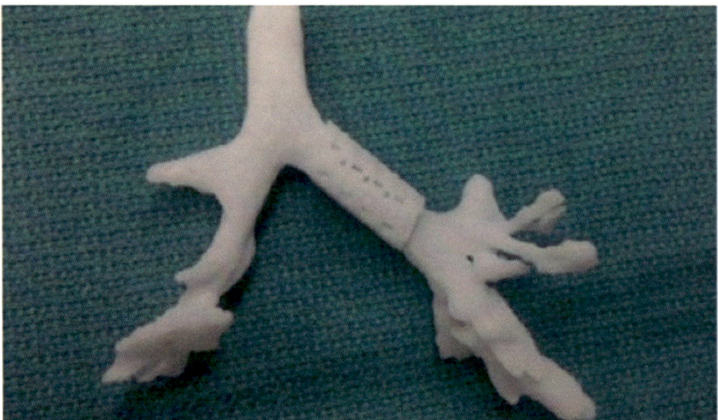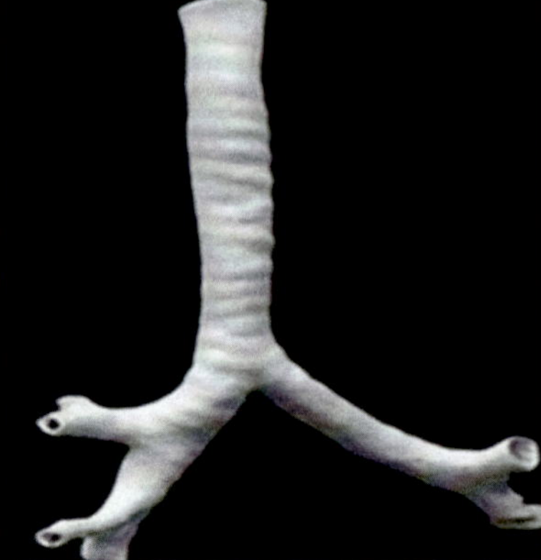

Fig. 8.12 3-D printed tracheal model, right and left main bronchus, and printed tracheal stent

3-D printed grafts can be reliably produced and have structural features that are more consistent with temporalis fascia. Such grafts have promising implications for clinical applications. With 3-D printing, we can rapidly create constructs with varying structural features and then answer these questions in a systematic way. It should help us generate a TM structure with the ideal features—a design that may one day be implanted into patients—and hopefully result in better outcomes.

8.9.4 Maxillofacial 3-D Printing

3-D design tools have enabled the virtual construction of 3-D-specific models to construct implants and guides to facilitate surgical procedures such as drilling and implant placement. The main applications of maxillofacial 3-D printing are dental implant surgery, mandibular reconstruction, mandibular pathology, orthognathic surgery, and midface reconstruction.

Please refer to Chap. 7 for more details.

8.9.5 3-D Printing in Preoperative Surgical Planning

The level of personalized care achieved through 3-D printing has been influential in increasing accuracy and efficiency in procedures, cutting down operating room time, and improving surgical outcomes. Working with patients who have cancer or radiation damage involving the mandible, we can use 3-D models to help prepare for and implement their surgical resections and reconstructions. We can use 3-D models for two reasons: to help plan where we will make our bone cuts around the tumor and to help streamline and optimize the reconstruction.

It starts with a CT scan that is turned into a 3-D image of the patient's face to determine where the bone cuts around the tumor will be and at what angles. Often times, there is a need to take part of the patient's fibula to create a new jawbone, and 3-D imaging is used to determine where fibula osteotomies will be. Once all of the cuts have been mapped out, the 3-D model is printed. These mod-

els are used to bend a titanium plate customized to the patient's native mandible, which is implanted during surgery. In some instances, the models are also shared with patients to give them a better understanding of what the surgery will look like.

Improved cosmetic outcomes have been another advantage to 3-D printing. Patients who have mandibles that are excessively deformed are now able to achieve a result that is much more symmetric than before. We can use the 3-D images to view the opposite side of the mandible, invert it, and make it an exact mirror image of the other side of the jaw.

From a point-of-view of bone reconstruction anywhere in the head and neck region, using 3-D models is going to become the standard way to go.

8.9.6 Reductions in Operation Room Time

Operating room time has usually been one of the huge debates for health care 3-D printing. Of the 227 articles, 42 explained the precise effect of utilizing 3-D printing innovation on OR time. For a large number of applications, 3-D printing resulted in time-saving. The outcomes are given in applications such as operative guides for maxillofacial surgical operation, models for vertebral and maxillofacial surgical preparation, and designs for forming implants utilized in maxillofacial surgery appear to benefit the more from the modern 3-D technology [17] (Fig. 8.13).

8.9.7 Resident Training

Quick prototyping is a developing innovation that has the possibility to transform health care learning. As plastic cosmetic surgeons, we are anticipated to recognize the touches of comprehensive human anatomical designs and their spatial relationship with one another. 3-D printing can enable an in-depth awareness of human anatomy that was generally obtained from text illustrations and years of operative expertise doing complex dissections. The future of plastic surgery learning is interesting because of the capability to take a

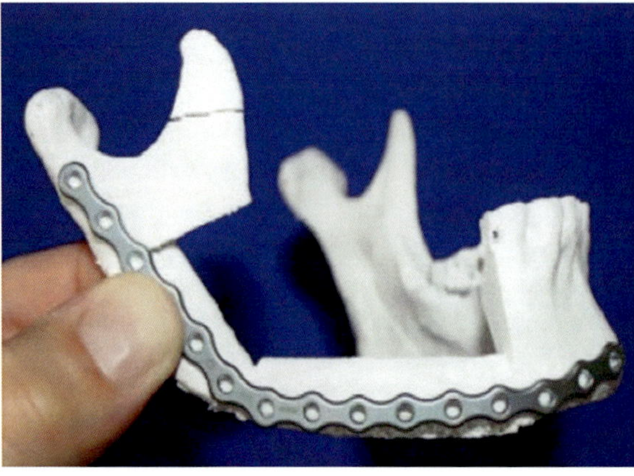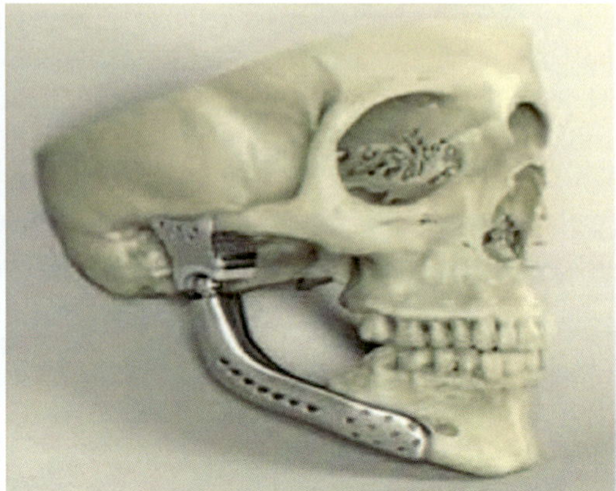

Fig. 8.13 3-D model print as a rehearsal and accurate measurement of the metallic plate and screws in a patient going to have right-sided hemimandibulectomy

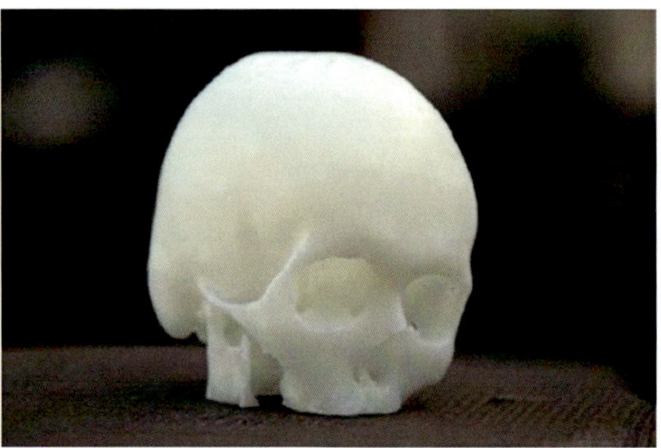

Fig. 8.14 3-D print model of the skull

2-dimensional (2-D) picture and carry it to way of life with a full-scale design (Fig. 8.14).

8.9.8 Patient Education of Head and Neck Surgery

Throughout (ENT) subspecialty, a somewhat minimal portion of patients follow through with elective procedures to fix ailments such as oral, head and neck tumors, or pathology. Patient awareness of their medical diagnosis and therapy plan is integral to compliance, which essentially generates enhanced health care results and far better quality of life. Here we report the usage of advanced, polyjet 3-D printing options to develop a multimaterial reproduction of human nasal sinus anatomy, derived from clinical X-ray computed tomography (CT) data, to be used as an educational aid during doctor assessment. The last patient education model was developed over several models to optimize material properties, anatomical reliability, and overall performance [18].

8.10 Future Applications

Incredible advances have been gained from 3-D reconstruction and printing; however, there is some concern that such claims may be exaggerated. There has been major dramatic and important discovery in tissue scaffolds and bio-printing in the last few years; however, many of these technologies, including organ printing, are in their primitive stage.

Three 3-D printed implantable models of auricular and nasal scaffolding have been assessed.

In such models, anatomic structure has been persevered and histologic appearance revealed cartilaginous growth within the territories of these scaffolds. The need to develop and present a vascular network to deliver oxygen and remove waste remains a considerable challenge to organ printing. Vascular structures could be constructed from biomaterials, using three-dimensional printing, which, thereafter, can be incorporated with endothelial cells. Vessel-like microfluidic channels flanked by tissue spheroids have also been proposed and may be a viable option in the future. The organ production steps also include separation and differentiation of stem cells, culturing the cells in support medium, checking for markers, and organogenesis in a bioreactor. Correcting congenital anomalies, reconstructing defects from resecting large tumors, and rebuilding traumatic injuries can be achieved from complex tissue and organ production. Vascular pathologies such as arteriovenous malformations can be created as well.

Ossicular reconstruction, cochlear and vestibular structures, turbinates, and laryngeal subunit reconstructing defects arising from large head and neck tumor resection can be some important future applications in the field of otolaryngology.

8.11 Conclusion

Surgical procedures in otolaryngology-head and neck surgery can be so challenging even to the most experienced surgeons during resection of infiltrative diseases and reconstruction of anatomical structures. These challenges arise from performing excision of lesions within critical and anatomically complex structures in the head and neck region. Virtual endoscopy (VE) and 3-D reconstructions have become more attractive imaging modalities used in head and neck surgical planning. 3-D reconstruction images and virtual endoscopy images have the potential to provide realistic and customizable environments for surgical trainees, enable the creation of patient-specific models for surgical planning and procedure simulation before starting the actual surgery, and facilitate technology development in an environment that mimics clinical practice.

References

1. Prisman E, Daly MJ, Chan H, Siewerdsen JH, Vescan A, Jaffray DA, et al. Real-time tracking and virtual endoscopy in cone-beam CT-guided surgery of the sinuses and skull base in a cadaver model. Int Forum Aller Rhinol. 2011;1(1):70.
2. Chan HHL, Siewerdsen JH, Vescan A, Daly MJ, Prisman E, Irish JC. 3D rapid prototyping for otolaryngology—head and neck surgery: applications in image-guidance, surgical simulation and patient-specific modeling. PLoS One. 2015;10(9):e0136370.
3. Canzi P, Magnetto M, Marconi S, Morbini P, Mauramati S, Aprile F, Avato I, Auricchio F, Benazzo M. New frontiers and emerging applications of 3D printing in ENT surgery: a systematic review of the literature Nuove frontiere applicazioni emergenti della stampa 3D in ORL: revisione sistematica della letteratura. Acta Otorhinolaryngol Ital. 2018;38(4):286–303.
4. Toro C, Robiony M, Costa F, et al. Feasibility of preoperative planning using anatomical facsimile models for mandibular reconstruction. Head Face Med. 2007;3:1–11.
5. Yeung R, Samman N, Cheung L, et al. Stereomodel-assisted fibula flap harvest and mandibular reconstruction. J Oral Maxillofac Surg. 2007;65:1128–34.
6. Singare S, Dichen L, Bingheng L, Yanpu L, Zhenyu G, Yaxiong L. Design and fabrication of custom mandible titanium tray based on rapid prototyping. Med Eng Phys. 2004;26(8):671–6. https://doi.org/10.1016/j.medengphy.2004.06.001.
7. Hallermann W, Olsen S, Bardyn T, et al. A new method for computer-aided operation planning for extensive mandibular reconstruction. Plast Reconstr Surg. 2006;117:2431–7.
8. Hannen E, Wiedermann J, Joshi A, Jamshidi A, et al. Utilization of a submental island flap and 3D printed model for skull base reconstruction: infantile giant cranio-cervicofacial teratoma. Int J Pediatr Otorhinolaryngol. 2017;92:143–5.
9. Paydarfar J, Wu X, Halter R. MRI-and CT-compatible polymer laryngoscope: a step toward image-guided transoral surgery. Otolaryngol Head Neck Surg. 2016;155:364–6.
10. Dorati R, De Trizio A, Marconi S, et al. Design of a Bioabsorbable multilayered patch for esophagus tissue engineering. Macromol Biosci. 2017;17:1–11.
11. Shallik N, Haidar H, Dogan Z, Enezi H, Rahman W, Arun N, Ishac N, Moustafa A. Circular hyoid bone: the first reported case in literature. Trends Anaesth Crit Care. 2017;16:27–8. https://doi.org/10.1016/j.tacc.2017.10.040.
12. Shallik N, Zaghw A, Dogan Z, Rahman A. The use of virtual endoscopy for diagnosis of traumatic supraglottic airway stenosis. JCAO. 2017;2(1):103.
13. Shallik N, Soliman M, Aboelhassan A, Hammad Y, Haidar H, Moustafa A. Does the surgical airway still the gold standard step in securing the airway in patients with obstructing laryngeal tumors? Trends Anesth Crit Care. 2018;23:42–3. https://doi.org/10.1016/j.tacc.2018.09.085.
14. Maragiannis D, Jackson MS, Igo SR, Schutt RC, Connell P, Grande-Allen J, Little SH. Replicating patient-specific severe aortic valve stenosis with functional 3-D modeling. Circulation: Cardiovascular Imaging, (10), e003626. three-dimensional, computer-assisted customized airway stent. Am J Respir Crit Care Med. 2015;195(7):e31–3.

15. Guibert N, Didier A, Moreno B, Mhanna L, Brouchet L, Plat G, Mazieres J. Treatment of post-transplant complex airway stenosis with a three-dimensional, computer-assisted customized airway stent. Am J Respir Crit Care Med. 2017;195(7):e31–3.
16. STI Laser, Stent manufacturing process. https://www.sti laser.com/products/stents/stent-manufacturing-process/.
17. Bauermeister AJ, Zuriarrain A, Newman MI. Three-dimensional printing in plastic and reconstructive surgery: a systematic review. Ann Plast Surg. 2016;77(5):569–76.
18. Van Lith R, Baker E, Ware H, Yang J, Farsheed AC, Sun C, Ameer G. 3-D-printing strong high-resolution antioxidant bioresorbable vascular stents. Adv Mat Technol. 2016;1(9):1600138.

Perspectives in the Current and Future Use of Augmented Reality Visualization in Thoracic Surgery and Pulmonary Interventions

Mohamed A. Elarref, Ahmed Aljabary, Nabil A. Shallik, Mohamed Abbas, and Noran Elarif

9.1 Introduction

Decision-making and preparation of the patient for surgical intervention take time, effort, and a lot of preparations by patient care team, and for the anaesthetist the most important step is airway assessment and for this mission to be accomplished multiple score indices and techniques were developed for proper assessment with variable degrees of sensitivity and accuracy.

Virtual bronchoscopy (VB) or virtual endoscopy (VE) is an animated 3-D CT post-processing practice that generates high-definition tracheobronchial tree photos and endobronchial views that mimic standard bronchoscopy reports.

While the procedure was defined in the mid-1990s, it created increasingly new actual interest due to advances in computer functionality and technology in multi-detector computed tomography (MDCT) advanced scan technology, which permit isotropic data acquisition [1].

Discussion of the current role of VB and 3-D MDCT imaging in clinical settings on the airways is very important. In fact, one of the latest techniques in the current medical practice to have an accurate idea about airway anatomy is fibre-optic scopes, which use a camera with either a flexible or rigid probe to visualize the anatomy and make accurate judgements; the use of this technique has revolutionized the practice of pulmonary medicine and anaesthesia and reduced the risk of unanticipated difficulties intraoperatively, but despite its huge benefits it has its own limitations and the most important is (1) inability to visualize the anatomy beyond significant obstruction through which the probe

Electronic Supplementary Material The online version of this chapter (https://doi.org/10.1007/978-3-030-23253-5_9) contains supplementary material, which is available to authorized users.

M. A. Elarref (✉) · N. A. Shallik
Department of Clinical Anesthesiology, Weill Cornell Medical College in Qatar (WCMQ), Doha, Qatar

Department of Anesthesiology, ICU and Perioperative Medicine, Hamad Medical Corporation, Doha, Qatar

Department of Anesthesiology and Surgical Intensive Care, Faculty of Medicine, Tanta University, Tanta, Egypt
e-mail: Melarref@hamad.qa

A. Aljabary
Department of Anesthesiology, ICU and Perioperative Medicine, Hamad Medical Corporation, Doha, Qatar

M. Abbas
Radiology Department, Detroit Medical Center, Detroit, MI, USA

N. Elarif
Cardiology Department, National Heart Institute, Cairo, Egypt

© Springer Nature Switzerland AG 2019
N. A. Shallik et al. (eds.), *Virtual Endoscopy and 3D Reconstruction in the Airways*,
https://doi.org/10.1007/978-3-030-23253-5_9

cannot pass and the next important is (2) the invasiveness and the advanced training and preparation that are needed for proper handling and accurate results; these drawbacks raised a strain to figure out a non-invasive technique that can overcome these limitations: these facts highlighted the role of non-invasive imaging techniques like CT and MRI in the assessment of tracheobronchial tree [2].

Virtual bronchoscopy (VB) is one of the most recent innovations in the field of post-processing technique. It visualizes inner structures using a perspective projection for easy navigation or to generate animations for the bronchial tree that illustrate the inner structures when it is indicated for diagnosis and assessment for any needed procedure [3].

In this chapter, we will try to explain more about the role of CT in airway assessment by implicating the images obtained by CT into specific computer-based software and analyse them to produce a real-time virtual 3-D image of the airway, hence producing a virtual bronchoscopy (VB) image.

9.2 Definition

Virtual bronchoscopy (VB) is a newly emerging technique; its clinical use started in the mid-1990s; at that time, CT imaging and computer software were not that well developed to produce a clinically significant 3-D model of the lung and airways; the current systems have improved their technological capabilities so that it can produce a dependable 3-D model based on 2-D image. Virtual bronchoscopy is a novel multi-detector computed tomography (MDCT) imaging technique that demonstrates a non-invasive intra- and extra-luminal evaluation of the tracheobronchial tree. Virtual bronchoscopy visualizes the inner structures through a perspective projection. To have an animated navigation tracking of the inner structures of the bronchial tree, a computer-generated path tracking is easier than using manual tracking [1].

Virtual bronchoscopy, as mentioned before, is CT image dependent, which means the final virtual images are dependent on the type of quality and the radiological specifications of the per-

formed images and also on the software program used to process the images [3].

9.3 Technique Implications

Please refer to Chap. 3 for more radiological background.

9.4 Clinical Uses

From a clinical point of view, this technique can aid in perioperative preparations and assessment of the patient in the following spectrum:

9.4.1 Preoperative

9.4.1.1 Visualization of Normal Anatomical Features and Variants

The proper identification of anatomical variants of tracheobronchial (T-B) tree is very crucial in multiple aspects that involves the diagnosis and the treatments of certain pathologies of the lung; the fibre-optic technique was and still is the basic tool for such evaluation, but its well-known limitations include inability to advance beyond the 4–5 dichotomous divisions and its invasiveness in high-risk patients, raising the need for multi-detector computed tomography (MDCT) (VB) for evaluation [4].

According to the article published in 2013 by *Polish Journal of Radiology* by Adamczyk et al., the atypical anatomical variation in the tracheobronchial tree ranges between 25% and 55%, for example, around 44% of the study population had atypical right upper lobe bronchus division, which was bifunctional rather than the normal trifurcation, and 1% of the B1 division arises from trachea directly; such results cannot be obtained previously by bronchoscopy alone with that much of accuracy; this study showed that CT virtual bronchoscopy is a fast and productive method to assess the bronchial branching down to the level of segmental bronchi, which is characterized by a huge anatomical variability [3] (Figs. 9.1, 9.2, and 9.3).

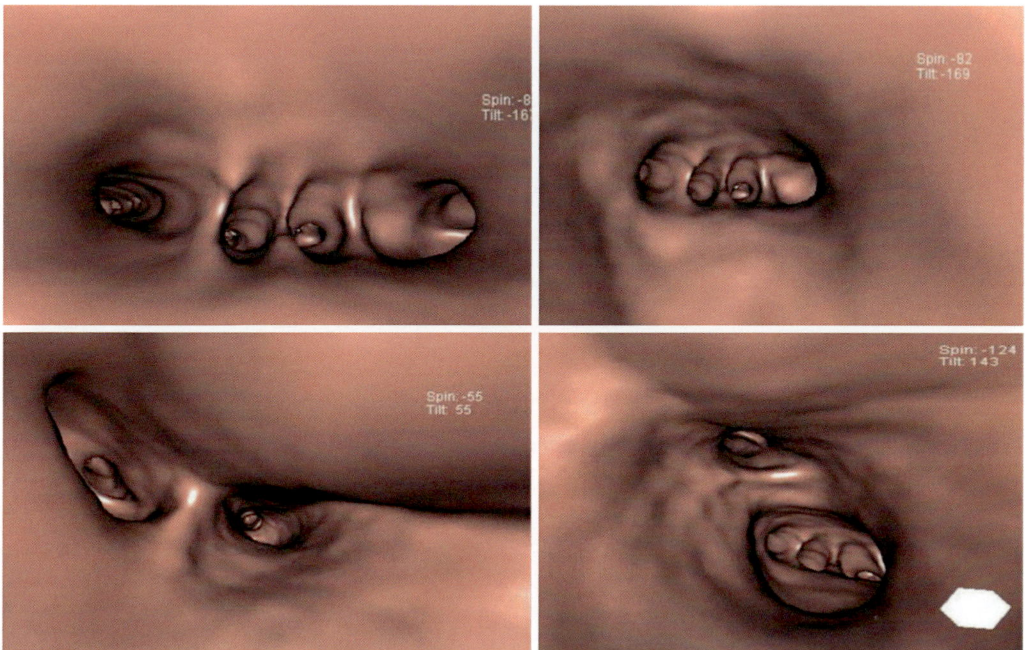

Fig. 9.1 Different levels of virtual bronchoscopic evaluation of the right lung; the two images at the top correspond to the two images at the bottom, which nicely demonstrate the endoluminal views of the bronchial segmentation

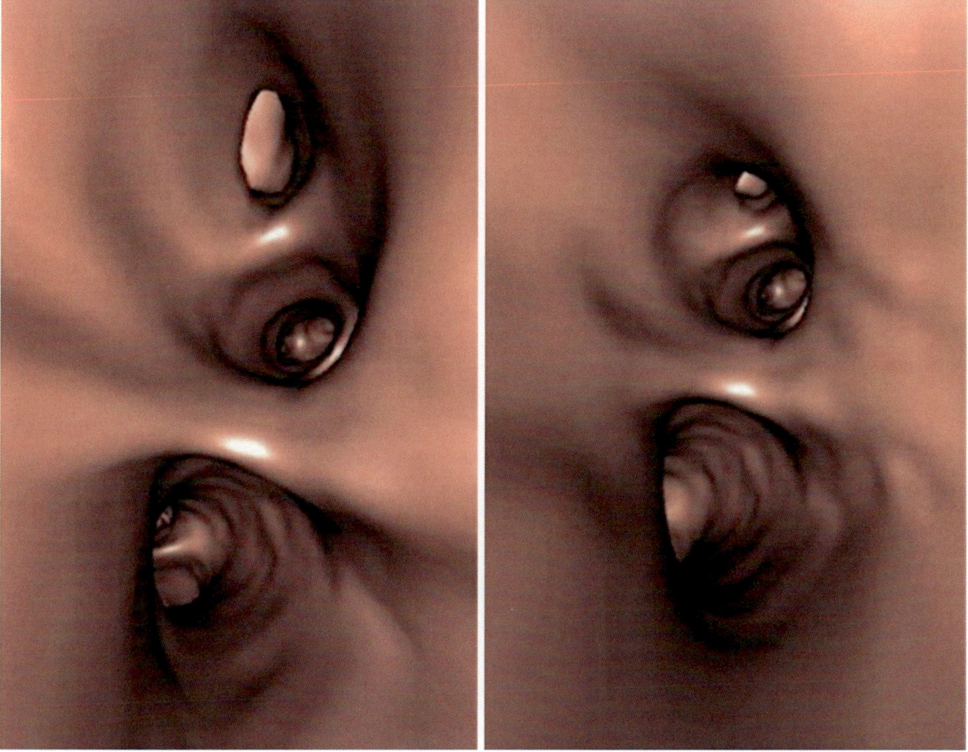

Fig. 9.2 Right-side VB views at the right main bronchus and the proximal part of the bronchus intermedius

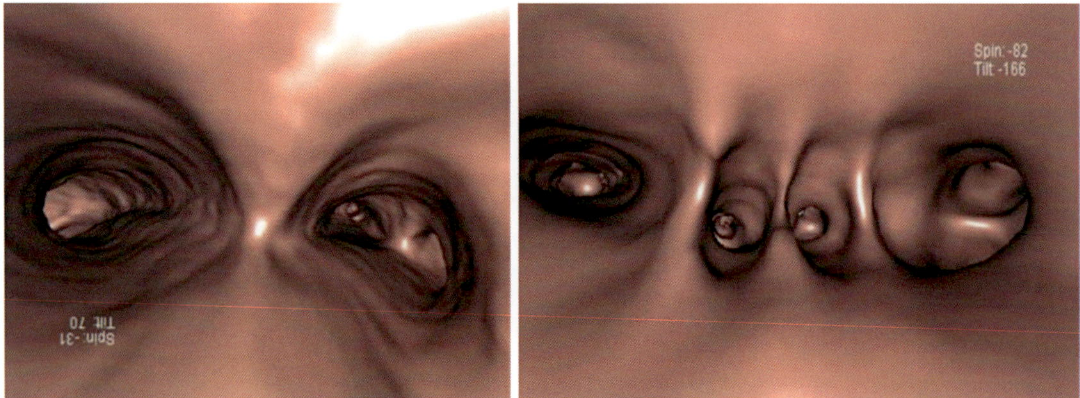

Fig. 9.3 The left-side image is VB at the level of the tracheal bifurcation (carina). The right-side image is the VB at the right main bronchus and bronchus intermedius

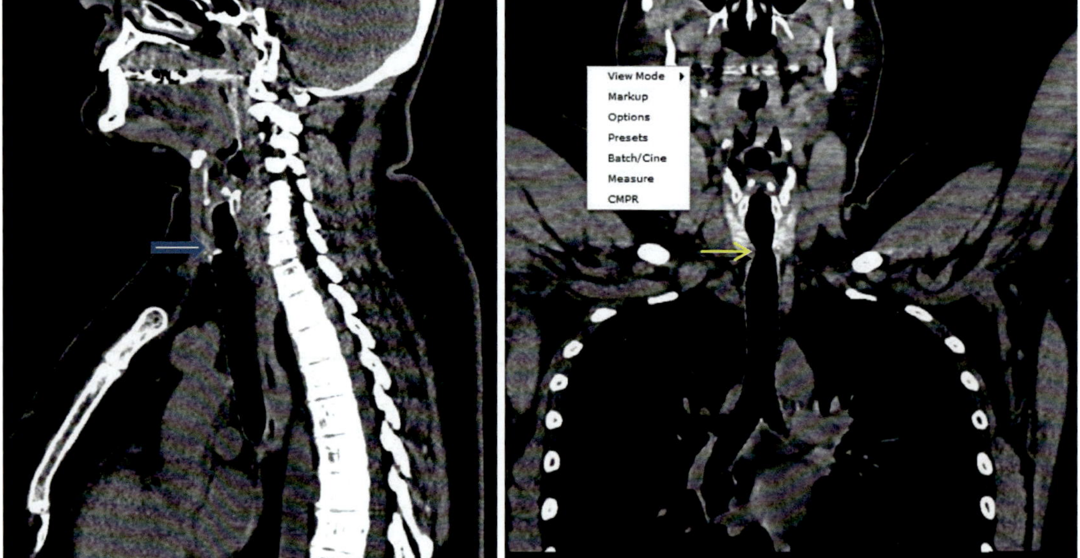

Fig. 9.4 Sagittal and coronal reformatted images showing stenotic segment/narrowing at the level of the thyroid gland (arrows)

9.4.1.2 Tracheobronchial Stenosis

The aetiology of tracheobronchial stenosis might be inflammatory, granulomatous, traumatic, or pressure from outside by adenopathy for instance. The positron emission tomography/computed tomography (PET/CT) scan seemed to be a highly valuable diagnostic modality. Englmeier and Seeman used virtual hybrid bronchoscopy by a low-dose diagnostic CT. The importance is that it can identify and diagnose the character of malignancy and can identify the tumour from atelectasis and has the ability to help in tumour staging, which may not be detectable by virtual CT-bronchoscopy. Virtual hybrid bronchoscopy can also replace fibre-optic bronchoscopy in the situation that it is contraindicated or not possible [5] (Figs. 9.4, 9.5, and 9.6).

Others compared different imaging modalities including virtual bronchoscopic images and flexible bronchoscopy for grading of tracheobronchial stenosis; the results were as predicted: virtual bronchoscopic findings of tracheobronchial tree revealed 98% accuracy rate and 91%

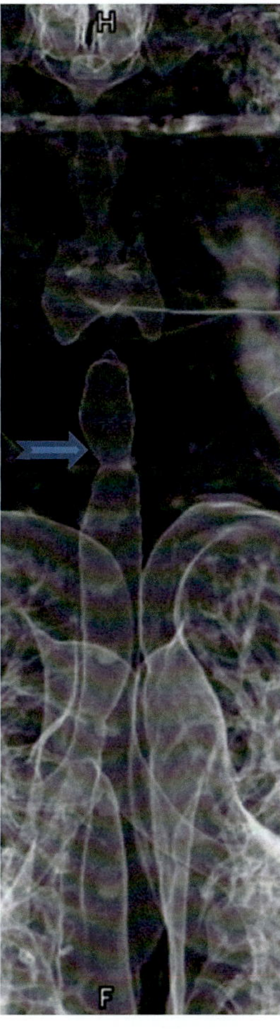

Fig. 9.5 Tissue transparent projection of the airway showing the narrow segment (arrow)

accuracy rate in grading of tracheobronchial stenosis compared with images obtained by flexible bronchoscopy [6].

These results also support the rising assumption of considering reliable virtual bronchoscopy as a non-invasive method that allows accurate grading of tracheobronchial stenosis [5] (Movie 9.1).

9.4.1.3 Endoluminal Lesions

Virtual bronchoscopy evaluation of malignant tumours of the thorax: lung cancers are considered one of the most common leading causes of death worldwide, and it is well known that the earlier the detection the better the prognosis; despite the advancements in lung cancer diagnosis, patients still present with signs and symptoms of airway narrowing or obstruction as a result of endoluminal lesion [5], while fibre-optic examination is still considered as one of the leading modalities to detect endoluminal lesions that can represent invasive pulmonary malignancy questions related to its invasiveness; its seriousness as a procedure that requires sedation and monitoring can hinder its use on widespread practice in addition to its adverse outcome in high-risk patients [7].

In 2002, an article by Finkelstein et al. was published in *The Journal of Thoracic and Cardiovascular Surgery* that compared the sensi-

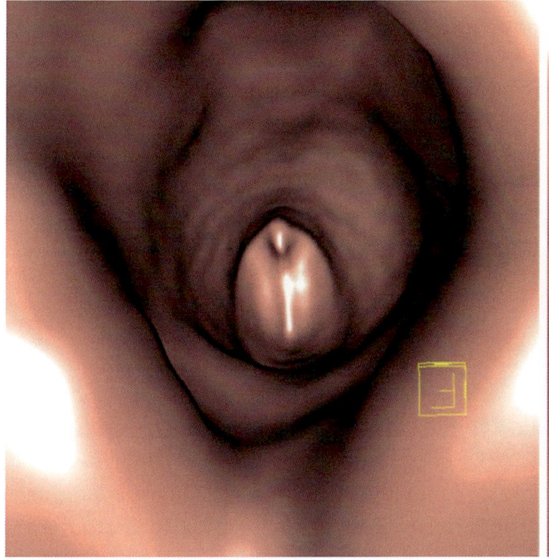

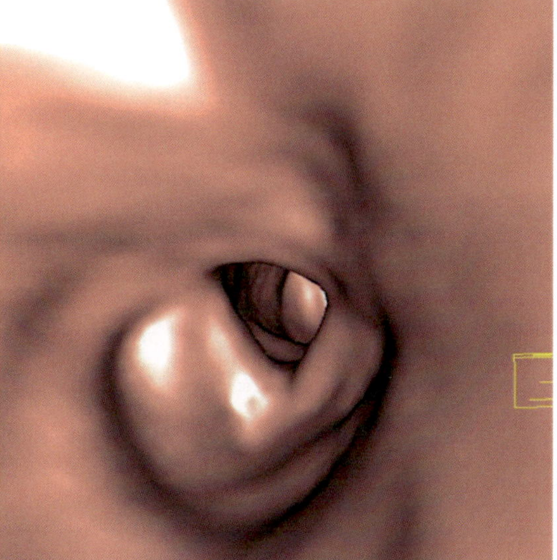

Fig. 9.6 VB views showing the appreciable narrow segment

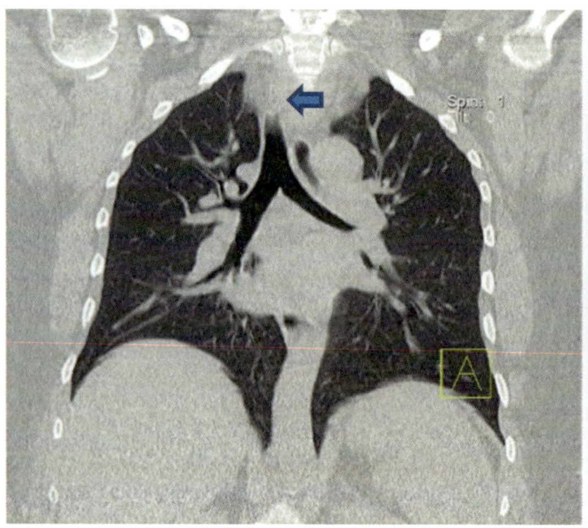

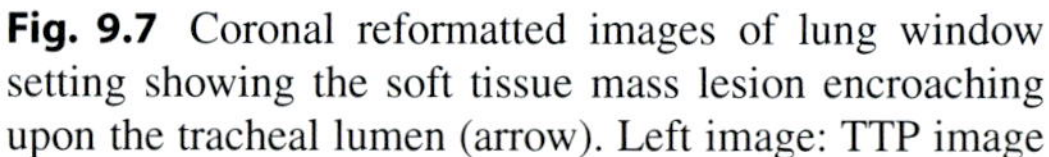

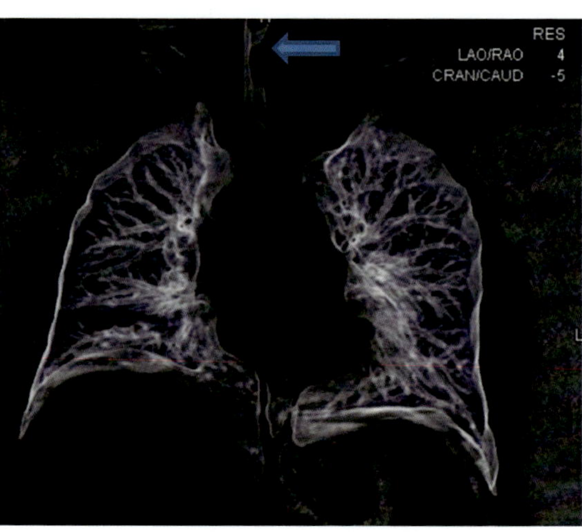

Fig. 9.7 Coronal reformatted images of lung window setting showing the soft tissue mass lesion encroaching upon the tracheal lumen (arrow). Left image: TTP image showing the violation and filling defect at the t\left side of the trachea (arrow). right-sided image

tivity and specificity of images obtained by fibre-optic and multi-detector computed tomography (MDCT) (VB) in the detection of endoluminal and obstructive lesions; although the study sample was not that big, the sensitivity of virtual bronchoscopy was 100% for obstructive lesions, 83% for endoluminal lesions, and 82% for all abnormalities; the specificity of virtual bronchoscopy was 100%; however, one interesting finding was the inability of multi-detector computed tomography (MDCT) (VB) to detect mucosal lesions which is considered a drawback to use this modality for the detection of minor mucosal lesions, and hence this modality may not be appropriate for identifying pre-malignant lesions in the respiratory tract [8].

For intra-tracheal thyroid mass case, please refer to Thyroid mass case in Chap. 12 (Fig. 9.7).

9.4.1.4 Evaluation of Inhalational Injury

There has been a significant morbidity and mortality in inhalation injury patients. Supportive treatment of inhalation injury remained the main management. Research has led to advances in recognizing the molecular pathophysiology of inhalation thermal injury. These new achievements in research on targeted therapies would improve the outcome [9].

Comparison of virtual bronchoscopy to fibre-optic bronchoscopy for the assessment of inhalation injury severity is important. The final product images of multi-detector computed tomography (VB) are based on processing software and the sensitivity of the CT machine. Inhalational injury most of the time produces mucosal changes that cannot be easily detected by ordinary CT imaging, especially in the acute phase of injury when there is no airway narrowing or obstruction secondary to fibrosis caused by the initial injury.

Evaluation of how reliable is multi-detector computed tomography (VB) to detect such injury is challenging not just on the technical aspect but also on the clinical aspect since MDCT (VB) is a new emerging modality in this field; the question will be are we as physician satisfied with grading system for inhalational injury totally dependent on MDCT (VB) images or will fibre-optic examination remain as the sole technique for such evaluation [4].

Herbert et al. tried to answer this question in his article "Comparison of virtual bronchoscopy to fibre-optic bronchoscopy for assessment of inhalation injury severity" which was published in 2014 in the *Burns* Journal; this trial showed " smoke inhalation injury score" as the grading system for respiratory injury and used both fibre-optic bronchoscopy and VB to detect the severity; the results of this trial were interesting in which VB provided a similar injury severity [4].

9.4.1.5 Specificity of Virtual Bronchoscopy (VB) Animated 3-D CT

Although FOB still has higher sensitivity and specificity than MDCT in the detection of inhalational injury as assumed from the trial result, per-forming a VB during admission CT may be a useful screening tool, especially to demonstrate airway narrowing induced by smoke injury [4].

9.4.1.6 TOF (Figs. 9.8, 9.9, 9.10, and 9.11)

9.4.1.7 Bronchogenic Carcinoma

CT is the principal imaging method intended for the diagnosis, staging, and proper diagnosis of

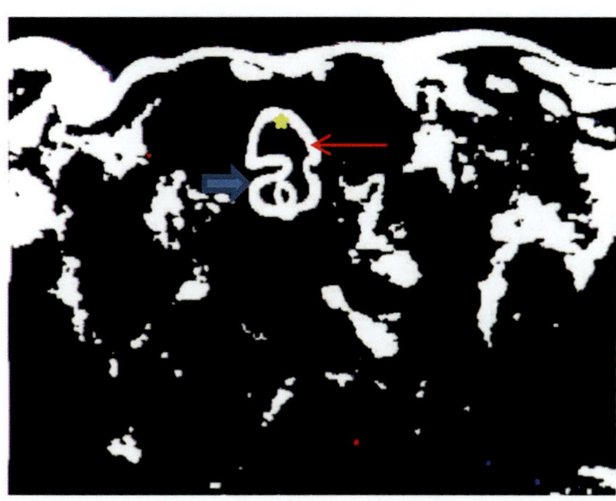
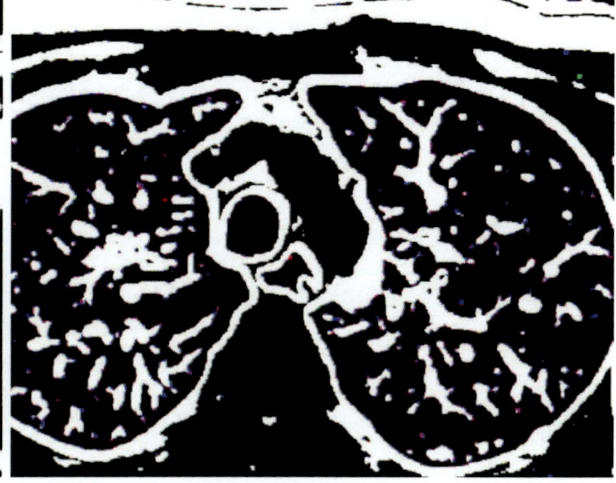

Fig. 9.8 Axial reformatted images showing the TOF-forming figure of "8" and the NGT is nicely demonstrated Astrics: Trachea, red arrow, is the fistulous track and light blue arrow wave to the oesophagus with the NGT seen inside. The right-sided image distal to the level of the TOF still showing the unduly dilated oesophagus

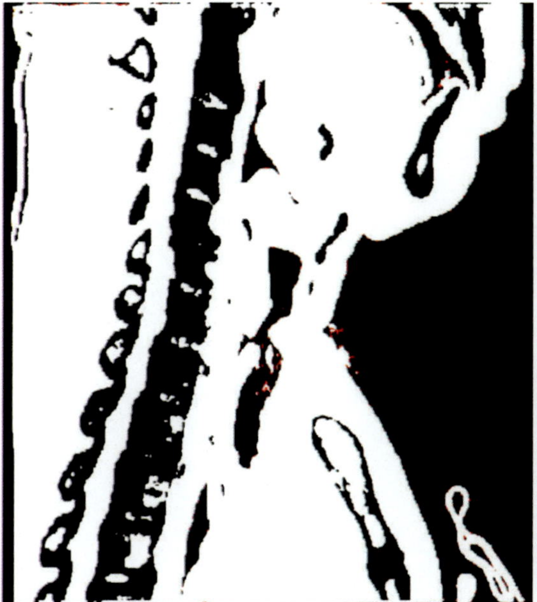
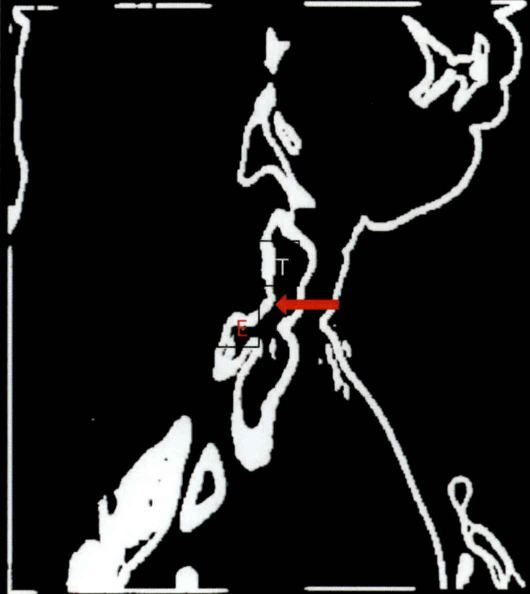

Fig. 9.9 Sagittal reformatted VRT images showing the TOF (arrow) T: Trachea, E: Esophagus, and red arrow: fistula

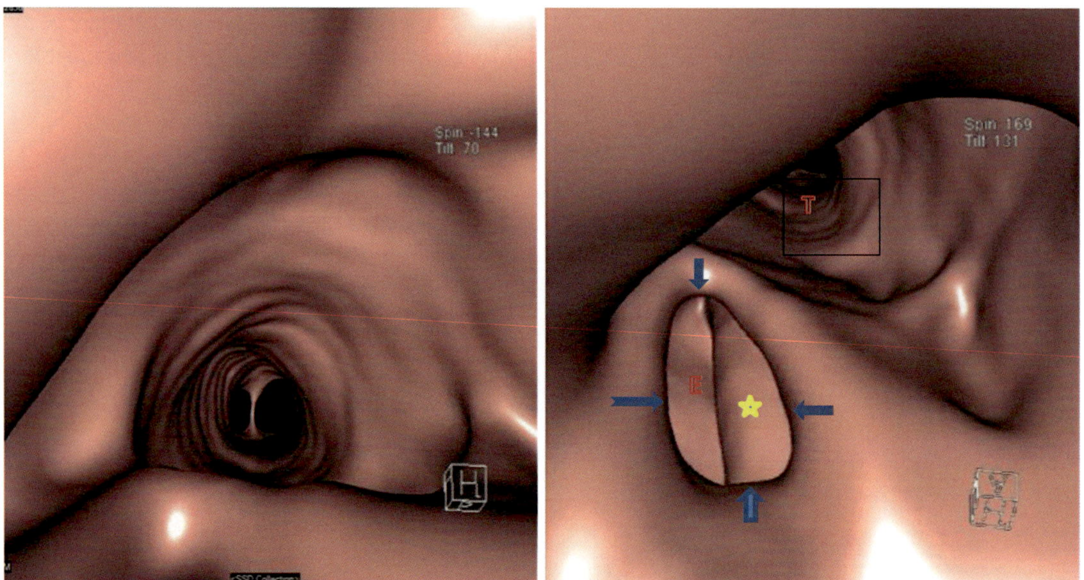

Fig. 9.10 VB showing the trachea bifurcation (left), and on the right the TOF is nicely demonstrated. T: Trachea, E: Esophagus, *: NGT and blue arrows show the TOF rent boundaries

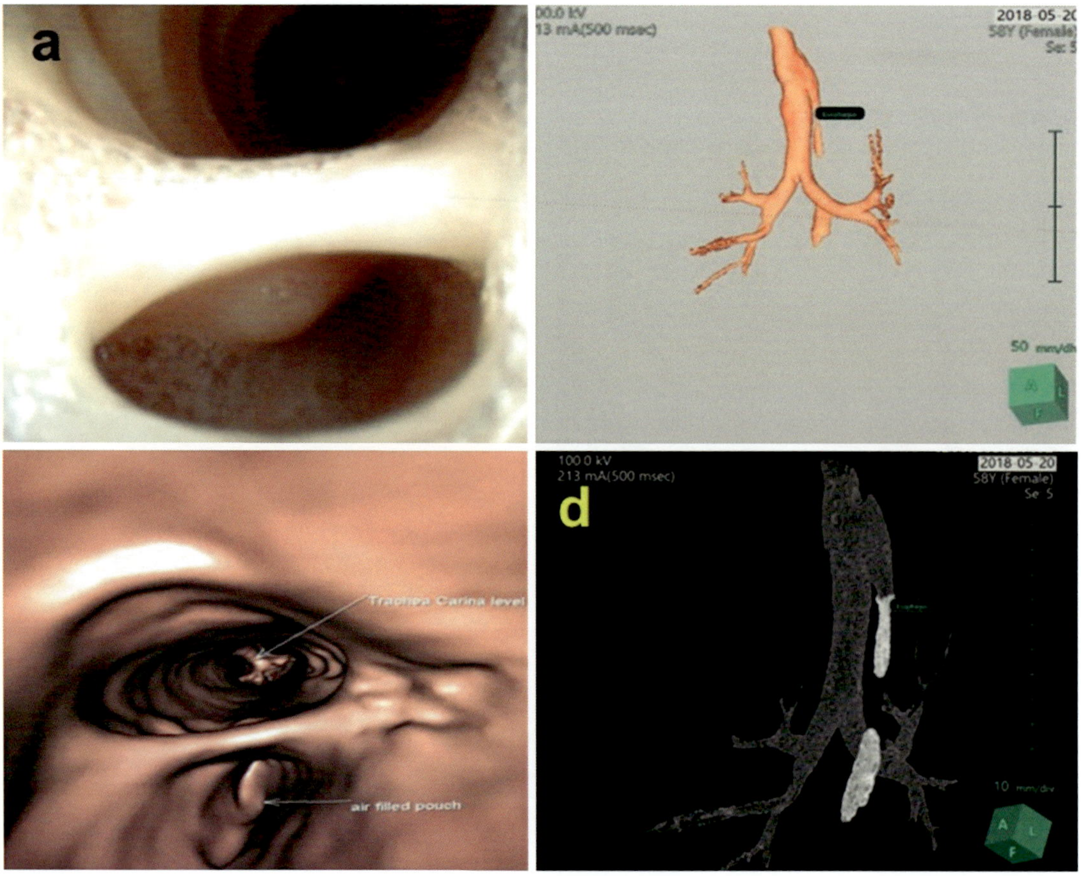

Fig. 9.11 TOF, a: conventional endoscopy showing the TOF and confirmed by the TTP and VRT images, as well as the virtual endoscopy evaluation

primary malignant tumours of the lung. Radiologists basically depend exclusively on axial images of those patients' group. Even so, researchers have already started to survey the possible value of VB for this medical utilization. Finkelstein et al. [8] studied and reviewed a series of 32 cases with pulmonary malignancy tumours and undiagnosed tracheobronchial pathology. The VB and the results of standard bronchoscopy were matched for 20 of the 32 patients. VB illustrated all 13 of occlusive pathology and five of the six endobronchial lesions but none of three mucosal lesions. Within that research study, the sensitivity of VB for all of the changes was 82%, and the specificity was 100% [10].

In a following study, Finkelstein et al. [11] discovered that CT with VB had a sensitivity of 100% for occlusive lesions, 16% for mucosal lesions, and 90% for endoluminal lesions. The overall sensitivity was 83% in patients with malignant tumours, and the specificity was 100%. In a related study, Liewald and colleagues [12] utilized VB and fibre-optic bronchoscopy to review 30 patients with pulmonary malignant tumours. All the 13 obstructive lesions were actually adequately viewed on VB, but no mucosal lesions were recognized on VB. An advantage of VB more than fibre-optic bronchoscopy is the capability to overcome the site of blockage and to see the smaller sized air passages, which in turn are not possible with fibre-optic bronchoscopy. For example, the study by Finkelstein et al. reported that in five patients, VB depicted peripheral obstructive lesions that were not possible to visualize further than the dimension restriction of the endoscope [8].

9.4.1.8 Tracheal Trauma

Moriwaki et al. had reported that 3-D CT along with VB was helpful for the diagnosis of tracheal trauma in people in hemodynamically stable condition. A small-variety CT showed a deficiency or depression in the wall structure at the location of the injury detected at bronchoscopy. CT depiction of the site and dimension of the trauma was similar to that of fibre-optic bronchoscopy [4].

VB can be actually utilized to guide transbronchial needle aspiration of mediastinal and hilar nodes and masses. The result for transbronchial biopsy is only 50% for nodes and tumours not visible to the bronchoscopist [13].

McAdams et al. reported significant success while utilizing VB as a quick guide for transbronchial needle aspiration in the course of fibre-optic bronchoscopy. All these authors discovered that the sensitivity for malignancy on a per node basis was 88%, significantly greater than the sensitivity reported for non-CT-guided transbronchial needle aspiration. They attributed their achievement to their capability to much better correspond node place and position of needle approach utilizing VB instead of traditional axial pictures. These authors similarly strongly believed that VB imaging gave them higher assurance in the examination of small nodes and nodes at inaccessible sites. In that study, the use of VB was time-saving. VB likewise may be actually used to guide biopsy of peripheral lesions. For example, Shinagawa et al. found that VB can be used to guide transbronchial biopsy along with an ultrathin bronchoscope. Minimal peripheral lesions (<20 mm) were effectively biopsied along with this method [14].

9.4.1.9 Single Lung

It is uncommon to diagnose patients with single lung. Case reports had documented that some cases presented as congenital lung aplasia, while others may have had previous surgery for pneumonectomy due to either malignancies or bronchiectasis (A).

Congenital anomalies in the lung may be found below the lung at a level down to carina; these include bronchogenic cyst, congenital lobar emphysema, alveolocapillary dysplasia and cystic adenomatoid malformation (B).

They may require surgical interventions to manage airway symptoms.

Mortality or morbidity of patients diagnosed as single-lung is significant. They may have a diminished pulmonary reserve. Assessment by bronchoscopy is commonly invaluable for the diagnosis of these patients. (A) But 3-D reconstruction and VE change the diagnosis and surgical management so we have the following case:

One patient came accidently for pre-employment routine check-up, and we found very interesting study results.

This male adult patient presented to the communicable disease centre referred from the medical commission with abnormal chest X-ray for the assessment of his medical fitness. History of previous surgical intervention to remove foreign body with left-sided intercostal scar on the skin. The plain radiographs suggested status post left lower lobectomy.

MDCT scan revealed absent left lung, obliterated left main bronchus with nippling, absent left pulmonary artery and significant hyperinflation of the right lung crossing to the left through the anterior mediastinum.

The compensatory overinflated right lung creeps to the left side via anterior mediastinum route filling the space of the left lung potential space, displacing the mediastinal structures to the left posteromedially. The left pulmonary artery is not visible as well as abrupt termination of the left main bronchus few centimetres following its origin with nippling noted. No metallic clips or dense sutures seen. No evidence of sternotomy or rib resections apart from subtle approximation of the left fifth and sixth ribs (Figs. 9.12, 9.13, 9.14, 9.15, and 9.16) (Movies 9.2, 9.3, 9.4, and 9.5).

9.4.2 Intraoperative

9.4.2.1 Foreign Body Aspiration (FBA)

Foreign body aspiration is one of the leading causes of mortality and morbidity in children, especially in those younger than 2 years of age. In the USA alone, FBA was responsible for 17,000 emergency department visits in children younger than 14 years in 2000 and in 2013 was responsible for about 4800 deaths, or about 1 death per 100,000 children aged 0–4 years with an estimated annual associated inpatient cost of nearly $13 million [15]. Before the era of bronchoscopy, aspiration of a foreign body had a 24% mortality rate. With the development of modern bronchoscopy techniques, mortality has fallen dramatically, and early intervention and diagnosis of fibre-optic bronchoscopy cases have a vital role in the prognosis and outcome.

Initial radiological evaluation reveals normal chest X-ray in nearly 30% of such patients, which means poor sensitivity and specificity of such techniques for the early diagnosis of foreign body aspiration. Tomography-generated virtual bronchoscopy (VB) can facilitate the early diagnosis and rapid management of these cases.

Traditionally, bronchoscopy is used for definitive diagnosis and management, but problems and complications associated with its use in the

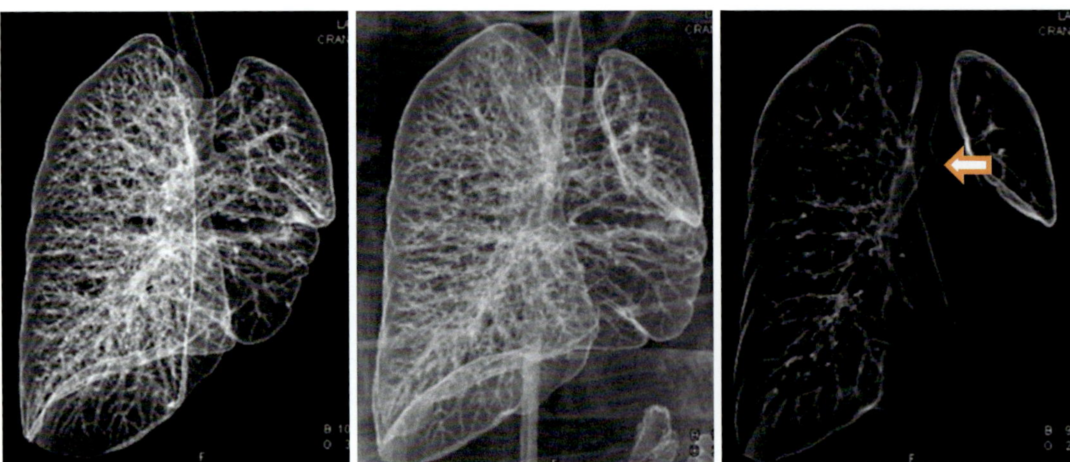

Fig. 9.12 TTP of the lungs, compensatory hyperinflation of the right lung, termination and nippling of the left main bronchus (arrow)

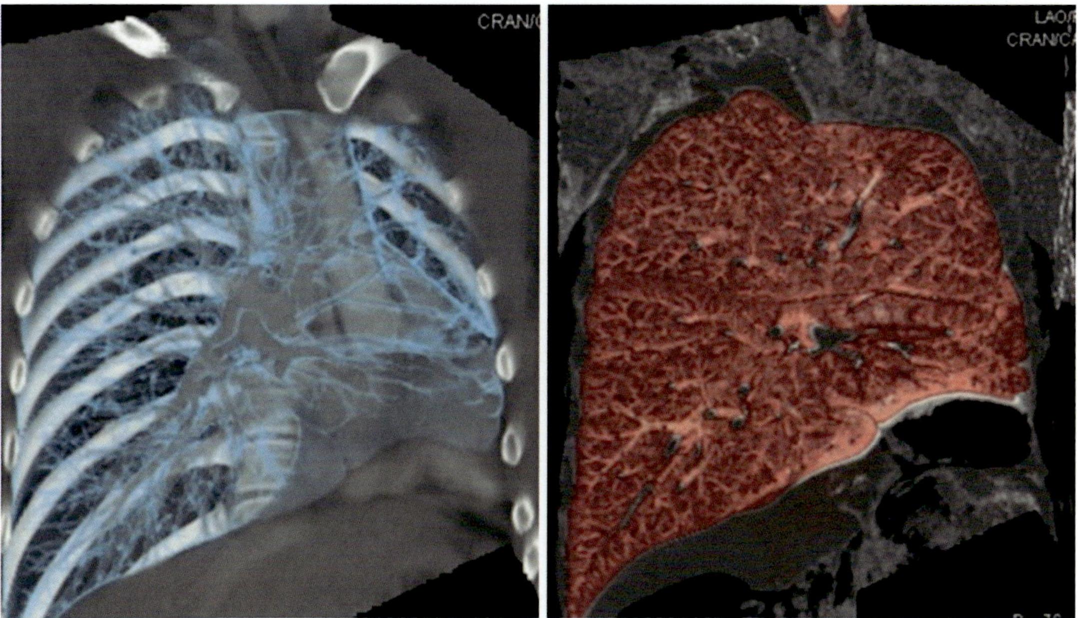

Fig. 9.13 VRT and SSD of the lungs, compensatory hyperinflation of the right lung, termination, and nippling of the left main bronchus

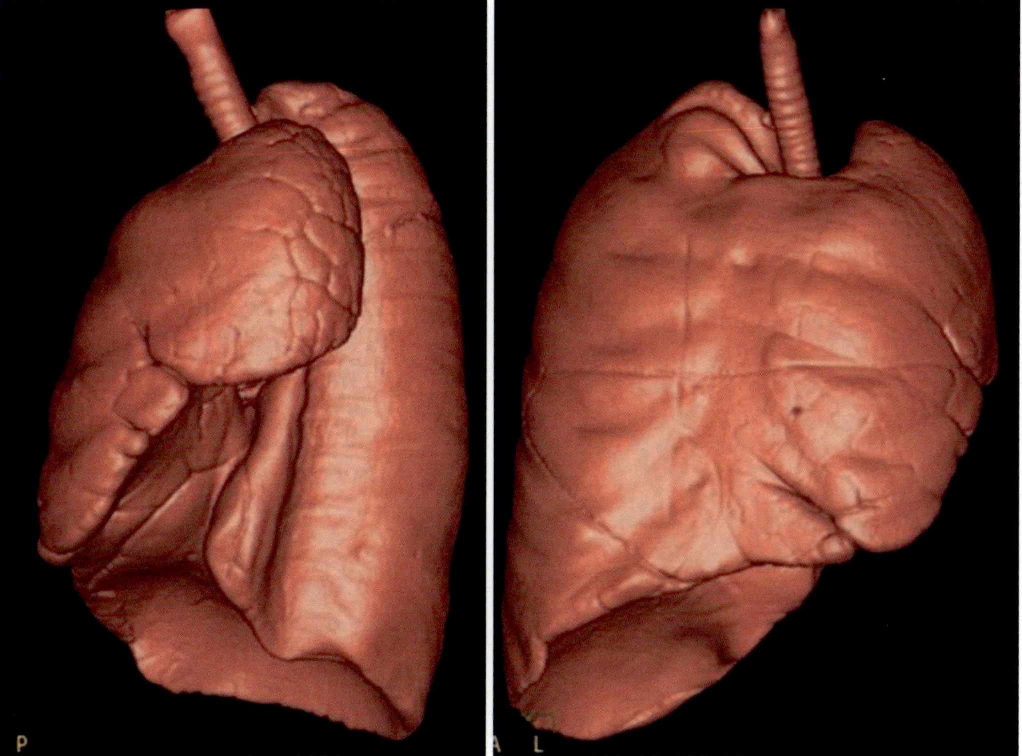

Fig. 9.14 VRT/SSD of the lungs, compensatory hyperinflation of the right lung, and it is seen creeping to the left side superiorly

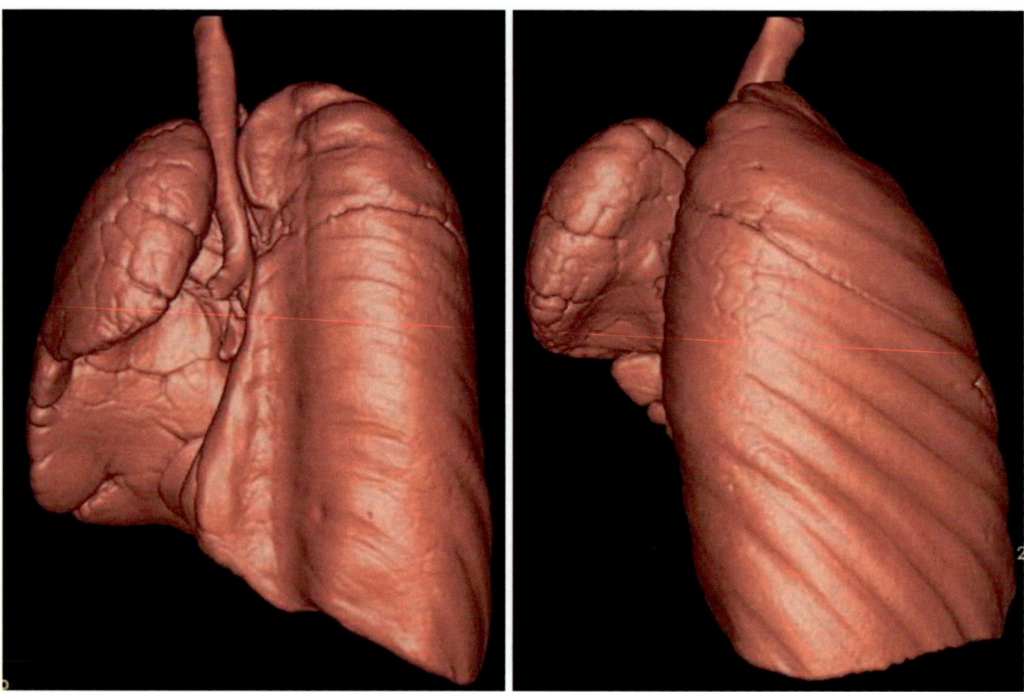

Fig. 9.15 VRT/SSD of the lungs, compensatory hyperinflation of the right lung, termination, and nippling of the left main bronchus

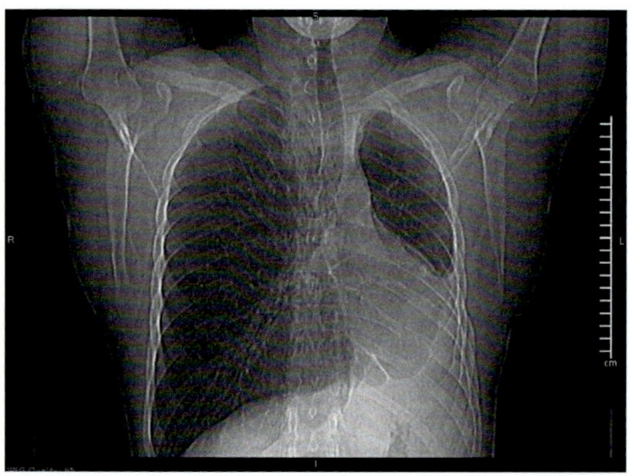

Fig. 9.16 Topogram of the CT chest showing the reduced volume of the left hemithorax with overinflated right lung, and superiorly it shows transmediastinal creeping to the left side with obliteration of the left costophrenic sinus and shift of the mediastinum to the left

pediatrics group including monitoring sedation and trauma raised a concern and emerged the need to use less invasive techniques like virtual bronchoscopy (VB) [16].

Comparison between the efficacy of traditional bronchoscopy and virtual bronchoscopy (VB) has proved that virtual bronchoscopy (VB) is as effective as bronchoscopy in the detection of FB, and it is a reliable method for definitive diagnosis of FB.

Images obtained by virtual bronchoscopy (VB) show not only the location of the FB but also other pathologies associated with aspiration like hyperaeration, atelectasis, infiltration, and bronchiectasis that cannot be detected by traditional bronchoscopy [17].

9.4.2.2 Stent Positioning and Endobronchial Stent Planning

MDCT CT evaluation of airway stents is important, and the use of airway stents is getting more popular to treat symptoms of patients with obstructive tracheobronchial diseases with non-resectable lesion or who have poor functional performance status preventing any surgical intervention to be done for them; primary lung cancer and metastatic disease comprise the majority of these conditions.

MDCT CT has gained a very important role in pre- and post-procedure assessment of airway stenting, and images captured by this technology provides accurate evaluation of the exact anatomy of the airways in the target area of the lung or outside the lung. Moreover, these images can show the relation between the airways and adjacent structures like main blood vessels which cannot be visualized by traditional bronchoscopy [18].

The scope of this chapter is beyond the discussion about the type of stents, but it is worth mentioning that MDCT provides information about the optimal position and number of potential stents, which requires considering the location and length of the obstruction.

9.4.2.3 Imaging Guidance

VB has been used for the direct aspiration of mediastinal as well as hilar lymph nodes and masses using transbronchial needles. For transbronchial biopsy, the success rate is only 50% for lymph nodes and tumours that are not visible to the bronchoscopist [13].

McAdams et al. reported great success by using VB as a transbronchial needle aspiration guide during fibre-optic bronchoscopy. They had reported that sensitivity to malignancy per node was 88% significantly higher than the sensitivity reported for transbronchial needle aspiration without CT guidance.

They significantly correlated node location and angle of needle approach with VB accurately rather than using basic axial photos.

They had also reported that VB photos enabled them to biopsy small nodes, especially those at inaccessible sites, and they found that the procedure time was less by using VB [17].

Furthermore, it had been reported that the VB biopsy guidance can be used for the peripheral lesions. Shinagawa et al. concluded that VB had been used to guide ultrathin bronchoscope for transbronchial biopsy. With this technique, they could achieve doing biopsies in lesions (<20 mm) successfully [19].

9.4.3 Postoperative

Masahiro Yanagiya and his colleagues reported the effectiveness of virtual bronchoscopic navigation to close the endobronchial fistula in post-operative bronchopleural fistula, by capturing images of virtual bronchoscopic navigation before, and they confirmed the position of the catheter by CT fluoroscopy [20].

In postoperative lung transplantation, there may be bronchial anastomosis stenosis, and VB has been used to diagnose any airflow obstruction. The importance of this decreased airflow is that it is clinically similar to some conditions like bronchiolitis obliterans, and the proper diagnosis leads to successful treatment.

By using the correlation between VB and pulmonary functions tests, VB is an important diagnostic screening tool in post-transplant patients when there is doubt of the presence of bronchial stenosis [21].

9.4.3.1 Lung Transplant

Organ transplantation is a lifesaving intervention that is needed when there is no other choice; the field of transplantation is growing dramatically in the last century because of the advancement of surgical technique and of course immunosuppressant use. The first lung transplant procedure was done in 1963, although the patient died after 18 days, but this attempt opened a new hope in this field.

Earlier, most of the early patient mortality cases were attributed to airway and vascular complications like bronchial anastomotic dehiscence and pulmonary artery anastomotic stenosis, which requires a sensitive imaging modality for early detection [22].

Multidetector CT provides an excellent assessment tool not just postoperatively but also for the preoperative preparation of the patient in terms of evaluating donor and recipient size and volume measurements and in alerting the surgeon about an incidental malignancy or infection that could possibly complicate the outcome [17]. The follow-up process of lung transplant (single lung transplantation, bilateral lung transplantation, or lobar transplants) is extensive and includes many steps and tests; maybe the most important of them is the daily chest radiography and the monthly surveillance biopsies that determines the rejection. Abnormal findings that cannot be fully explained needs CT imaging evaluation, and MDCT VB provides invaluable information in the diagnosis, evaluation, and post-treatment assessment of those abnormalities either central airway or vascular complications in lung transplant recipients [23].

9.5 Summary and Future Directions

Virtual bronchoscopy generates high-definition tracheobronchial tree pictures and endobronchial views which mimic traditional bronchoscopy conclusions.

However, the increasing involvement of virtual bronchoscopy rises as computer virtualization advancements and innovations in MDCT permit isotropic data to be obtained [24].

Although both three-dimensional CT with VB had been used for over 10 years, radiological and respiratory clinical specialties are indeed increasingly excited about the technique due to advances in CT scanner operating systems. VB can clearly be a useful addition to conventional axial CT in the assessment of patients with suspected pulmonary disorders [1].

Medical imaging has created and developed augmented reality (AR) that facilitates clinicians to understand what is produced by the machines and helps in minimally invasive surgery. A variety of conditions could benefit the most from AR. Different innovation tools will be tailored for different problems [24].

The technique reported by Salama and Kolb, opacity peeling for direct volume rendering, had described the implementation of real-time volume visualization technique in the medical field. It has shown to be particularly useful in emergency situations, that is, in the operating room [25].

Augmented reality-guided techniques should be developed for clinical integration. Developers who are interested in the field of medical AR techniques would achieve a good progress that covers the physician's needs and the patients would get the benefits in the future [26].

Segmented pulmonary airway branches cast architecture and medical imaging in situ is an effective way using three-dimensional micro-CT imaging to view the airway tree beyond what would be similarly seen in CT images. Imaged casts are then easily and quickly divided for utilization in computational fluid dynamics (CFD) simulations or morphometric parameters. Researchers have shown that small changes in the airway branching angles implemented by the casting process can be adjusted using the cast-to-total lung capacity image directory [27].

Data sets from MDCT that are used for VB can also be used to obtain volumetric data that can be utilized to produce in vivo airway casts and anatomic 3-D models that can be used for 3-D printing. 3-D printed airway models and airway casts are invaluable in understanding and teaching the complex airway anatomy, and pathophysiology, pharmacological effects on the airway, mechanics of various airway diseases, and also aid in preoperative planning. Current ongoing research has proved that 3-D printing is a promising technique that will help provide personalized patient care with great outcome at a relatively low cost [28, 29].

References

1. Honnef D, Wildberger JE, Das M, et al. Value of virtual trachea-bronchoscopy and bronchography from 16-slice multidetector-row helical CT for assessment of suspected tracheobronchial stenosis in children. Eur Radiol. 2006;16:1684–91.
2. Fetita CI, Preteux F, Beigelman-Aubry C, Grenier P. Pulmonary airways: 3-D reconstruction from MDCT and clinical investigation. IEEE Trans Med Imaging. 2004;23:1353–64.
3. Adamczyk M, Tomaszewski G, Naumczyk P, Kluczewska E, Walecki J. Usefulness of computed tomography virtual bronchoscopy in the evaluation of bronchi divisions. Pol J Radiol. 2013;78(1):30–41.
4. Kwon HP, Zanders TB, Regn DD, Burkett SE, Batchinsky AI. Comparison of virtual bronchoscopy to fiber-optic bronchoscopy for assessment of inhalation injury severity. Burns. 2014;40(7):1308–15.
5. Englmeier KH, Seemann MD. Multimodal virtual bronchoscopy using PET/CT images. Comput Aided Surg Mar. 2008;13(2):106–13.
6. Hoppe H, Dinkel HP, Walder B, von Allmen G, Gugger M, Vock P. Grading airway stenosis down to the segmental level using virtual bronchoscopy. Chest. 2004;125:704–11.
7. Koşucu P, Ahmetoğlu A, Koramaz I, Orhan F, Özdemir O, Dinç H, Ökten A, Gümele HR. Low-dose MDCT and virtual bronchoscopy in pediatric patients

with foreign body aspiration. Am J Roentgenol. 2004;183:1771–7.

8. Finkelstein SE, Summers RM, Nguyen DM, Stewart JH, Tretler JA, Schrump DS. Virtual bronchoscopy for evaluation of malignant tumors of the thorax. J Thorac Cardiovasc Surg. 2002;123:967–72.

9. Walker PF, Buehner MF, Wood LA, Boyer NL, Driscoll IR, Lundy JB, Cancio LC, Chung KK. Diagnosis and management of inhalation injury: an updated review. Crit Care. 2015;19:351.

10. Gore MA, Joshi AR, Nagarajan G, Iyer SP, Kulkarni T, Khandelwal A. Virtual bronchoscopy for diagnosis of inhalation injury in burnt patients. Burns. 2004;30(2):165–8.

11. Finkelstein SE, Schrump DS, Nguven DM, Hewitt SM, Kunsl TF, Summers RM. Comparative evaluation of super high-resolution CT scan and virtual bronchoscopy for the detection of tracheobronchial malignancies. Chest. 2003;124:1834–40.

12. Liewald F, Lang G, Fleiter T, Sokiranski R, Halter G, Orend KH. Comparison of virtual and fiberoptic bronchoscopy. Thorac Cardiovasc Surg. 1998;46:361–4.

13. Moriwaki Y, Sugiyama M, Matsuda G, et al. Usefulness of the 3-D-tracheography. World J Surg. 2005;29:102–5.

14. McAdams HP, Goodman PC, Kussin P. Virtual bronchoscopy for directing transbronchial needle aspiration of hilar and mediastinal lymph nodes: a pilot study. AJR. 1998;170:1361–4.

15. Marescaux J, Diana M. Next step in minimally invasive surgery: hybrid image-guided surgery. J Paediatr Surg. 2015;50(1):30–6.

16. Sultan TA, van As AB. Review of tracheobronchial foreign body aspiration in the south African paediatric age group. J Thorac Dis. 2016;8(12):3787–96.

17. Godoy MC, Saldana DA, Rao PP, Vlahos I, Naidich DP, Benveniste MF, Erasmus JJ, Marom EM, Ost D. Multidetector CT evaluation of airway stents: what the radiologist should know. Radiographics. 2014;34(7):1793–806. https://doi.org/10.1148/rg.347130063.

18. Gill RR, Poh AC, Camp PC, Allen JM. MDCT evaluation of central airway and vascular complications of lung transplantation. Am J Roentgenol. 2008;191(4):1046–56.

19. Shinagawa N, Yamazaki K, Onodera Y, et al. CT-guided transbronchial biopsy using an ultrathin bronchoscope with virtual bronchoscopic navigation. Chest. 2004;125:1138–43.

20. Yanagiya M, Matsumoto J, Nagano M, Kusakabe M, Matsumoto Y, Furukawa R, Ohara S, Usui K. Endoscopic bronchial occlusion for postoperative persistent bronchopleural fistula with computed tomography fluoroscopy guidance and virtual bronchoscopic navigation.A case report. Medicine (Baltimore). 2018;97(7):e9921.

21. Shitrit D, Valdsislav P, Grubstein A, Bendayan D, Cohen M, Kramer MR. Accuracy of virtual bronchoscopy for grading tracheobronchial stenosis∗ correlation with pulmonary function test and Fiberoptic bronchoscopy. Chest. 2005;128(5):3545.

22. Cho EN, Haam SJ, Kim SY, Chang YS, Paik HC. Anastomotic airway complications after lung transplantation. Yonsei Med J. 2015;56(5):1372–8.

23. Luecke K, Trujillo C, Ford J, Decker S, Pelaez A, Hazelton TR, Rojas CA. Anastomotic airway complications after lung transplant clinical, bronchoscopic and CT correlation. J Thorac Imaging. 2016;31:W62–71.

24. Horton KM, Horton MR, Fishman EK. Advanced visualization of airways with 64-MDCT: 3-D mapping and virtual bronchoscopy. Am J Roentgenol. 2007;189(6):1387–96.

25. Rezk-Salama C, Kolb A. Opacity peeling for direct volume rendering. Comp Graph Forum. 2006;25(3):597–606.

26. Wacker FK, Vogt S, Khamene A, Jesberger JA, Nour SG, Elgort DR, Sauer F, Duerk JL, Lewin JS. An augmented reality system for MRI image guided needle biopsy: initial results in a swine model. Radiology. 2006;238(2):497–504.

27. Jacob RE, Colby SM, Kabilan S, Einstein DR, Carson JP. In situ casting and imaging of the rat airway tree for accurate 3D reconstruction. Exp Lung Res. 2013;39:249–57. https://doi.org/10.3109/01902148.2013.801535.

28. Cheng GZ, Folch E, Wilson A, et al. 3D printing and personalized airway stents. Pulm Ther. 2017;3:59–66. https://doi.org/10.1007/s41030-016-0026-y.

29. Van de Moortele T, Wendt CH, Coletti F. Morphological and functional properties of the conducting human airways investigated by in vivo computed tomography and in vitro MRI. J Appl Physiol. 2017;124:400–13. https://doi.org/10.1152/japplphysiol.00490.2017.

10

Role of Virtual Endoscopy and 3-D Reconstruction in Airway Assessment of Critically Ill Patients

Adel E. Ahmed Ganaw, Moad Ehfeda, Nissar Shaikh,
Marcus Lance, Arshad Hussain Chanda,
Ali O. Mohamed Belkair,
Muhammad Zubair Labathkhan,
and Gamal Abdullah

10.1 Introduction

Virtual endoscopy (VE) is a technique which generates computer simulations of anatomy from radiological image data and shows these simulations in a manner similar to conventional endoscopy. Advancement in computer technology has created numerous advancements in noninvasive diagnostic imaging. For instance, introduction of helical computed tomography (CT) has allowed the acquisition of bulks of CT records from which three-dimensional (3-D) images can precisely be generated.

VE uses such 3-D images in real time to mimic the visions achieved with conventional endoscopy. The most important advantages of VE over actual endoscopy in intensive care units are that it is noninvasive, and it can be used safely for unstable and critically ill patient. Furthermore, VE can generate exceptional views like retrograde view of intraluminal tract of tracheobronchial tree as well as extra-

Electronic Supplementary Material The online version of this chapter (https://doi.org/10.1007/978-3-030-23253-5_10) contains supplementary material, which is available to authorized users.

A. E. A. Ganaw (✉) · M. Ehfeda · N. Shaikh · M. Lance
A. H. Chanda · A. O. M. Belkair · M. Z. Labathkhan
G. Abdullah
Department of Anesthesiology, ICU and Perioperative Medicine, Hamad Medical Corporation, Doha, Qatar
e-mail: AGanaw@hamad.qa

luminal anatomy. Moreover, the airway could be examined from all angles, extracted from its surroundings, and the precise association of surrounding anatomy can be reviewed. This chapter reviews the present role of VE and 3-D reconstruction in airway assessment of critically ill patients [1–3].

10.2 Imaging Technique

In contrast to virtual colonoscopy, no pre-procedural patient preparation is required to assess airway and tracheobronchial tree. For routine airway assessment, administration of contrast is not needed. However, the intravenous contrast is essential for assessment of airway invasion by tumors or queried patients with a vascular ring or sling; non-ionic iodinated contrast is typically administered (1 mL/kg for adults) through peripheral intravenous cannula at a rate of 3 mL/s. Thin-slice axial images can be attained in a single breath hold. Scanning takes only a few seconds; hence, children and newborns can be scanned without sedation. Moreover, this relieves intubated patients from interrupting ventilation and changes in airway pressures which might be important for oxygenation.

The cross-sectional images transferred to single graphic computer and reconstruction are completed with using standard visualization software. The acquired near-isotropic data is used to

© Springer Nature Switzerland AG 2019
N. A. Shallik et al. (eds.), *Virtual Endoscopy and 3D Reconstruction in the Airways*,
https://doi.org/10.1007/978-3-030-23253-5_10

create minimum intensity projections (MinIPs), multiplanar reformations (MPRs), and volume-rendered images for 3-D reconstruction [3, 4] (for more details please refer to Chap. 3).

10.3 Tracheobronchial Stenosis

Tracheal stenosis in critically ill patients most commonly results in traumatic intubation, prolonged intubation, and tracheostomy. Furthermore, malignant and benign tumors, inflammatory disease, and systemic autoimmune diseases can cause tracheal stenosis in adult patients. Currently, with increase in tendency to use low-pressure cuffs, the incidence of tracheal stenosis has decreased to less than 1%. Tracheal stenosis following tracheostomy or prolonged intubation frequently occurs at two locations: At the level of the cuff of the endotracheal tube and at the stoma site. High cuff pressure leads to damage of tracheal mucosa, followed by tissue necrosis, scarring, and eventually stenosis of the tracheal lumen. Rarely, compression from structures outside the airway could lead to obstruction (e.g., enlarged goiter, aortic aneurysms). The most frequent CT finding in post-intubation stenosis is a confined part of constriction of tracheal lumen. These circumferential constrictions generate typical hourglass structures (Fig. 10.1). Sometimes the CT shows a thin membrane projection in the trachea. Additionally, damage of tracheal mucosa may lead to creation of multiple synechiae which compromises the tracheal lumen (Figs. 10.2 and 10.3) [4, 5, 6].

Accurate mapping of the stenosis is very important to plan the right management, and it is very important to assess the degree and length of the stenosis, status of the peri-tracheal anatomy, and function of the vocal cords [5].

The usual diagnostic investigations for the assessment of tracheobronchial stenosis are computed tomography (CT) and flexible tracheobronchoscopy (FT). Even though these investigations are very accurate, they have technical limits which might affect the accuracy of the description of tracheobronchial pathology. Conventional

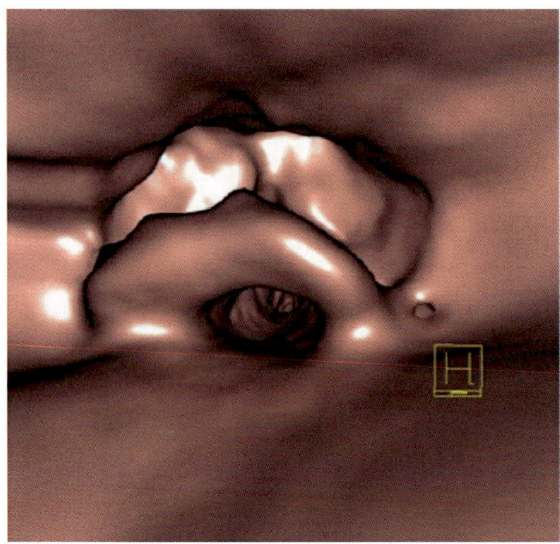

Fig. 10.1 VB of a CT finding in post-intubation stenosis is a confined part of constriction of tracheal lumen. These circumferential constrictions generate typical hourglass structures at the epiglottis level

endoscopy has been considered as the investigation of choice for the recognition and categorization of tracheobronchial pathology or tracheal stenosis. Endoscopy, though, may fail to provide necessary details when the stenosis is very severe or the lesion totally obstructing bronchi; consequently, the assessment of distal segments becomes impossible [5].

Diagnostic flexible bronchoscopy is minimally invasive and a safe intervention. Survey of flexible bronchoscope in the United Kingdom stated a fatality rate of 0.045% out of 60,100 bronchoscopies. Other references report different percentages: 0.01% out of 2452 procedures, and 0.02% out of 48,000 bronchoscopies, still showing a minimal risk of death when performing bronchoscopy to critically ill patients [7, 8].

Minor and major complications occur at a very low rate as well; however, the risks may significantly increase in critically ill patients. Furthermore, flexible tracheobronchoscopy in critically ill patients is constricted to perform or complete due to severe hypoxia, arrhythmia, bleeding, or coagulopathy. Table 10.1 summarizes the most common complications associated with bronchoscopy [7].

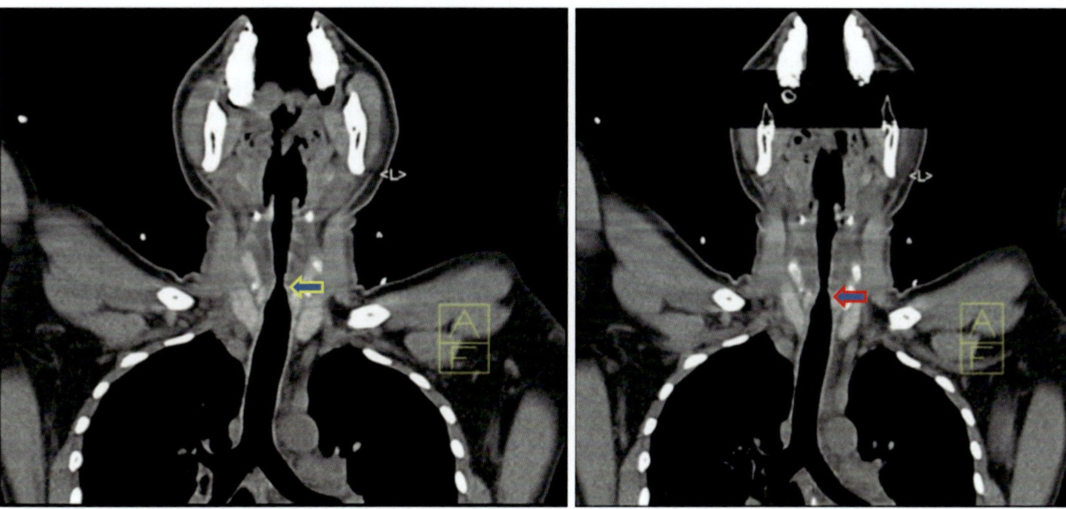

Fig. 10.2 Tracheal smooth short-segment narrowing is noted at the thyroid gland level (arrow) (status post tracheostomy) in coronal reformatted images

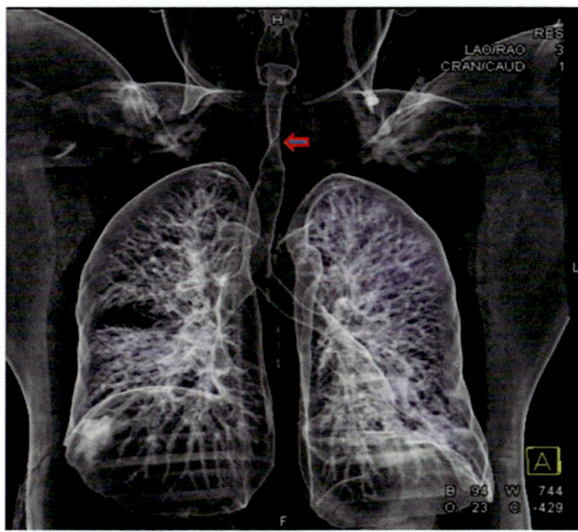

Fig. 10.3 Tracheal smooth short-segment narrowing is noted at the thyroid gland level (arrow) in TTP VRT image

10.3.1 Comparison between Virtual Bronchoscopy and Conventional Fiber-Optic Bronchoscopy [9]

Virtual bronchoscopy (VB) is a noninvasive technique for intraluminal assessment of the tracheobronchial tree. Many trials have revealed that VB can precisely assess tracheal lumen, right and left main stem bronchi, as well as lumen of bronchial tree down to the fourth order of bronchial orifices and branches. VB is operator independent. Reports have proved that the sensitivity of VB in the identification of central stenosis ranges between 63% and 100%, and the specificity ranges between 61% and 99% [3, 5].

A main advantage of VB in comparison with flexible tracheobronchoscopy (FT) is its noninvasiveness; therefore, it can be used safely in critically ill patients or in case of contraindication for conventional endoscopy. Due to the noninvasiveness, there is no additional risk of infection which may be important in immunocompromised patients. Another advantage is the protection of any surgical suture after fresh operation (e.g., tracheal surgery). Moreover, VB can describe passageway through very severe stenosis, which allows assessment of the post-stenotic tracheobronchial tree. Moreover, VB evidenced to be marginally more precise than CT for the recognition of critically significant narrowing at bronchial anastomoses in lung transplant patients [6]. Furthermore, VB may help treating physicians in visualizing external nonmucosal compressions on the bronchial wall that cause bronchial stenosis and stridor, especially in children (Movie 10.1). These compressions may be caused by normal anatomic structures (esophagus or aortic arch) (Movie 10.2) or due to pathologic structures (enlarged lymph nodes, fibrotic masses, and extra-luminal tumor) [3, 4, 5] (Movie 10.3).

Pleural effusion and vascular anomlies cause tracheal compression (Fig. 10.4).

Moreover, VB can be complementary to FT in the interventional setting such as stent implementations or tracheostomy. VB can accurately assess the extent and severity of stenosis; therefore, it is very useful treatment planning for stent placement and subsequent follow-up. In patients who have had stents inserted, CT and VB can be used in the assessment of stent patency and migration [4, 5] (Fig. 10.5).

Table 10.1 Most common complications associated with fiber-optic bronchoscopy [7, 9]

1. Systemic complications	1. Procedure related (vasovagal syncope, nausea/vomiting, aspiration, hypoxia, and hypercarbia).
	2. Medication related (sedation, nonsedative medications)
	3. Comorbid illness (myocardial dysfunction/arrhythmia, pulmonary insufficiency, elevated intracranial pressure, death)
2. Mechanical complications	1. Trauma (oropharyngeal, nasopharyngeal, glottic structure, vocal cord)
	2. Bronchospasm/laryngospasm
	3. Infection
	4. Atelectasis/de-recruitment
	5. Elevated airway pressure
	6. Hemorrhage

10.4 Tracheostomy Cannula Placement in Patients with Abnormal Anatomy

Tracheostomy is a common invasive procedure in critical care, aimed to maintain a patent airway in critically ill patients. Usually commercially available, manufactured tracheostomy cannulas are used to keep the tracheostomy patent. These tracheostomy cannulas have fixed distinctions in size, diameter, radius, and curvature. Nevertheless, in patients with abnormal anatomy of the neck or thorax such as morbidly obese patients, patients with extreme scoliosis, and patients with Duchenne muscular dystrophy, the selection of the appropriate tracheostomy site with the matching cannula type can be extremely difficult; the commercially available cannulas frequently do not fit, which may lead to suboptimal cannula placement and inflammation of the trachea, ultimately causing airway obstruction due to granulation tissue formation (Fig. 10.6).

Several case reports have presented patients who had a fistula of the trachea and innominate artery causing a fatal hemorrhage. For that reason, appropriate and careful cannula selection is vital to decrease these risks. In general, cannula placement is totally dependent on the assessment of the surgeons during the tracheostomy; in case of aberrant anatomy, this appraisement is very difficult.

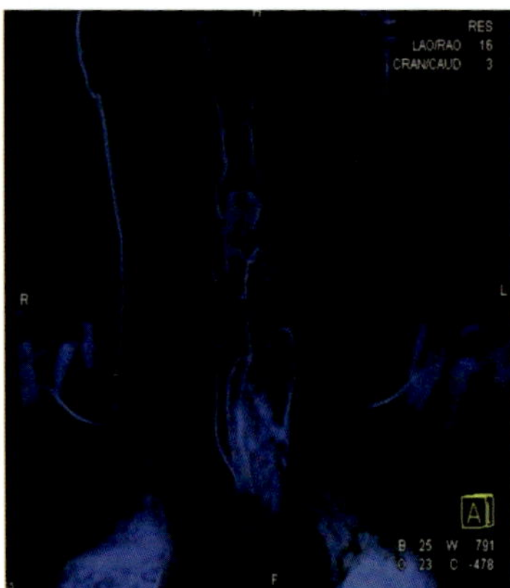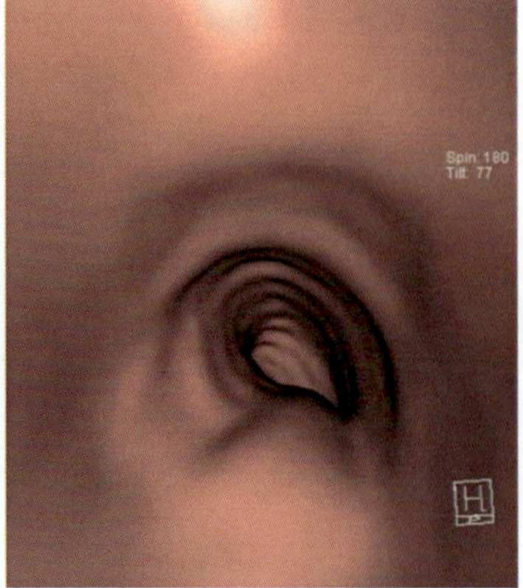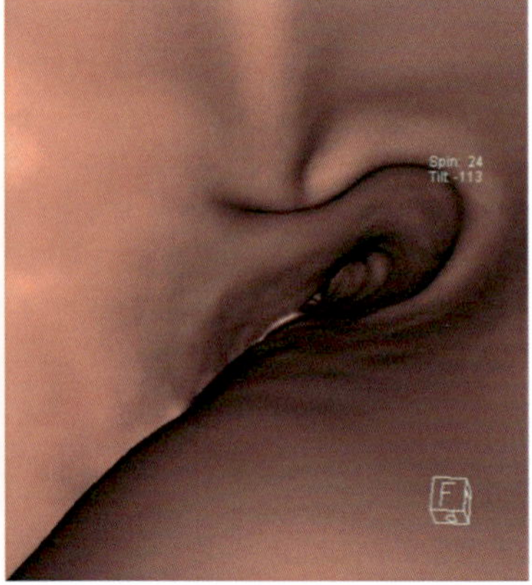

Fig. 10.4 VRT and VB images showing the different levels of the narrow segment caused by external indentations by combined vascular lesion and pleural effusion

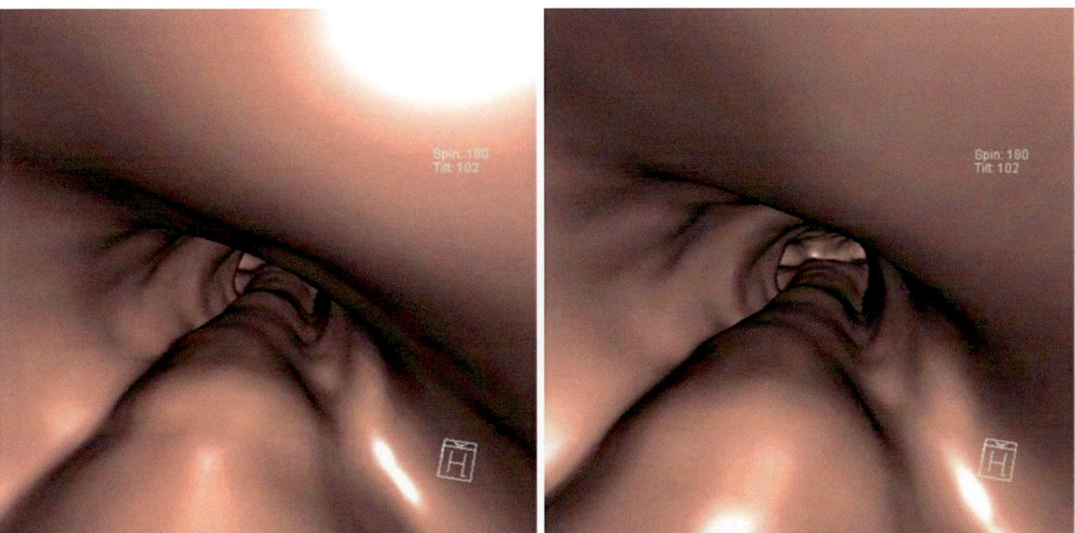

Fig. 10.5 VB navigation within the trachea with relative reduction of its caliber (anteroposteriorly); kindly note the posterior wall indentation upon the membranous part by the effect of the esophagus

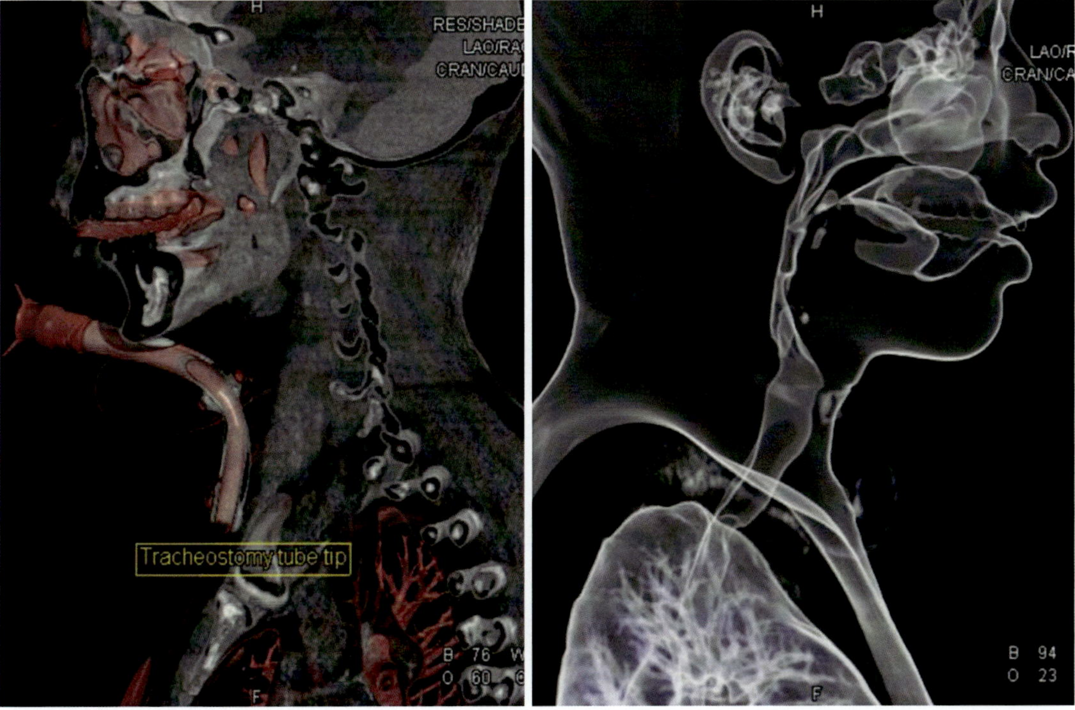

Fig. 10.6 Sagittal VRT and SSD images showing the slipped tracheostomy tube outside the trachea in a subcutaneous location. The right-hand-side images clearly visualize that there are no tubes within the tracheal lumen

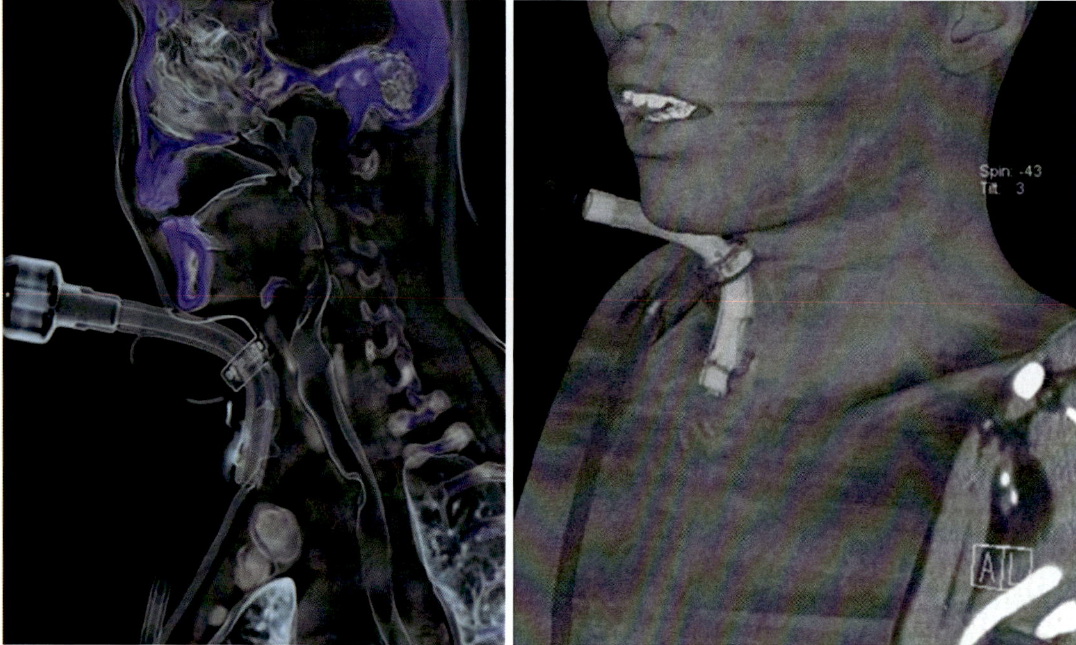

Fig. 10.7 Slipped extraluminal tracheostomy tube. The airway is nicely demonstrated with the tip of the tracheostomy tube seen in a subcutaneous ligation outside the skin tracheostomy orifice/vent

Therefore, outcome is subjective and extremely dependent on the experience of the surgeon [10].

In patients with aberrant neck anatomy, virtual 3-D can be theoretically useful in preoperative assessment of the upper airway and determination of the optimal stoma site which may help the surgeons in surgical planning and choose proper standard cannula or custom- made cannula. (Figs. 10.6 and 10.7) [11].

10.5 Tracheo-Esophageal Fistula (TOF)

Tracheo-esophageal fistula or broncho-esophageal fistula is an abnormal direct communication between tracheobronchial tree and the digestive system; this communication causes frequent and permanent pulmonary contamination by food and digestive secretions which may lead to disastrous and fatal complications. Please refer to Chap. 12 for challenge case discussion. TOF is either congenital or acquired.

The pathophysiology of congenital TOF is not clear; it may be the result of unidentified intrauterine insult during the stage of separation of embryonic foregut into esophagus and trachea. Acquired TOF most commonly occurs as a consequence of prolonged tracheal intubation; however, introduction of high-volume and low-pressure endotracheal tube cuffs decreases the incidence of this complication. The incidence of trachea-esophageal fistula is between 0.3% and 3% in prolonged ventilated patients. Acquired tracheo-esophageal fistula was also reported as result of tracheostomy and trauma [4, 12] (Movie 10.4).

Post-prolonged intubation of tracheo-esophageal fistula is usually associated with tracheal stenosis. Current usefulness of multidetector computed tomography (MDCT) and VB in the diagnosis and assessment of TOF is debatable. They offer inadequate details about the fistulous tract in comparison to endoscopy. Therefore, the usage of CT scan and VB is not consistently suggested. However, they may be

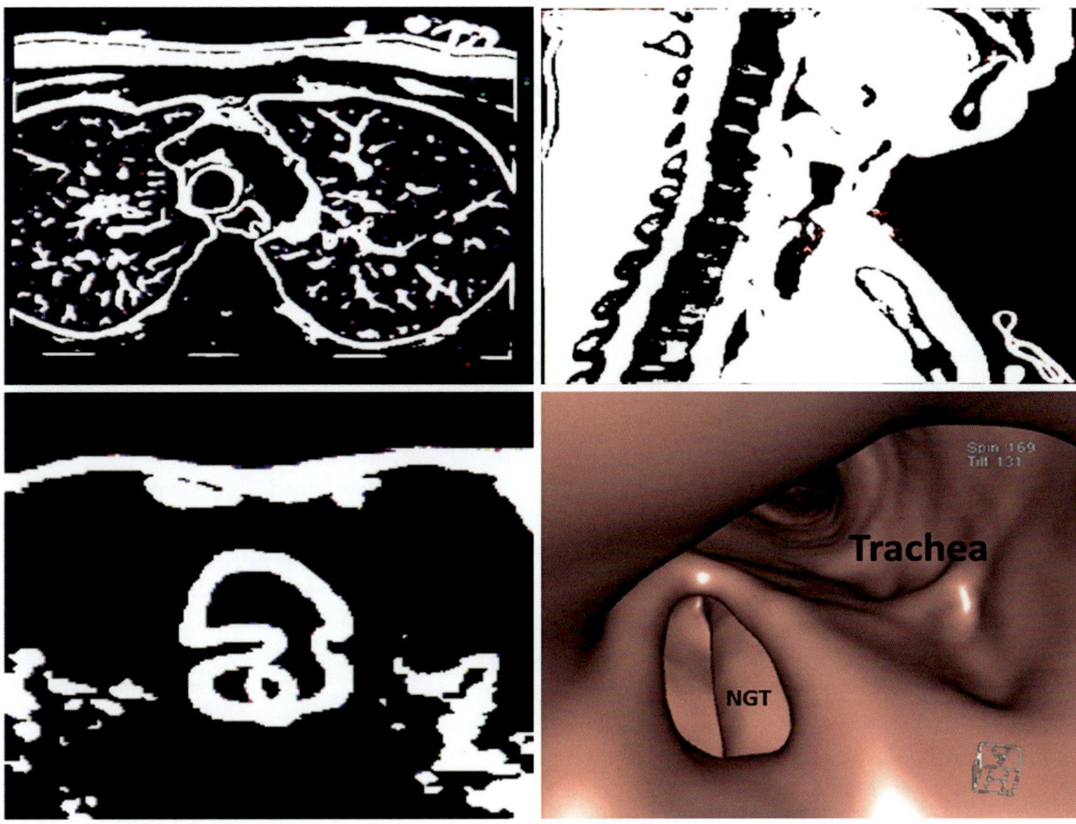

Fig. 10.8 TOF with the findings of the conventional and virtual endoscopies are identical and also the value of modified Valsalva maneuver is demonstrated

very useful to provide important details about the coexisting tracheal stenosis such as the distance of segmental stenosis from the vocal cord, degree of the stenosis, length of stenotic segment, and stent placement (Fig. 10.8) [13].

10.6 Bronchopleural Fistula (BPF)

Bronchopleural fistula is a fistulous connection between the bronchial tree and pleural space. BPF is the severest life-threatening postoperative complication post a pneumonectomy and a lobectomy. A central BPF is sinus tract between pleural space and trachea or bronchial segments, and it results from pneumonectomy or lobectomy or arises from traumatic injury of tracheobronchial tree. A peripheral BPF is the direct passageway connection between pleural space and the airway distal to bronchial segments or lung parenchyma; it may arise due to the rupture of emphysematous bullae, post-necrotizing pneumonia, after radiotherapy and invasive thoracic interventions, empyema, and tuberculosis. The incidence of BPF ranges as 0.5–3% after lobectomy and 2–20% post-pneumonectomy [14].

Bronchoscopy is the investigation of choice used by intensivists or cardiothoracic surgeons to diagnose and localize a BPF; it permits the treating intensivists to assess the apposition of the cartilaginous and membranous walls of the bronchial stump and distinguish between stump dehiscence secondary to tumor recurrence, surgical site infection, and necrosis. Nevertheless, the false-negative rate in the identification of BPF with bronchoscopy has been high. Failure of early diagnosis of BPF will delay initiation of lifesaving therapy, resulting in deterioration of respiratory function, sepsis, and aspiration and increase in mortality [14].

In patients with a doubted BPF, numerous enquiries need to be clarified to properly manage the patients. The initial step is to ascertain the location and size of the fistulae and its relationship with the tracheobronchial tree, nearby mediastinal structures and major vessels. Moreover, the pleural space should be controlled with closed drainage or decortication. Lastly, the etiology of BPF such as tumor recurrence, stump necrosis, or infections must be recognized and properly addressed [14].

VB simulates the tracheobronchial tree; the imagings can be magnified and shown as 3-D constructs to determine the precise location, size, and fluid collection in relation to the fistulae.

Being a noninvasive investigation, VB can be used safely in critically ill patients and can be repeated for post-treatment control evaluation and assessment of healing process [14, 15].

Moreover, VB can be used to study acute angle of tracheobronchial tree before stent implementation, and evaluate airway complications following stent placement. VB can also be used to evaluate internal diameter of the stumps for different sealants [14].

The most important limitations of VB is that it may provide a false-negative result of a BPF if a fistulous lumen has been blocked with mucus or the image has been misregistered during respiration [14].

10.7 Trauma: VB and MDCT Play Important Role in Diagnosis and Assessment of Tracheal and Laryngeal Injury

10.7.1 Traumatic Tracheobronchial Injury (TBI)

Tracheobronchial injury (TBI) including iatrogenic and traumatic is very rare; the TBI represents only 0.5%–2.8% of blunt thoracic injury, although it is associated with high mortality and morbidity if not immediately diagnosed and treated. Iatrogenic TBI may result from traumatic

intubation or tracheostomy. Prompt diagnosis of TBI depends on the clinical manifestations, radiographic findings, and bronchoscopy [16].

The most important clinical findings of TBI are dyspnea, cyanosis, hemoptysis, flail chest, stridor, aphonia, hoarseness of the voice, and subcutaneous emphysema. Yet these findings may not be obvious or remain undetected at initial presentation, especially in severally injured patients [16].

Bronchoscopy is the investigation of choice to assess TBI. It permits visualization of the site and extent of the injury and guarantees that the cuff of the endotracheal tube has been inflated distal to the site of the airway defect; the most frequent findings of TBI are laceration of the tracheobronchial wall. Occasionally, the view might be compromised due to presence of blood clots and tissue debris; furthermore, if severe tracheobronchial stenosis occurs, the bronchoscope can block the airway, and evaluation of tracheobronchial tree distal to stenosis becomes impossible [17].

Hypoxic and/or hypotensive critically ill patients might not collaborate with the intensivists to complete the bronchoscopy without sedation. In these circumstances, rigid bronchoscopy under inhalation anesthesia with preserving spontaneous ventilation should be considered; it permits removal of blood, secretions, and necrotic tissue with good assessment of the tracheobronchial injury. The most important disadvantage of rigid bronchoscopy is the necessity to manipulate the neck which is contraindicated in case of cervical spine injury [17].

The radiographic findings of TBI are nonspecific and depend on the site and extent of injury. The most important radiographic findings are subcutaneous emphysema, pneumomediastinum, pneumothorax, pneumopericardium, disrupted or blurred major airway, abnormal endotracheal tube, and the "fallen-lung" sign, although some patients have no radiographic evidence of TBI [17]. CT can identify all the signs for tracheobronchial injury. Chen et al. stated that CT imaging assisted authors to detect more than 70% of tracheobronchial injuries [18]. Recent evidence shows that multi-slice detector CT imaging with MPR/3-D reconstruction of the images may improve the diagnostic precision of the technique up to 100%. VB mimics the view of conventional bronchoscopy; thus, it may be a suitable alternative for detection as well as assessment of TBI [17].

10.7.2 Laryngeal Trauma

Laryngeal trauma (blunt or penetrating) is very rare; the incidence fluctuates between 1:5000 and 1:137000 trauma patients. Nonetheless, laryngeal injury is very dangerous in the severely injured patient; it might lead to disastrous long-term functional sequelae. The fatality of laryngeal injury is directly associated with the ability to maintain patent airways and cervical spine protection; it may reach up to 80% before hospitalization. However, as soon as the airways are protected and the laryngeal trauma is properly evaluated, the fatality rate falls to 5%. Accurate diagnosis and early management of laryngeal trauma are vital to save the patient and prevent longstanding impairment of breathing, swallowing, and speaking [19].

Patient with doubted laryngeal injury should be assessed with proper clinical examination, endoscopic evaluation, and radiological investigation (CT scan or MRI) to approve the doubted injury as well as to accurately evaluate its extent before treatment.

MDCT is the best investigation to assess laryngeal trauma and related injuries because it permits quick scanning and evaluation of huge anatomical areas with excellent quality, exceptional-resolution imagings. It allows trustworthy assessment of the critically ill, tachypnic, or mechanically ventilated in acute state and routine imaging [19].

Moderate and severe laryngeal trauma may cause laryngeal hematoma, edema, and mucosal laceration. The elastic larynx could absorb shock, although the thyroarytenoid muscle or the vocal ligament might damage. Therefore, injury of the vocal ligament and thyroarytenoid muscle must be assumed whenever thickening or bulging of the vocal cords into the airway lumen is noticed on MDCT. Small hematoma is easily missed at

MDCT, but recognition of a large one is straightforward [19].

Laryngeal edema generally causes soft tissue swelling with reduction of airway lumen on CT, while laryngeal laceration is identified whenever air in the paraglottic space with or without disruption of the laryngeal mucosa is noticed. Mucosal injury is very hard to identify on axial CT imagings, and 2-D MPR, 3-D VR, and VE are very useful by showing asymmetrical, air-filled pouches interconnecting with the laryngeal cavity [20].

Major trauma may cause fractures of laryngeal cartilage with or without fragment displacement. Fractures are detected when the continuousness of ossified or nonossified cartilages is disturbed. Generally, the identification of ossified cartilage ruptures is much simpler on CT than the identification of nonossified cartilage ruptures [19].

The thyroid cartilage is frequently fractured in laryngeal injury. It can be unilateral or bilateral, horizontal or vertical. Horizontal fractures are usually seen in strangulation cases, typically bilateral and affect upper edge of the thyroid laminae as well as superior horns of the thyroid cartilage. They are frequently accompanied with fracture of hyoid bone and hypo-pharyngeal hematoma [19].

Horizontal thyroid cartilage fractures and hyoid bone fractures tend to be missed axial CT imagings; therefore, coronal ± sagittal oblique 2-D MPR or 3-DVR should be done. The advantage of 3-D VR in recognizing these fractures has been proofed in a postmortem study that compared the performance of MDCT with autopsy of strangling victims; MDCT with 3-D VR recognized fractures originally undiagnosed at autopsy [19].

Fractures of the cricoid cartilage are usually two-sided, and it might lead to abrupt airway obstruction. An isolated cricoid cartilage fractures are very rare, and they are frequently accompanied with fractures of other cartilages. Because the cricoid cartilage is poorly ossified, these fractures are usually unnoticed at MDCT; therefore, soft tissue windows should be cautiously analyzed or MRI should be requested.

3-D VR has a limited role in diagnosis cricoid fractures; it does not afford extra-diagnostic information in these fractures [19].

10.8 Foreign Body Aspiration

Foreign body aspiration into tracheobronchial tree is very common and an important cause of airway obstruction and respiratory distress in children, particularly those younger than 36 months. Many patients of foreign body aspiration are misdiagnosed at presentation; they are usually diagnosed as asthma or respiratory tract infections. Applegate et al. reported that the recognition of foreign body aspiration is made correctly in 59% of patients on day one after aspiration [20]. Early diagnosis of foreign body aspiration is extremely important for proper management and avoiding disastrous pulmonary complications like infection, pneumonia, lung abscess, and life-threatening airway obstruction [21, 22]. When foreign body aspiration is suspected, chest X-ray is frequently requested, which is very useful sometimes. However, chest X-ray findings are frequently normal in about 30% of patients. Most of aspirated foreign body is radiolucent, and it is estimated that 90% of aspirated foreign bodies are radiolucent. Moreover, the presence of pulmonary infiltrates might confuse treating physician and makes timely recognition of foreign body aspiration extremely difficult. The chest X-ray sensitivity and specificity for foreign body recognition are 68% and 67%, respectively [23–25].

Therefore, CT is very helpful in the detection of aspirated radiolucent foreign bodies such as food and plastic objects. Hence, it is kept for the diagnosis of vague patients of a foreign body aspiration to avoid hazards of radiation exposure. Moreover, CT shows the secondary signs of foreign body aspiration such as segmental pulmonary changes and air trapping [22, 24].

VB offers clear description of the tracheobronchial lumen as well as tracheobronchial walls. High-performance workstations allow computer post-processing of complex algorithms and virtual reality techniques. Due to perspective-rendering algorithm, VB mimics an endoscopist's vision of the interior surface of the tracheobronchial tree. These procedures allow precise imitation of main intra-luminal defects with an outstanding correlation with fiber-optic findings about the site, severity, and shape of tracheobronchial tree pathology including aspirated foreign body [22, 24].

Soo-long Hong et al. reported that CT scan and VB have diagnosed and recognized the site of aspirated foreign bodies with sensitivity of 100% and specificity of 67%, it is most likely due to the presence of endoluminal secretions and artifacts [25]. Another important limitation of VB is the inability to show the sub-segmental parts of the tracheobronchial tree [22, 24].

VB can be used in the identification of the exact location of aspirated foreign body before the endoscopy and in excluding the presence of foreign bodies in patients with a low level of doubt and normal or nonspecific findings on chest X-ray which may prevent unnecessary exposure to anesthesia and invasive procedures [22, 26].

10.9 Inhalation Injuries

Inhalation injury diagnosis is very important in the management of burn patients because the presence of inhalation injury increases fatality by 20–60% above that expected by degree and surface area of burn. Assessment of severity and extent of inhalation injuries is challenging because chest X-ray, arterial blood gas, and chest examinations are nondiagnostic for inhalation injuries. The fiber-optic bronchoscopy is the investigation of choice for inhalation injuries diagnosis and assessment. It provides direct evaluation of the tracheobronchial tree within the field of view as well as it is useful in taking biopsies, performing pulmonary toilet, and removing casts which could improve ventilation and oxygenation and prevent airway obstruction. However, fiber-optic bronchoscopy is invasive intervention, and it is associated with high rate of false negatives, especially if performed in the first few hours after the injuries; thus, serial assessments are usually required. Furthermore, it is a risky procedure in patients with laryngeal edema, hypoxia, or hemodynamically unstable patients. Moreover, fiber-optic bronchoscopy has limitations such as discrepancy in grading, subjectivity, and limits of diameter of the endotracheal tube versus fiber-optic bronchoscope diameter, torturous anatomy, and skills level of the operator [26].

Gore et al. reported that VB can be very useful in the diagnosis of inhalation injuries in burn patients with doubted airway involvement. Ten burn patients suspected to have inhalation injury underwent CT examination, and in eight patients the inhalation injury was identified on the VB images [27].

Animal studies showed that VB showed comparable injury severity scores to fiber-optic bronchoscopy correlated with PaO_2-to-FiO_2 ratios (PFR) and reliably identified airway stenosis [28].

Further studies are required to support these studies. However, in scenarios when a burn patient has had admission CTs, VB may rule out airway obstruction, hence extracting supplementary details from previously performed diagnostic investigation; therefore, unnecessary immediate diagnostic fiber-optic bronchoscopy can be avoided, especially when the patient is critically ill or when the expert provider is not available [29].

10.10 Limitations of VB

There are few limitations of VB: the presence of retained mucus or blood can mimic tracheobronchial stenosis or foreign body. Furthermore, the diameter of tracheobronchial tree on the CT changes with inspiration and expiration; therefore, stenosis of tracheobronchial tree may be underestimated on inspiration, and it is very important to perform VB during the correct cycle of respiration, e.g., expiration to assess stenosis of tracheobronchial tree or in few scenarios such as tracheomalacia during both expiration and inspiration. Performing CT during inspiration and expiration can be very challenging in examinations of infants and children. Moreover, VB cannot be used to assess mucosa, perform biopsies, and therapeutic maneuvers [30].

Additionally, VB does not show segmental and sub-segmental part of tracheobronchial tree.

Transport of critically ill patients to radiology department is very challenging, and the adverse events during transport are very common and may expose patients to additional risks. These major risks must be estimated by the intensivists before requesting the CT scan; based on benefit/risk assessment in which the risk of transport and radiology exposure, it must be put in balance with predictable benefit of the CT scan.

Finally, it can be very hard to detect some dynamic tracheobronchial tree pathologies, for example immobile vocal cords [3, 31].

10.11 Conclusion

VE is a noninvasive technique that generates computer simulations of anatomy from radiological image data. Its simulations are close to conventional endoscopy. Due to advancements in CT scanner hardware and software, passion for the VE is growing in radiologists and pulmonary physicians.

It is obvious that VE can be a beneficial adjunct to conventional axial CT in the airway assessment of critically ill patients. It is highly accurate in the evaluation of airway stenosis, obstruction, vascular abnormalities, and tracheobronchial wall defects. Moreover, virtual endoscopy can be used as an exceptional research tool for understanding and teaching normal and abnormal pathology, as well as for surgical planning, all without requirement of added radiation exposure or distress to the patients if staging CT images have already performed.

VE does not replace fiber-optic bronchoscopy in critical care because it gives opportunity to sample material for diagnostic purpose or to treat the problem immediately.

Hence, VE can be used to extract supplementary data from an already completed diagnostic procedure; so, unnecessary diagnostic fiber-optic bronchoscopy can be avoided, especially when the patient is respiratory unstable.

References

1. Burke AJ, et al. Evaluation of Airway Obstruction Using Virtual Endoscopy. Laryngoscope 110: January 2000. Lippincott Williams & Wilkins, Inc. Philadelphia: The American Laryngological, Rhinological and Otological Society, Inc; 2000.

2. Brink JA, Heiken JP, Wang G, et al. Helical CT: principles and technical considerations. Radiographies. 1994;14:887–93.

3. Horton, et al. Advanced visualization of airways with 64-MDCT: 3-D mapping and virtual bronchoscopy. AJR. 2007;189 https://doi.org/10.2214/AJR.07.2824.

4. Tejeshwar Singh Jugpal et al Multi-detector computed tomography imaging of large airway pathology: A pictorial review. World J Radiol 2015; 7(12): 459–474. https://doi.org/10.4329/wjr.v7.i12.459.

5. Morshed K, et al. Evaluation of tracheal stenosis: comparison between computed tomography virtual tracheobronchoscopy with multiplanar reformatting, flexible tracheofiberoscopy and intra-operative findings. Eur Arch Otorhinolaryngol. 2011;268:591–7. https://doi.org/10.1007/s00405-010-1380-2.

6. Thomas BP, et al. CT virtual endoscopy in the evaluation of large airway disease: review. AJR. 2009;192 https://doi.org/10.2214/AJR.07.7077.

7. Díaz-Jimenez P, Rodriguez AN, editors. flrxible bronchoscopy. Interventions in Pulmonary Medicine. New York: Springer; 2013. https://doi.org/10.1007/978-1-4614-6009-1_2.

8. Smyth CM, Stead RJ. Survey of flexible bronchoscopy in the United Kingdom. Eur Respir J. 2002;19:458–6.

9. Stahl DL, Richard KM, Papadimos TJ. Complications of bronchoscopy: A concise synopsis. Int J Crit Illn Inj Sci. 2015;5(3):189–95. https://doi.org/10.4103/2229-5151.164995.

10. Sodhi K. Anticipated difficult tracheostomy: should CT scan be a pre-requisite. J Emerg Intern Med. 2017;1(2):14.

11. de Kleijn BJ, et al. Virtual 3-D planning of tracheostomy placement and clinical applicability of 3-D cannula design: a three-step study. Eur Arch Otorhinolaryngol. 2018;275:451–7. https://doi.org/10.1007/s00405-017-4819-x.

12. Paraschiv M. Tracheoesophageal fistula - a complication of prolonged tracheal intubation. J Med Life. 2014;7(4):516–21.

13. Hegde RG, et al. Esophagobronchial fi stulae: Diagnosis by MDCT with oral contrast swallow examination of a benign and a malignant cause. Ind J Radiol Imag. 2013;23(2)

14. Gaur, et al. Bronchopleural fistula and the role of contemporary imaging. J Thorac Cardiovasc Surg. 2014;148:341.

15. Shitrit D, Valdsislav P, Grubstein A, Bendayan D, Cohen M, Kramer MR. Accuracy of virtual bronchoscopy for grading tracheobronchial stenosis: correlation with pulmonary function test and fiber-optic bronchoscopy. Chest. 2005;128:3545–50.

16. Lim KE, et al. Tracheal Injury Diagnosed with Three-Dimensional Imaging Using Multidetector Row Computed Tomography. Chang Gung Med J. 2004;27(3)

17. Prokakis, et al. Airway trauma: a review on epidemiology, mechanisms of injury, diagnosis and treatment. J Cardiothorac Surg. 2014;9:117.

18. Chen JD, Shanmuganathan K, Mirvis SE, Killeen KL, Dutton RP. Using CT to diagnose tracheal rupture. AJR Am J Roentgenol. 2001;176:1273–80.

19. Becker M, et al. Imaging of laryngeal trauma. Eur J Radiol. 2014;83:142–54.

20. Applegate KE, Dardinger JT, Lieber ML, et al. Spiral CT scanning technique in the detection of aspiration of LEGO foreign bodies. Pediatr Radiol. 2001;31:836–40.

21. Scaglione M, Romano S, Pinto A, Sparano A, Scialpi M, Rotondo A. Acutetracheobronchial injuries: impact of imaging on diagnosis and managementimplications. Eur J Radiol. 2006;59(3):336–43.

22. Kosucu, et al. Low-Dose MDCT and Virtual Bronchoscopy in Pediatric Patients with Foreign Body Aspiration. AJR. 2004;183:1771–7.

23. Tan HKK, Brown K, McGill T, Kenna MA, Lund DP, Healy GB. Airway foreign bodies (FB): a 10- year review. Int J Pediatr Otorhinolaryngol. 2000;56:91–9.

24. Abd-ElGawad EA, et al. Tracheobronchial foreign body aspiration in infants & children: Diagnostic utility of multidetector CT with emphasis on virtual bronchoscopy. Egypt J Radiol Nucl Med. 2014;45:1141–6.

25. Soo-long H, Woo GH, Jong-Lyel R. Utility of spiral and cine CT scans in pediatric patients suspected of aspirating radiolucent foreign bodies. J Otolaryngol Head Neck Surg. 2008;138:5576–80.

26. Shin S-M, Kim WS, Cheon J-E, Jung AY, Youn BJ, Kim I-O, Yeon KM. CT in children with suspected residual foreign body in airway after bronchoscopy. AJR. 2009;192:1744–51.

27. Gore MA, Joshi AR, Nagarajan G, Iyer SP, Kulkarni T, Khandelwal A. Virtual bronchoscopy for diagnosis of inhalation injury in burnt patients. Burns. 2004;30:165–8.

28. Tsitouridis I, et al. Endotracheal and tracheostomy tube-related complications: imaging with three-dimensional spiral computed tomography. Hippokratia. 2009;13(2):97–100.

29. George A, et al. Virtual endoscopy for evaluation of tracheal laceration. Emerg Radiol. 2002;9:162–4. https://doi.org/10.1007/s10140-002-0210-2.

30. Kwon HP, et al. Comparison of virtual bronchoscopy to fiber-optic bronchoscopy for assessment of inhalation injury severity. Burns. 2014;40:1308–15.

31. Finkelstein SE, Summers RM, Nguyen DM, Stewart JH, Tretler JA, Schrump DS. Virtual bronchoscopy for evaluation of malignant tumors of the thorax. J Thorac Cardiovasc Surg. 2002;123:967–72.

Three-Dimensional Printing and Its Implication on Airway Management

Yasser Al-Hamidi, Abdulla Baobeid, and Nabil A. Shallik

11.1 Introduction

The advancement of rapid manufacturing technologies known as 3-D printing is transforming several medical practices and solutions. In contrast to traditional mass production technologies of manufacturing, 3-D printing prevails in terms of low-volume production cost saving, introducing flexibility and personalization. This means that the manufacturer can change the design of the produced parts at will, without the time and effort associated with tooling change in other production methods. Furthermore, 3-D printing has a better ability of producing models with complex geometries, such as the patient-specific anatomical models.

In its core, 3-D printing is an automated manufacturing technique that aims to reduce the human manual labor. Operation of 3-D printers is rarely associated with safety concerns and has a small footprint in comparison to other high-volume methods. This introduced to using 3-D printing in the medical field and improved accessibility to research and development of patient-specific solutions, especially to address solutions for rare pathologies.

The improved understanding of 3-D printing and its technologies is allowing researchers and developers to fully control the process, down to the microstructure of the produced parts, to ensure the best results. This resulted in the use of 3-D printing not only for prototyping (Fig. 11.1) but also to produce finished parts that can be used as treatment for patients. Consequently, 3-D printing is profoundly impacting medical practice by providing a more diverse solutions arsenal to medical practitioners.

With 3-D printing, the experimentation of new designs and concepts is easier than before. Accessibility to design and digital prototyping tools and shared databases [1] has greatly improved and expanded the know-how of a niche industry, spurring innovation and development in medical routines and medical education and training in many fields [2, 3]. In this chapter, a basic description and classification of the technology is offered; then we introduce a glimpse into a few of

Electronic Supplementary Material The online version of this chapter (https://doi.org/10.1007/978-3-030-23253-5_11) contains supplementary material, which is available to authorized users.

Y. Al-Hamidi (✉) · A. Baobeid
Texas A and M University at Qatar, Doha, Qatar
e-mail: yasser.al-hamidi@qatar.tamu.edu

N. A. Shallik
Department of Anesthesiology, ICU and Perioperative Medicine, Hamad Medical Corporation, Doha, Qatar

Department of Clinical Anesthesiology, Weill Cornell Medical College in Qatar (WCMQ), Doha, Qatar

Department of Anesthesiology and Surgical Intensive Care, Faculty of Medicine, Tanta University, Tanta, Egypt
e-mail: Nshallik@hamad.qa

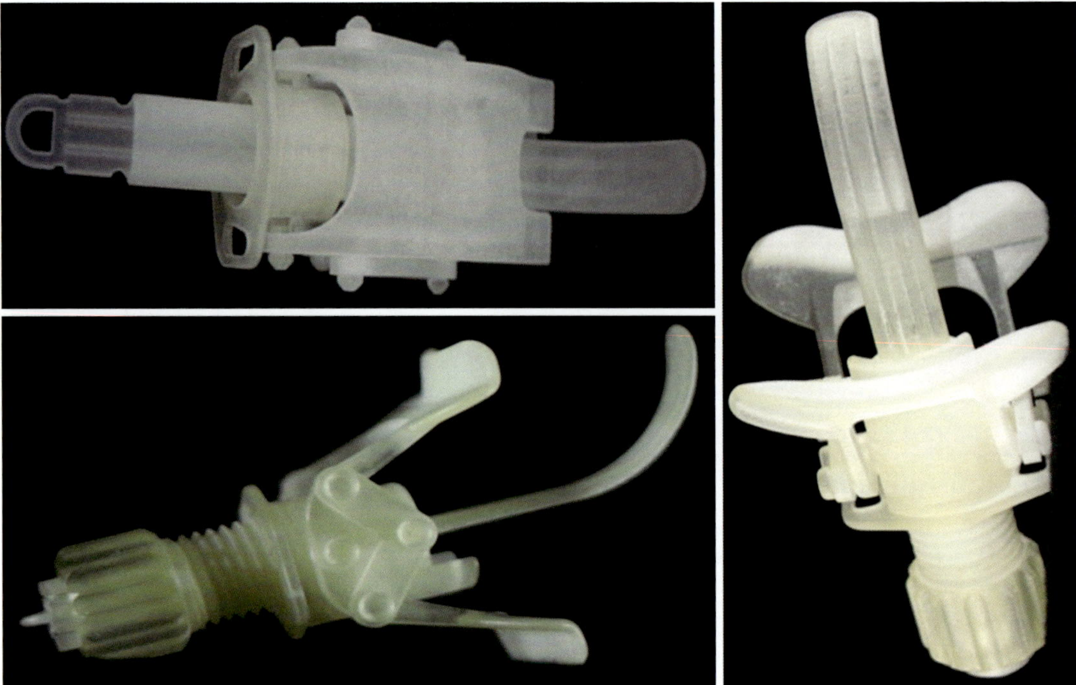

Fig. 11.1 Novel airway device prototype printed by 3D printer in Texas A&M, Qatar

the use cases of 3-D printing and the exploding creativity of use cases in the medical field.

11.2 Classification of 3-D Printing Techniques

Understanding different processes is essential for the user to expect the different behaviors of the diverse nuances of the produced output. 3-D printing is a direct digital manufacturing technique, which means that the user has control over most of the virtual process variables to produce parts with certain engineering properties.

Materials used in 3-D printing can generally be classified into three categories, namely polymers, metals, and ceramics. Polymers such as polylactic acid (PLA), acrylonitrile butadiene styrene (ABS), polyamide (nylon), and polyether ether ketone (PEEK) are commonly used in 3-D printing [4]. Many of these polymers are biodegradable and biocompatible; however, they are hard to sterilize and more intricate procedures must be followed to ensure that. Metals used in

3-D printing include, but not limited to, alloys of gold, titanium, steel, aluminum cobalt, and chrome. Metals have high strengths and are generally easy to sterilize. Ceramics are used for bioactive orthopedic implants and have an excellent compressive strength and can be used for drug delivery applications [5].

These materials are being utilized currently in several manufacturing processes; their basic physics are explained briefly.

11.2.1 Material Extrusion, Including Fused Deposition Material (FDM)

The material is drawn, mostly, and pushed through a heated nozzle in a fashion similar to that of a hot melt adhesive, colloquially known as glue guns. The nozzle assembly and the platform are arranged to cover the entire build volume, either by a gantry x, y, and z coordinates or by using polar coordinates. The model is built by depositing the extruded material, layer by layer.

The melted material fused together as soon as they are deposited [6].

This method is currently the most popular 3-D printing technique due to the hobbyist and consumer 3-D printing movement. FDM 3-D printing is the cheapest method, and it is possible to select the printing material out of a variety of polymers such as ABS, PLA, and nylons [6].

11.2.2 Vat Photo Polymerization

In vat polymerization, a photosensitive resin placed in a vat is exposed to an accurately focused light source of a certain power and wavelength. This triggers a chemical curing process of the polymer from the liquid to the solid state. There are two popular variations of vat polymerization: the first is stereolithography apparatus (SLA), where an ultraviolet light LASER is continuously manipulated through a reflective mirror to cure the resin according to the desired geometry; the other variation is direct light processing (DLP), where light is directly shot to the resin [7].

The produced parts using vat polymerization have high levels of accuracy and good finish, which make this process, along with material jetting, which will be discussed later, the favorite option for jewelry manufacturing. However, the materials are limited to photo resins, which limits the other functional applications of this process. In addition, building the structures requires the use of supports, which calls for some postprocessing procedures.

Vat polymerization includes stereolithography process (SLA) and direct light processing (DLP) for polymers. There are variations of materials where it targets the manufacturing of ceramics and metals by using the photo polymer as the binding material and subjects the parts to sintering to remove the binding material [8].

11.2.3 Powder Bed Fusion (PBF)

Powder bed fusion (PBF) processing utilizes the production of high end of powder materials by projecting concentrated LASER or electron beams to the bed filled with powder printing material. PBF techniques require spreading the powder layer by layer [9].

Powder bed fusion techniques include, but not limited to, direct metal LASER sintering, electron beam melting (EBM), selective heat sintering (SHS), and selective LASER sintering (SLS). These are considered professional to industrial production tools, although SLS is witnessing recent attempts to be delivered to the hobbyist 3-D printing consumer [9].

Powder bed fusion techniques are witnessing an increase in popularity due to the higher mechanical properties of the produced parts. The powder bed fusion process is used to 3-D print metals, polymers, and ceramics [9].

11.2.4 Binder Jetting

The binder jetting process uses two materials: a powder-based material and a binder. The binder is usually in liquid form and the build material in powder form. A print head moves horizontally along the x and y axes of the machine and deposits alternating layers of the build material and the binding material [9].

Producing models of a variety of colors or textures is easier by using the different binding materials. In addition, the production of porous, bone-like form of triphosphate calcium is possible.

11.2.5 Direct Energy Deposition (DED)

This process fosters several complex methods of additive manufacturing methods, and it is popular to fabricate metals, although it has variations of use in ceramics and polymers. This process has been widely adopted for repairs and adding details to the existing structure in a fashion like welding. A classic DED machine consists of a nozzle processing, wire, or powder materials, installed on a 6 DOF arm, depositing molten materials to solidify on in specific building surfaces. This arrangement allows much more dimensional freedom and not confined to the layer-by-layer approach [10].

11.2.6 Material Jetting

Material jetting is a 3-D printing method inspired by 2-D paper ink jetting printing, where the material is sprayed on the building platform either in a continuous jet approach or in a Drop on Demand (DOD) approach. The extremely accurate models are built layer by layer, and in the case of polymers and waxes, the materials are cured to solidify using ultraviolet (UV) light. Due to the physics of the process, the process is limited to viscous materials that can be rapidly cured after dropping, such as polymer resins and waxes [11].

11.3 Workflow of 3-D Printing in Medical Applications

In 3-D printing of patient-specific models, the digital images acquired by either magnetic resonance imaging (MRI) or computed tomography (CT) scans are segmented, pre-processed, and simulated using 3-D software packages. Such software packages are available either as an open source or as a licensed software package. A very popular one is the proprietary software, Mimics® (image processing software for 3-D design and modeling, developed by Materialise NV, a Belgian company specialized in additive manufacturing software and technology for medical, dental, and additive manufacturing industries), which is approved for clinical and research uses. 3-D Slicer® (Slicer is a free and open-source software package used for image analysis and scientific visualization; slicer is used in a variety of medical applications) is another open-source software but approved only for research purposes. All these software packages are used to process, segment, and/or repair. Digital Imaging and Communications in Medicine (DICOM) based files into printable formats such as Standard Tessellation Language (STL).

Some of the challenges facing 3-D printing originate from the data acquisition of images. The acquired images are mainly static version that captures only a snapshot of the dynamic geometry of organism. For example, researchers have reported that the medical images of tracheal models, acquired at the supine position, were not necessarily representative of the true intubation conditions in the semi-recumbent position [12].

The process of designing the 3-D printed part varies with the application. All workflows start with CT and MRI medical imaging, converting the medical images to 3-D images, and processing the 3-D images according to the medical application before printing. For example, the 3-D scanned organ acts as a reference for the new implants (Fig. 11.2). The printing process entails control of parameters such as the selection of an individual or multiple material, the microstructure of the printed parts, and engineering the postprocessing stage of the part [13–15].

11.4 3-D Printed Implants

3-D printing is currently used to manufacture implants and replacements for several organs with structural physiological function such as spinal implants [20], sarectomy [21, 22] spinal guides 3-D [9], craniofacial implants [10, 11] (Fig. 11.3), maxillofacial surgeries (Fig. 11.4) [12], and pelvis and hip deformaties [23, 24] [13] (Figs. 11.5 and 11.6). As the use of 3-D printed implants is expanding, the clinical impact and long-term

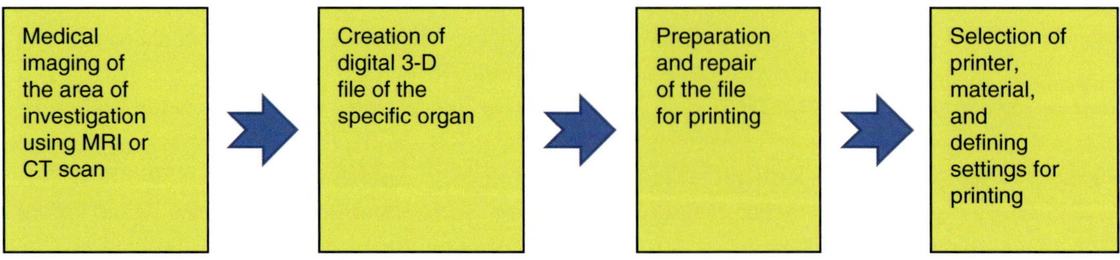

Fig. 11.2 Generalized workflow of medical 3-D printing

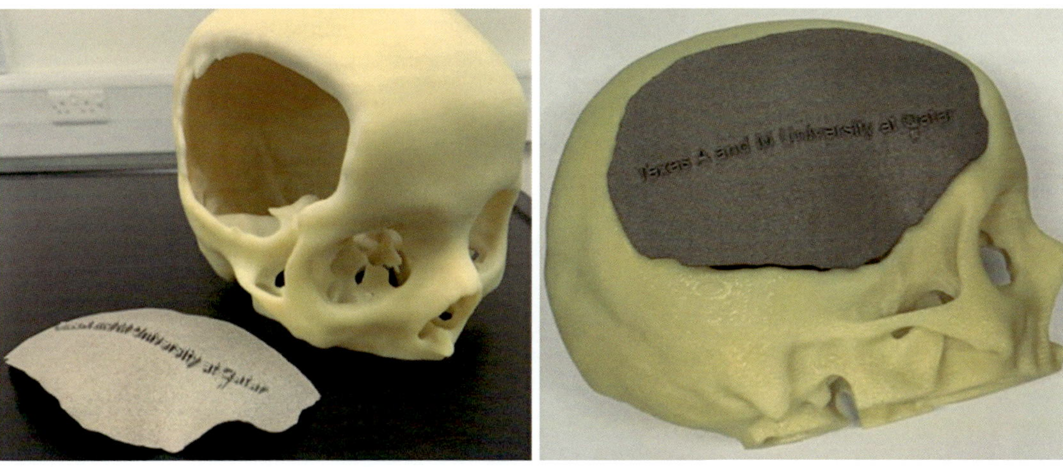

Fig. 11.3 3D printed cranioplasty part to fill a skull defect

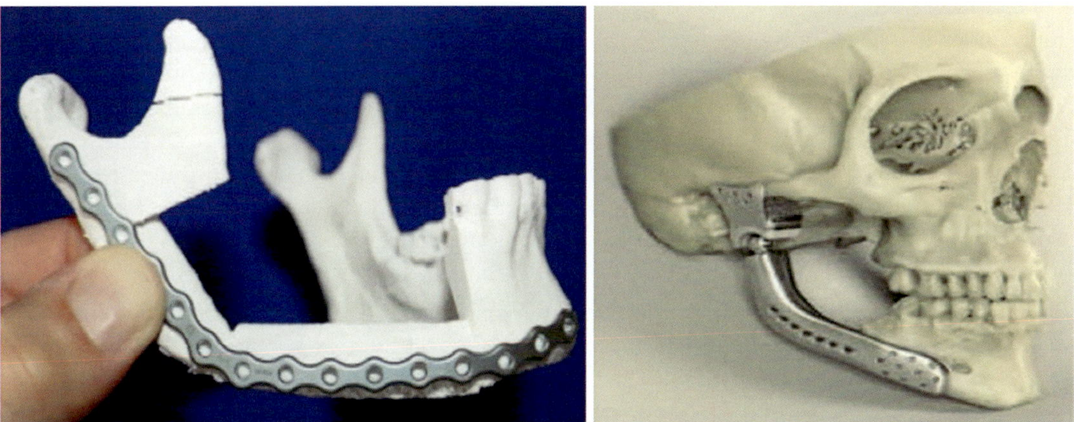

Fig. 11.4 A 3-D printed model for the mandible is of utmost benefit for planning for the reconstruction and plate and screw fixation in a step prior to the real surgical intervention. Rehearsal, measurement evaluation, and functional assessment will help the surgeons for better surgical outcome and it is of high impact upon the teaching part for the junior staff colleagues

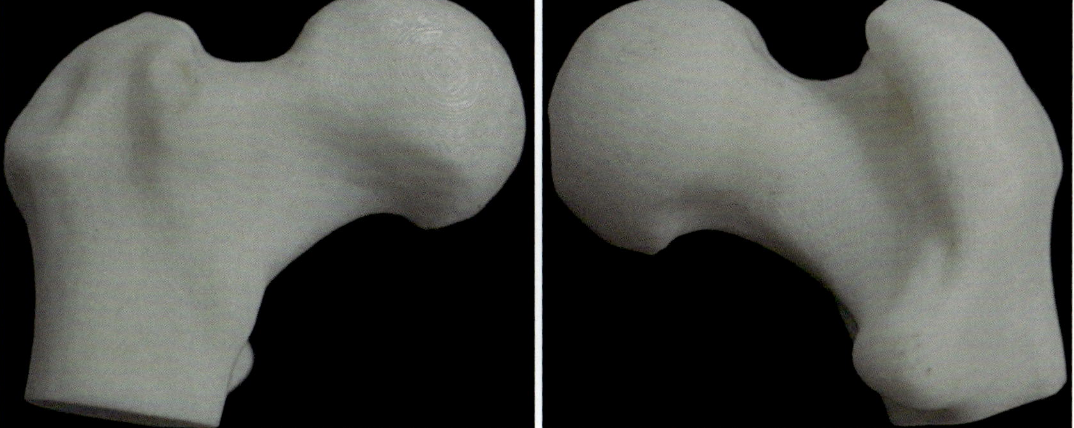

Fig. 11.5 A 3-D printed model for neck femur

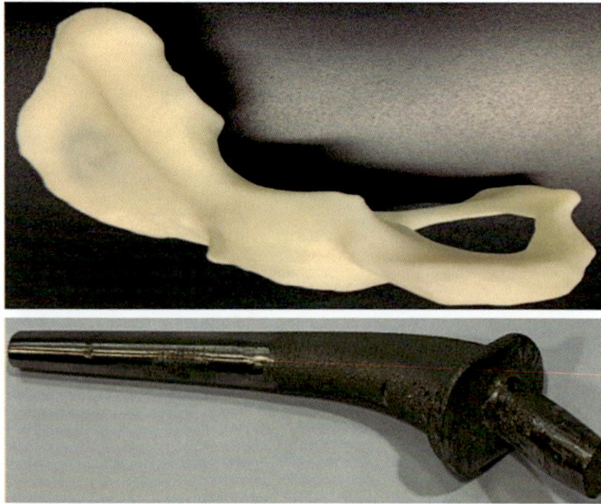

Fig. 11.6 A 3-D printed model for a pelvis and a neck femur implant

complications will be revealed and assessed with long-term follow-ups. For people waiting on transplants, 3-D techniques are a significant game changer where it mitigates the effects of issues such as tissue compatibility, tissue rejection, or a lifetime of immunosuppressive treatments and decreases waiting time [14].

11.5 3-D Printing Applications in the Clinical Field

The ability to fully control the geometry to reconstruct patient-specific geometry dictated based on CT and MRI medical imaging. Another factor stimulating the adaptation of the 3-D printing was the ability to manufacture complex internal patterns, using strong bio-compatible metals such as stainless steel, titanium alloys, and cobalt chromium alloys to minimize weight.

The freedom of design provided by 3-D printing is giving the opportunity to address anatomically challenging cases and treat rare pathologies and cases.

11.5.1 Splints and Stents for Trachea

Recently, researchers and clinicians are investigating the use of 3-D printing for more delicate and critical implants such as tracheobronchial splint [21] for pediatric patients, where the challenge is to create an external splint responsive to geometry changes. The case proves that 3-D printing can be useful to accommodate physiological behavior of the patients over time, in what many started to coin as four-dimension (4-D) printing, in which materials with thermomechanical properties with shape-morphing behavior.

Surgeons succeeded in treating airway stenosis with customizable 3-D printed airway stent [22]. 3-D printing proved useful in this case due to the complexity of the geometry of the stenosis. In this case, the patient suffering from a complex case of a complete stenosis of the bronchus intermedius (BI) with partial dehiscence of the bronchial anastomosis after lung transplanta-

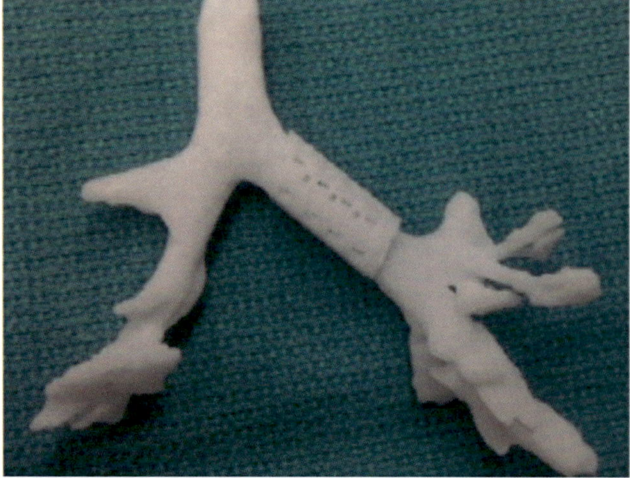
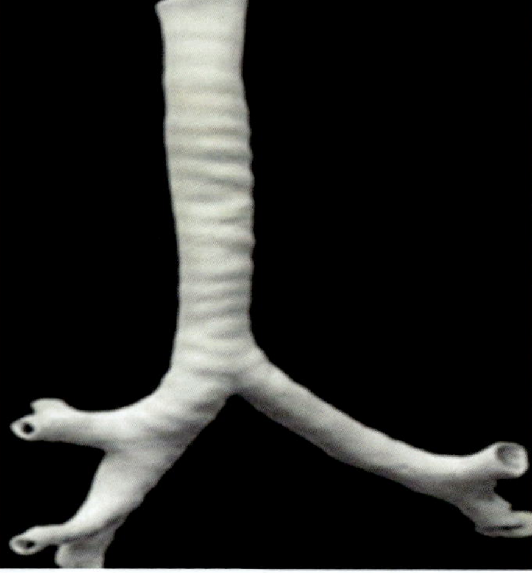

Fig. 11.7 A 3D printed tracheal model, right and left main bronchi and printed tracheal stent

tion [23]. The complexity of the case excluded the use of conventional airway stents (Fig. 11.7).

By using computer-assisted segmentation, by conducting a virtual operation, the stenosis and dehiscence were treated and a 3-D stent was designed.

11.5.2 Use of 3-D Printing in the Manufacturing of Nasal Stents

Nasoalveolar molding of the cleft lip, nose, and alveolar palate has been an effective technique for the reconstruction of oro-nasal function and look, but it has a few disadvantages. The short-term implant, which is placed before operative restoration, is a large appliance demanding various modifications, and it can irritate delicate soft tissues and obstruct with the infant's capability to nurse or nourish. In the early postoperative time and for months after cleft lip repair, clients use standard silicone stents that come in several dimensions but require considerable sculpting to match the unique cleft defect. Three-dimensional (3-D) reproduction offers the possibility of extremely individualized and patient-specific treatment. People created a technique that generates a personalized 3-D printed stent that fit the contours and unique functions of each patient and permits customization and adjustments in measurement and shape as the patient ages. With 3-D scanning innovation, the unit can be designed at the first visit to produce a device that could be put on sequentially with very little trauma, does not disrupt feeding, and a prosthesis that will enhance compliance. The device will be worn intraorally to help shape the alveolus, lip, and nose before surgical repair. Furthermore, the stent can be doped with medications as each patient's case measurements [24] (Fig. 11.8).

11.5.3 Maxillofacial 3-D Printing

3-D design tools have enabled the virtual construction of 3-D-specific models to construct

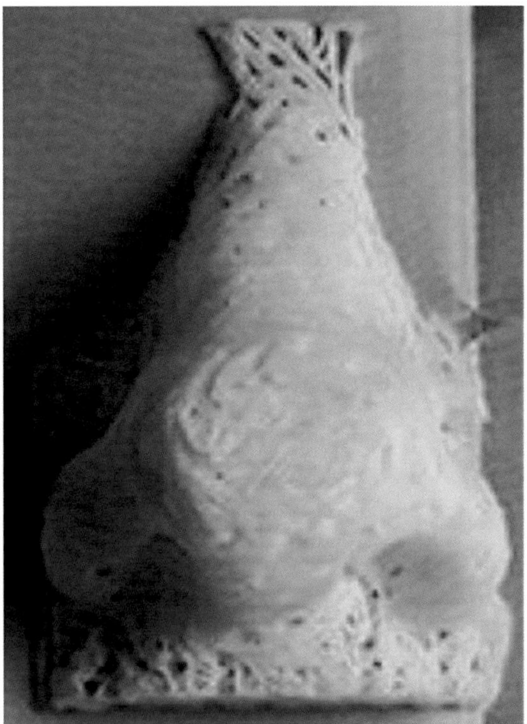

Fig. 11.8 3D printed nose surgical planning, intraoperative guidance, and surgical simulation

implants and guides to facilitate surgical procedures such as drilling and implant placement. The main applications of maxillofacial 3-D printing are dental implant surgery, mandibular reconstruction, mandibular pathology (Fig. 11.9), orthognathic surgery, and midface reconstruction. Please refer to Chap. 7.

11.5.4 Bio-absorbable Polymers Vascular Stents in Head and Neck Area

Currently, most vascular stents, which are used as flow diverters or to treat stenosis, are manufactured using a multi-step manufacturing processes that include, but not limited to, LASER precision micro-sheet and tube machining and micro-wire braiding. Essential postprocessing includes heat treatment to dispose internal stresses and manufacturing defects, as well as surface electrochemical treatments. Materials used for stent

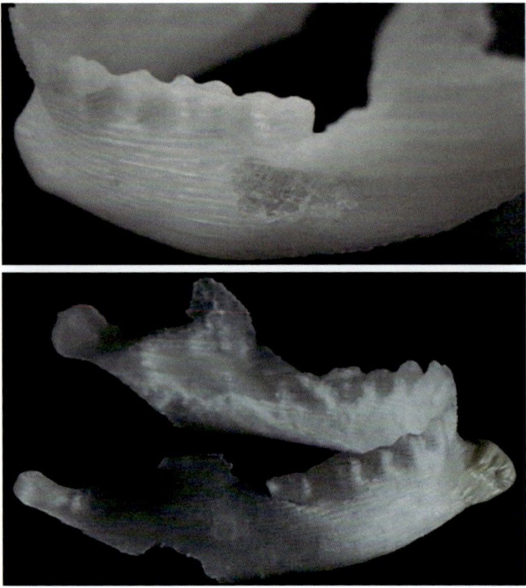

Fig. 11.9 3-D printed models for the mandible from different perspectives and showing bony lesions due to bone pathology

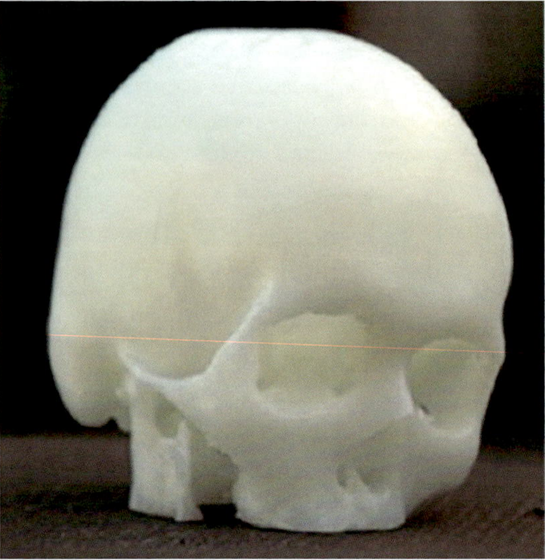

Fig. 11.10 A skull and mandible 3-D reconstruction-printed model shuttered into two segments, namely, the bony calvarium, orbits, and nasal bone and part of the maxilla

manufacturing include nickel titanium (NiTi) and cobalt chromium (CoCr) [25]. 3-D printing seemed to be unsuccessful to present any added value to the clean room manufacturing of stents. However, many are investigating 3-D printing for direct digital manufacturing of stents that can better fit with complex geometries of critical vessels in head and neck, thus reducing the probability of failure. Furthermore, 3-D printed flexible, biodegradable polymer stents, which are customized to patient-specific geometries, can be coated with drugs that aim to reduce complications and expedite the healing process [25].

1. Rhinoplasty: Please refer to Chap. 6.
2. Skull base: Please refer to Chap. 6.

11.5.5 Training Education and Surgical Planning

3-D printing is extensively used for training, education, and patient-specific surgical planning. 3-D printing of anatomical models, which are not used in the surgery room, is not costly and easy, and there is not a lot of requirements related to

patient safety at question. The medical images are used to produce 3-D printed models that are meant to simulate case-specific anatomical complexities and difficulties, evaluate, and negotiate surgical strategies and conduct preoperative dry runs. Here are some applications of 3-D printing in training, education, and surgical planning (Fig. 11.10).

11.5.5.1 Patient Education for Endoscopic Sinus Surgery

Throughout (ENT) subspecialty, a somewhat minimal portion of patients follow through with elective procedures to fix ailments such as a deviated septum or occluded sinus passage. Patient awareness of their medical diagnosis and therapy plan is integral to compliance, which essentially generates enhanced health care results and far better quality of life. Here we report the usage of advanced, polyjet 3-D printing options to develop a multi-material reproduction of human nasal sinus anatomy, derived from clinical X-ray computed tomography (CT) data, to be used as an educational aid during doctor assessment. The last patient education model was developed over several models to optimize material properties, anatomical reliability, and overall show [26].

11.5.5.2 Resident Training

Quick prototyping is a developing innovation that has the potential to transform health care learning. As plastic cosmetic surgeons, we are anticipated to recognize the touches of comprehensive human anatomical designs and their spatial relationship with one another. 3-D printing can enable an in-depth awareness of human anatomy that was generally obtained from text illustrations and years of operative expertise doing complex dissections. The future of plastic surgery learning is interesting because of the capability to take a 2-dimensional (2-D) picture and carry it to way of life with a full-scale design [27] (Fig. 11.11).

11.5.5.3 Reductions in Operation Room Time

Operating room time has usually been one of the huge debates for health care 3-D printing. Of the 227 articles, 42 explained the precise effect of utilizing 3-D printing innovation on OR time. For a large number of applications, 3-D printing results in time saving. The outcomes are given in applications such as operative guides for maxillofacial surgical operation, models for vertebral and maxillofacial surgical preparation, and designs for forming implants utilized in maxillofacial surgery appear to benefit the more from modern 3-D technology [28].

11.5.5.4 3-D Printing in Preoperative Surgical Planning

The level of personalized care achieved through 3-D printing has been influential in increasing accuracy and efficiency in procedures, cutting down operating room time, and improving surgical outcomes. Working with patients who have cancer or radiation damage involving the mandible, we can use 3-D models to help prepare for and implement their surgical resections and reconstructions. We can use 3-D models for two

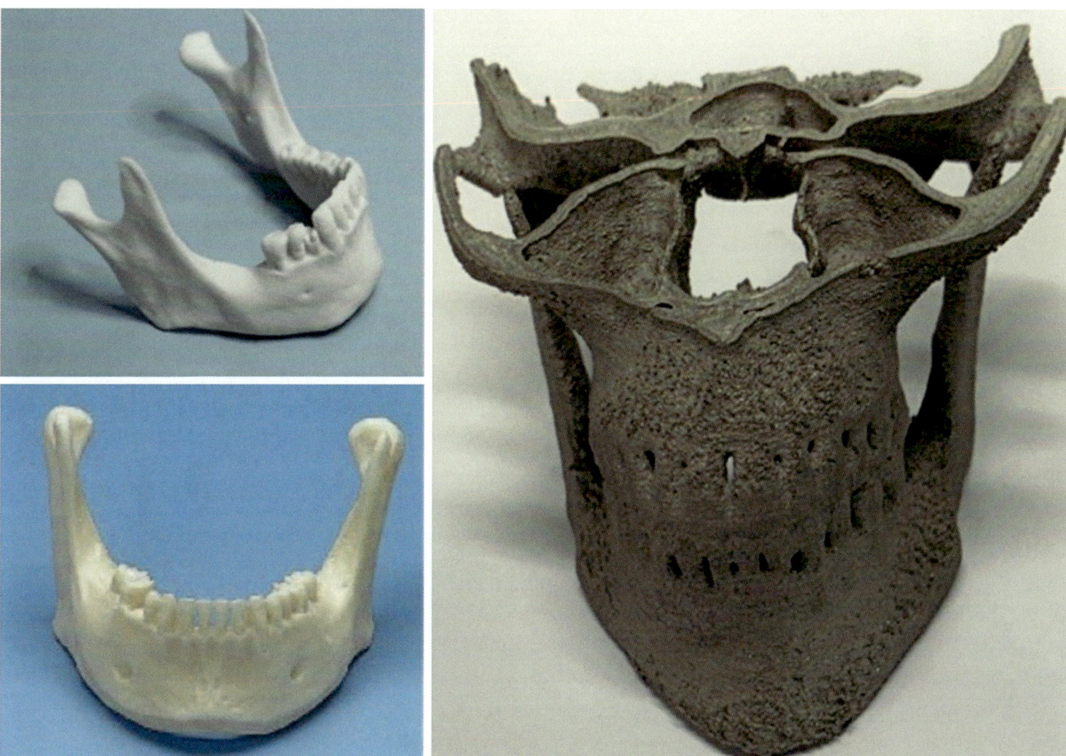

Fig. 11.11 3-D printed models for the mandible from different perspectives

reasons: to help plan where we will make our bone cuts around the cancer and to help streamline and optimize the reconstruction.

It starts with a CT scan that is turned into a 3-D image of the patient's face to determine where the bone cuts around the cancer will be and at what angles. Oftentimes, there is a need to take part of the patient's fibula to create a new jawbone, and 3-D imaging is used to determine where fibula osteotomies will be. Once all of the cuts have been mapped out, the 3-D model is printed. These models are used to bend a titanium plate customized to the patient's native mandible, which is implanted during surgery. In some instances, the models are also shared with patients to give them a better understanding of what the surgery will look like.

Improved cosmetic outcomes have been another advantage to 3-D printing. Patients who have mandibles that are excessively deformed are now able to achieve a result that is much more symmetric than before. We can use the 3-D images to take the opposite side of the mandible, invert it, and make it an exact mirror image of the other side of the jaw.

From the point-of-view of bone reconstruction anywhere in the head and neck region, using 3-D models will be the standard way to go.

11.5.5.5 3-D Printing for Design and Manufacture of Implantable Devices

Advances in 3-D printing now allow for the creation of biocompatible structures with impressive complexity.

We have begun exploring the feasibility of printing a multi-material biomimetic tympanic membrane (TM) grafts that could be implanted into a patient.

The goal is to overcome the limitations of current graft materials to improve the outcomes following tympanoplasty. If we could design a graft material from the ground up and include optimized features, this would be a huge step forward. I think 3-D printing may now offer the means to produce such a graft.

Currently, physicians use materials such as temporalis fascia, perichondrium, and cartilage for TM grafts. The problem with these materials is that they do not possess similar structural features as those of the native TM, and this can leave the patient susceptible to chronic otitis media, a longstanding infection of the middle ear. 3-D printers can fabricate biomimetic TM grafts.

Using non-absorbable materials, as well as biologics, such as collagen and fibrin, tympanic membrane grafts have been created with acoustic properties that can be tuned to restore the sound-induced motion patterns of the human TM.

3-D printed grafts can be reliably produced and have structural features that are more consistent to those of the temporalis fascia. Such grafts have promising implications for clinical applications. With 3-D printing, we can rapidly create constructs with varying structural features and then answer these questions in a systematic way. It should help us generate a TM structure with ideal features—a design that may one day be implanted into patients—and hopefully result in better outcomes.

11.6 Design of New Devices and Prototypes

11.6.1 Improving Endotracheal Intubation

In anesthesia, 3-D printed bronchoscopy uses simulators and trainers [12]. The trainers simulating the human subjects used for training help practitioners develop strategies for 3-D printing, and these are extensively used to prototype and develop new medical tools of video-laryngoscopy for endotracheal intubation. The process allows designers to add more complexity functionality and nuance to laryngoscopy, for example, different variations of the blades of laryngoscopy (Figs. 11.12 and 11.13 and Movie 11.1). Another application is the improvement of oropharyngeal airway (Fig. 11.14) with more advanced and complex functionality, seeking to allow the practitioner to move the jaw along with the intubation swiftly.

11.6.2 Design of New Devices and Prototypes

In addition to critical implants, surgical tools are easily customizable to patient's specific cases, giving clinicians the opportunity to take design initiatives when necessary. An example of design initiatives is 3-D printing of laparoscopic trocars and ureteric stents, oropharyngeal airways, Shalliscope with dimensions that are different than those of off-the-shelf products, designed to address specific patient challenges shown in (Figs. 11.12, 11.13, and 11.14). 3-D printing has been used to assess the different urological strategies as well as patient-specific solutions [29].

11.7 Limitations

3-D printed projects are expensive, but prices continue to decline, however, and there is evidence that using 3-D printed materials can be a cost-saving measure.

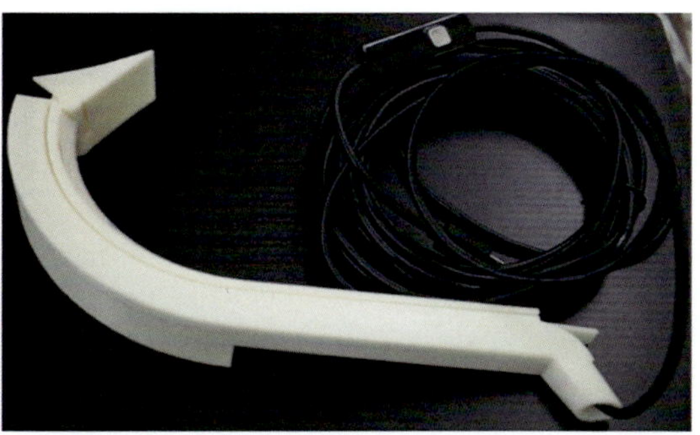

Fig. 11.12 Novel videoscope (Shalliscope) first prototype printed by 3D printer in Texas A&M, Qatar

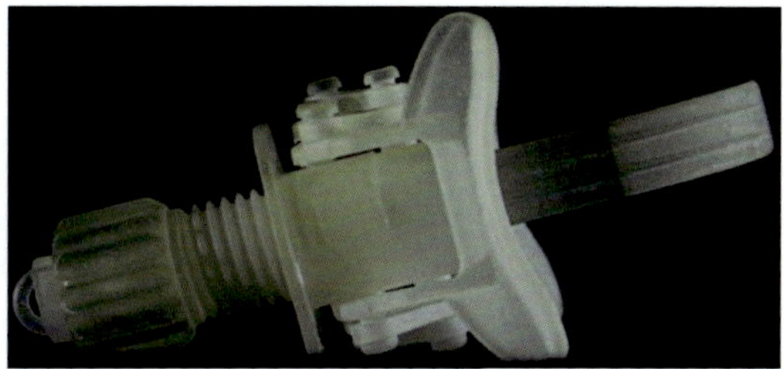

Fig. 11.14 Novel airway device prototype printed by 3D printer in Texas A&M, Qatar

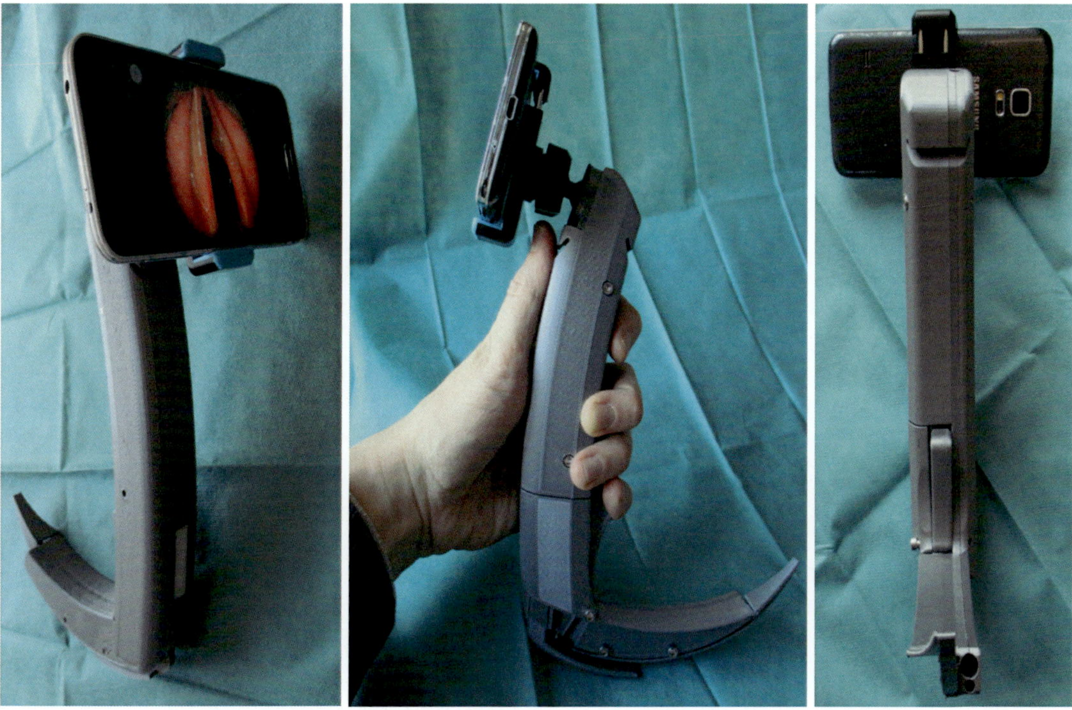

Fig. 11.13 Novel videoscope (Shalliscope) second prototype printed by 3D printer as proof of concept

For medical purposes, there remains a limited number of Food and Drug Administration–approved materials, which results in higher material costs. While the materials used to 3D print educational models are becoming more and more accessible, many educators have ongoing concerns that no true substitute exists for the human tissue.

The use of 3D-printed models, however, potentially reduces reliance on the acquisition of cadaveric bone. Research has shown that these models are an acceptable alternative.

Other concerns with 3D-printing implementation include the time required to obtain proper imaging formats, dedicated personnel for printer programming and troubleshooting, and the physical space and time required for printing high-fidelity models.

Another cost-saving measure is the in-house printing of surgical instruments such as retractors. This can be done at a discounted rate when compared with purchasing stainless-steel alternatives from a bulk supplier, and instruments can be printed in an optimal size or dimension to fit the situation. Polylactic acid is a commonly utilized material that can be sterilized and reused while withstanding enough force to retract human tissues during surgery. If costs still remain an issue, collaboration may be the solution. At academic medical centers, it is possible to share 3D printers and the required software among several departments.

11.8 Future Directions in 3-D Printing and the Next Step

In the future, bio-printing might allow us to integrate tissue engineering and materials to create functional implant to repair nasal turbinate tissue and trachea. Zhong and Zhao also suggest that further studies should be carried out to create 3-D printing models impregnated with airway epithelial cells or stem cells which could be used for functional disorders of nasal cavity such as empty nose syndrome and atrophic rhinitis [30]. Furthermore, three-dimensional printing opens up another exciting possibility for patient-specific customized instrumentation. Incorporating 3-D

printing models to mimic anterior skull base pathologies could be used for surgical training, allowing trainees to practice drilling through the endonasal approach. Based on current research, Zhong and Zhao predict that it might be possible to develop bio-printed nerve grafts to repair facial nerve and recurrent laryngeal nerve, in the future. The use of 3-D printing to form soft structures has not been fully explored. In neurosurgery and skull base surgery, 3-D printed models using the combination of hard and soft materials would allow exact simulation of skull base and the underlying dura and brain tissue [30].

11.9 Summary and Conclusion

In conclusion, there is a healthy prognosis for 3-D printing in surgery and medicine as it plays into both the highly technical and creative aspects of our work, says Dr. Remenschneider and Dr. Kozin. Three-dimensional printing is already directly affecting patient care, and it is easy to see how 3-D printers will play an important role in surgical planning and prosthetic design in the future. By being able to rapidly replicate anatomic scans or manipulate the structural features of implanted devices, surgeons are now the ones in control of the production line. "Three-dimensional printing is exciting as it provides surgeons the ability to rapidly study, design, and modify anatomic structures on a micron scale. Three-dimensional printing is democratizing the design and fabrication process. Surgeons can now think and act outside the box in terms of what is possible," said Dr. Kozin. "Whether it is being used to optimize operative techniques or to create new implantable constructs, 3-D printing is revolutionizing surgery and is here to stay." The applications of 3-D printing in the surgical field are going to continue to expand—discovering new medical questions to explore and finding more ways to improve procedures. Having insights that are made possible with 3-D printing will also continue to lead to better surgical successes, solutions to unsolved problems, and enhanced patient care. "The greatest thing about 3-D printing is that if you can imagine it, you can create it," said Dr. Remenschneider.

References

1. Tack P, Victor J, Gemmel P, Annemans L. 3-D-printing techniques in a medical setting: a systematic literature review. Biomed Eng Online. 2016;15(1):115.
2. Chao I, Young J, Coles-Black J, Chuen J, Weinberg L, Rachbuch C. The application of three-dimensional printing technology in anaesthesia: a systematic review. Anaesthesia. 2017;72(5):641–50.
3. Dodziuk H. Applications of 3-D printing in healthcare. Polish J Cardio-thoracic Surg. 2016; 13(3):283.
4. Chia HN, Wu BM. Recent advances in 3-D printing of biomaterials. J Biol Eng. 2015;9(1):4.
5. Tappa K, Jammalamadaka U. Novel biomaterials used in medical 3-D printing techniques. J Funct Biomater. 2018;9(1):17.
6. Dizon JRC, Espera AH, Chen Q, Advincula RC. Mechanical characterization of 3-D-printed polymers. Additive Manuf; 2017.
7. Gibson I, Rosen DW, Stucker B. Additive manufacturing technologies. Berlin: Springer; 2010.
8. de Blas Romero A, Lantada AD, Schwentenwein M, Jellinek C, Homa J. Lithogeraphy-based Ceramic Manufacture.
9. Loughborough University Research Group. 7 Categories of additive manufacturing. http://www.lboro.ac.uk/research/amrg/about/the7categoriesofadditivemanufacturing/.
10. Gibson I, Rosen D, Stucker B. Directed energy deposition processes. In: Additive manufacturing technologies. New York, NY: Springer; 2015.
11. Gay P, Blanco D, Pelayo F, Noriega A, Fernández P. Analysis of factors influencing the mechanical properties of flat PolyJet manufactured parts. Procedia Eng. 2015;132:70–7.
12. Pedersen TH, Gysin J, Wegmann A, Osswald M, Ott SR, Theiler L, Greif R. A randomised, controlled trial evaluating a low cost, 3-D-printed bronchoscopy simulator. Anaesthesia. 2017;72(8):1005–9.
13. Vukicevic M, Mosadegh B, Min JK, Little SH. Cardiac 3-D printing and its future directions. JACC Cardiovasc Imaging. 2017;10(2):171–84.
14. Giannopoulos AA, Mitsouras D, Yoo SJ, Liu PP, Chatzizisis YS, Rybicki FJ. Applications of 3-D printing in cardiovascular diseases. Nat Rev Cardiol. 2016;13(12):701.
15. Maragiannis D, Jackson MS, Igo SR, Schutt RC, Connell P, Grande-Allen J, Little SH. Replicating patient-specific severe aortic valve stenosis with functional 3-D modeling. Circ Cardiovasc Imaging. 2015;8(10):e003626.
16. Morrison RJ, et al. Mitigation of tracheobronchomalacia with 3D-printed personalized medical devices in pediatric patients. Sci Transl Med. 2015;7(285):285ra64–4.
17. Wei R, Guo W, Ji T, Zhang Y, Liang H. One-step reconstruction with a 3-D-printed, custom-made prosthesis after total en bloc sacrectomy: a technical note. Eur Spine J. 2017;26(7):1902–9.
18. Kim D, Lim JY, Shim KW, Han JW, Yi S, Yoon DH, Shin DA. Sacral reconstruction with a 3-D-printed implant after hemisacrectomy in a patient with sacral osteosarcoma: 1-year follow-up result. Yonsei Med J. 2017;58(2):453–7.
19. Wang S, Wang L, Liu Y, Ren Y, Jiang L, Li Y, Li H. 3-D printing technology used in severe hip deformity. Exp Ther Med. 2017;14(3):2595–9.
20. Liang H, Ji T, Zhang Y, Wang Y, Guo W. Reconstruction with 3-D-printed pelvic endoprostheses after resection of a pelvic tumour. Bone Joint J. 2017;99(2):267–75.
21. Morrison, Robert J., et al. Mitigation of tracheobronchomalacia with 3D-printed personalized medical devices in pediatric patients. Science translational medicine 2015;7.285 285ra64-285ra64.
22. Maragiannis D, Jackson MS, Igo SR, Schutt RC, Connell P, Grande-Allen J, Little SH. Replicating patient-specific severe aortic valve stenosis with functional 3-D modeling. Circ Cardiovasc Imaging. 2015;10:e003626.
23. Guibert N, Didier A, Moreno B, Mhanna L, Brouchet L, Plat G, Mazieres J. Treatment of post-transplant complex airway stenosis with a three-dimensional, computer-assisted customized airway stent. Am J Respir Crit Care Med. 2017;195(7):e31–3.
24. Mills D, Tappa K, Jammalamadaka U, Weisman J, Woerner J. The use of 3-D printing in the fabrication of nasal stents. Inventions. 2017;3(1):1.
25. STI Laser, Stent manufacturing process. https://www.sti-laser.com/products/stents/stent-manufacturing-process/.
26. Van Lith R, Baker E, Ware H, Yang J, Farsheed AC, Sun C, Ameer G. 3-D-printing strong high-resolution antioxidant bioresorbable vascular stents. Adv Mater Technol. 2016;1(9):1600138.
27. Sander I, Liepert T, Doney E, Leevy W, Liepert D. Patient education for endoscopic sinus surgery: preliminary experience using 3-D-printed clinical imaging data. J Funct Biomater. 2017;8(2):13.
28. Bauermeister AJ, Zuriarrain A, Newman MI. Three-dimensional printing in plastic and reconstructive surgery: a systematic review. Ann Plast Surg. 2016;77(5):569–76.
29. Youssef RF, Spradling K, Yoon R, Dolan B, Chamberlin J, Okhunov Z, Landman J. Applications of three-dimensional printing technology in urological practice. BJU Int. 2015;116(5):697–702.
30. Zhong N, Zhao X. 3-D printing for clinical application in otorhinolaryngology. Eur Arch Otorhinolaryngol. 2017;274(12):4079–89.

Challenging Clinical Cases Discussion

12

Nabil A. Shallik, Abbas H. Moustafa, and Amr Elhakeem

12.1 "Know-How" Chapter

This book addresses the "know what" (facts) and the "know why" (Science) and utilizes concepts by pairing the use of knowledge with technology, and then concludes with the "know how to do" chapter. This chapter aims to enable clinicians in solving everyday clinical encounters.

We have collected numerous simple, complex and interesting airway management clinical cases and presented them in a simple and practical way.

We hope that this may assist in better management of these cases and will inspire our colleagues to push the boundaries to make treatment safer and successful and safe life of our pateints.

Electronic Supplementary Material The online version of this chapter (https://doi.org/10.1007/978-3-030-23253-5_12) contains supplementary material, which is available to authorized users.

So, we will discuss the following items for each case:

- Clinical picture
- Examination
- Investigations
- Conventional radiological diagnosis
- Radiological 3-D and VE effects on:
  - Diagnosis
  - Surgical intervention
  - Airway management

12.2 Challenging Cases Discussion

12.2.1 Case Reference Number 1

A 27-year-old male was admitted in the hospital after suffering traumatic brain injury due to a road traffic accident. The full extent of his injuries included moderate right frontotemporal subgaleal haematoma. Minimal traces of subarachnoid haemorrhage are seen in the frontal regions bilat-

N. A. Shallik (✉)
Department of Clinical Anesthesiology, Weill Cornell Medical College in Qatar (WCMQ), Doha, Qatar

Department of Anesthesiology, ICU and Perioperative Medicine, Hamad Medical Corporation, Doha, Qatar

Department of Anesthesiology and Surgical Intensive Care, Tanta University, Tanta, Egypt
e-mail: Nshallik@hamad.qa

A. H. Moustafa
Department of Radiology and Clinical Imaging, Hamad Medical Corporation, Doha, Qatar

Diagnostic Radiology and Medical Imaging, El Minia University, El Minia, Egypt

A. Elhakeem
(ORL-HNS) Department, Hamad Medical Corporation, Doha, Qatar

© Springer Nature Switzerland AG 2019 143
N. A. Shallik et al. (eds.), *Virtual Endoscopy and 3D Reconstruction in the Airways*,
https://doi.org/10.1007/978-3-030-23253-5_12

erally and multiple small haemorrhagic contusions are also seen in the frontal regions bilaterally. There is a non-displaced fracture of the right frontal bone extending to the right superior orbital wall. There is a minimal pneumocephalus seen in the right frontal region. There is a fracture of the right superior orbital wall with a bone fragment seen displaced within the orbit. There is associated small intra-orbital haematoma and fat stranding. Subcutaneous emphysema and air loculi are seen in the right orbit. The right eye globe is intact. There is also fracture of the anterior and medial walls of the right maxillary sinus. There is fracture of the superior and inferior walls of the left sphenoid sinus.

During his stay, he had a tracheostomy done.

Few weeks later, he developed acute onset of desaturation which improved gradually; the in-charge nurse noticed that the tracheotomy tube suction could not be passed distally through the tube.

The ENT doctor was called to assess the patient. On arrival, he performed a fibre-optic examination through the tracheostomy opening which showed a large granulation tissue below the end of the tracheostomy tube and occluding almost 80% of the tracheostomy tube lumen.

CT of the neck was done, from which it was evident that soft tissue lesion seen in the subcutaneous location above the level of the sternoclavicular joint on the right side just lateral to the entrance of the tracheostomy tube (the tube is seen outside the airway proper) was irregular, dense and encroaching upon the related portion of the trachea resulting in a relative reduction of its diameter averaged about 2.2 × 0.9 cm in its maximum cross-sectional dimension, while its height averaged about 1.6 cm.

The transverse measurement of the airway above the lesion was 1.9 × 1.7 cm on average, while that of the lesion was around 1.3 × 1.4 cm on average.

The diameter of the airways both proximally and distally including the oro-pharyngeal airway, nasopharyngeal airway, hypopharyngeal airway and laryngeal airway proper, as well as the rest of the trachea beyond the level of the discussed lesion, was normal.

The diameter of the visualized portion of the tracheal bifurcation including the main bronchi was normal.

The curved MPR, TTP and virtual endoscopy (VE) with 3-D reconstruction were done, which confirm the diagnosis of dislodgement of tracheostomy tube into the subcutaneous tissues. They also showed granulation tissue at the mid-trachea (at the level of tracheostomy), resulting in significant narrowing of the airway lumen (Figs. 12.1 and 12.2). The patient's tracheotomy tube was repositioned back.

Surface-shaded display of the head, neck, and proximal chest region demonstrating the improper positioning of the slipped tracheostomy tube outside the normal tracheal lumen attaining subcutaneous location. Virtual endoscopy revealed the granulation tissue indenting, violating, and compromising the tracheal airway lumen at its right anterolateral aspect opposite to the assumed tracheostomy level confirmed by virtual endoscopy and TTP image frontal projection (Figs. 12.3 and 12.4).

12.2.2 Case Reference Number 2

The patient presented earlier with a recent diagnosis of thyroid carcinoma for preoperative anaesthesia assessment. Clinical evaluation was carried out and preoperative naso-endoscopic evaluation revealed the presence of an abnormal mucosal-lined drumstick-shaped structure of odd presentation, yet with no signs of malignancy or hypervascularity.

Its exact aetiology origin was unclear until this point. Subsequently, 3-D reconstruction was carried out, which solves this mystery as the aetiology being due to the displaced blade of the hypoid bone, and the thyroid mass lesion was clearly visualized (kindly refer to Chap. 8, Movies 8.5 and 8.6) (Fig. 12.5).

The anaesthesiology plan was dramatically changing upon the obtained data from the 3-D reconstruction which is considered to have a pivotal role in patient management; awake fibre-optic intubation using VAFI video-assisted

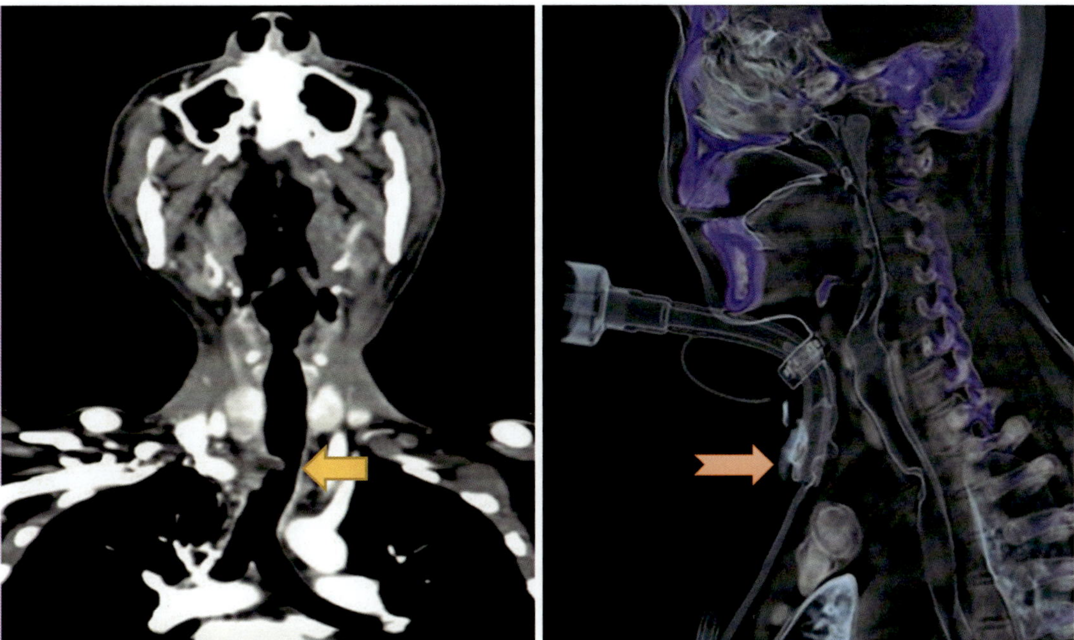

Fig. 12.1 Curved MPR of the airway (left-side image) showing the site of tracheostomy (yellow arrow) with no obvious intraluminal tubes. Sagittal VRT image showing that the tracheostomy tube slipped out with its tip (pink arrow) seen in a subcutaneous location

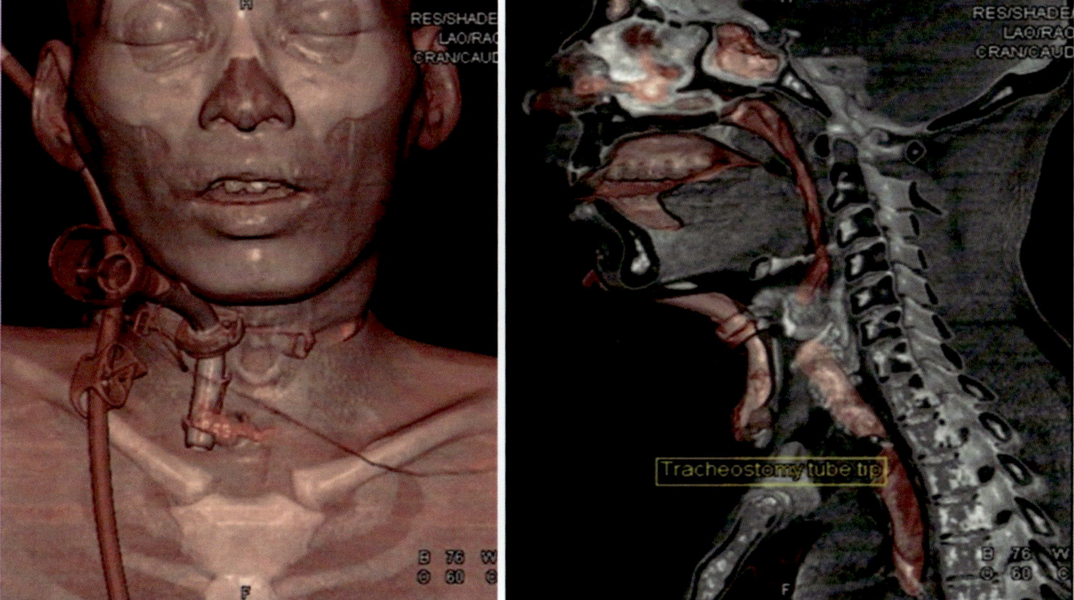

Fig. 12.2 VRT skin surface image showing the tip of the tracheostomy tube totally outside the tracheostomy skin orifice and documented by the sagittal cropped reformatted image

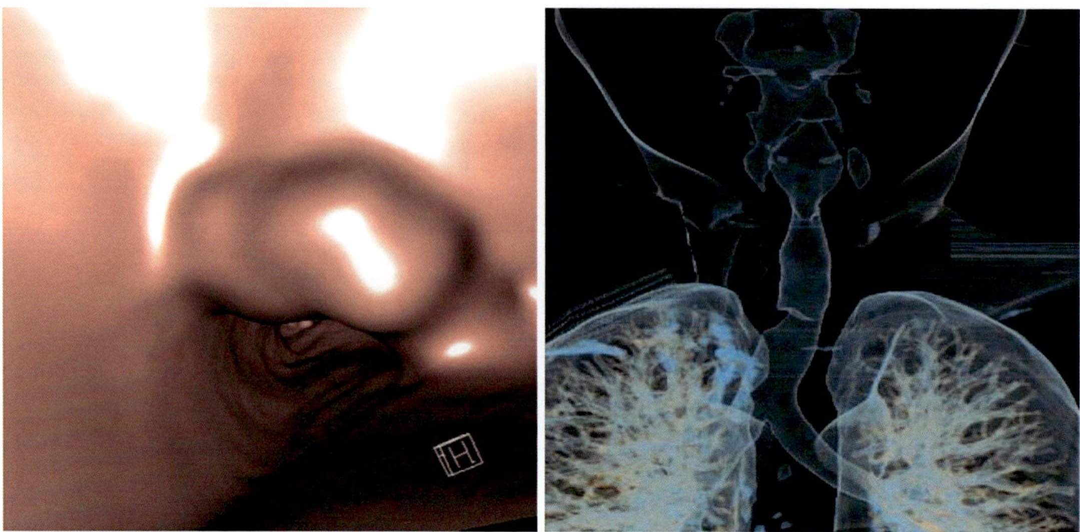

Fig. 12.3 VE shows the site of tracheostomy with no obvious intraluminal tubes

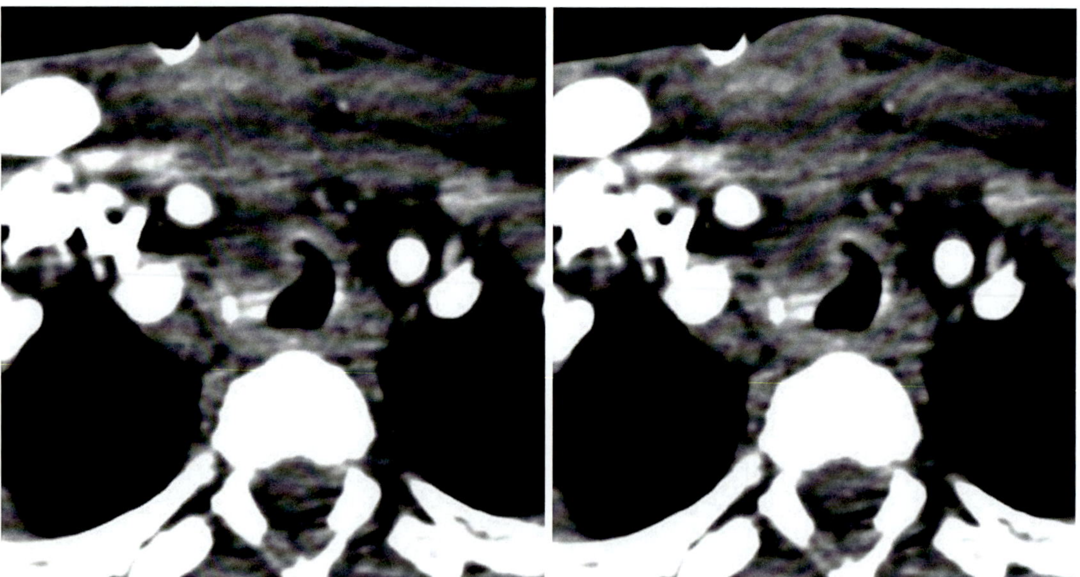

Fig. 12.4 Cross-section selected images showing the site of tracheostomy at the anterior neck/chest wall presented as a notch with the tracheostomy tube slipped outside its normal track. Granulation tissue is noted encroaching upon the tracheal lumen at its right anterolateral aspect

fibre-optic intubation was resorted to instead of the previous plan of classical intubation technique for the sake of the patient's safety.

Upon the second visit, the patient presented with recurrent tumour mass lesion-related symptoms and difficult tracheostomy de-cannulation.

The second CT evaluation reveals the presence of recurrent thyroid mass lesion as well as left-sided cervical lymphadenopathy both significantly violating and displacing the related airway column to the right and reducing its calibre; kindly refer to the TTP and VE images with the indentation upon

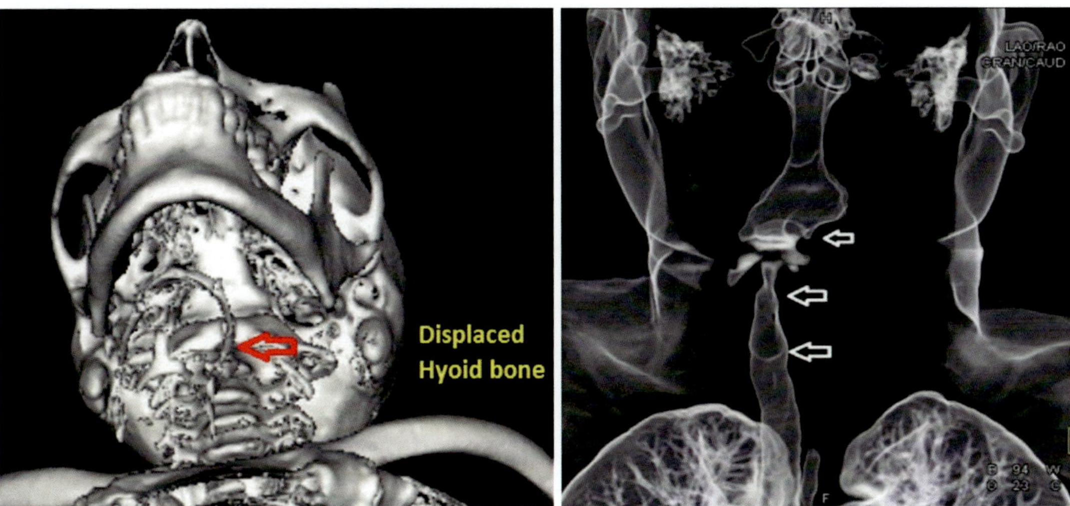

Fig. 12.5 Displaced and rotated hyoid bone (red arrow) with significant encroachment upon the airway which is violated and displaced by a soft tissue mass lesion (white arrows)

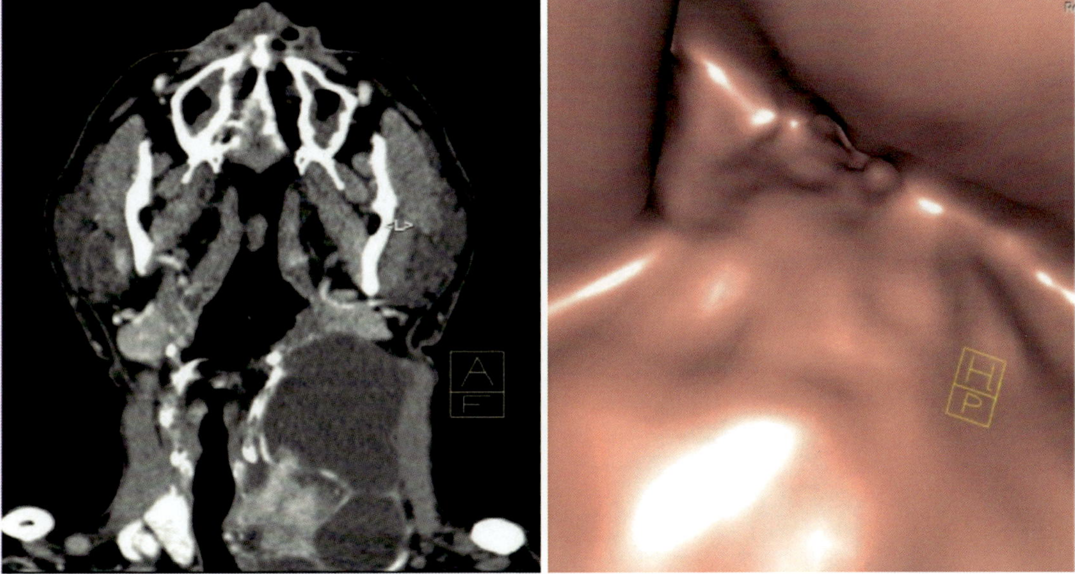

Fig. 12.6 Curved MPR and VE images of displaced and rotated hyoid bone due to mass effect in the airway

the displaced airway to the right "Arrows" (kindly refer to Chap. 8, Movie 8.6 and Fig. 12.6).

12.2.3 Case Reference Number 3

A 52-year-old male presented to the emergency department with a history of acute onset of chest pain. Further evaluation had revealed an inferior wall myocardial infarction for which he had to undergo cardiac catheterization and stenting.

The procedure was complicated by cardiac arrest. He was successfully resuscitated but required endotracheal intubation, tracheostomy tube insertion, and insertion of nasogastric tube (NGT) for few months.

He was later weaned from the tracheostomy and decannulated.

At the peri-extubation period, the patient continued suffering from episodes of choking attacks and aspiration.

Two months later, during a follow-up visit, a chest X-ray was done, which revealed findings suggestive of tracheoesophageal fistula (TOF) (Figs. 12.7, 12.8, and 12.9).

The barium swallow study was done but was inconclusive.

Attempted CT with oral contrast was abandoned, as the patient developed aspiration and arrhythmia.

A second CT examination was done using a modified Valsalva technique which confirmed the diagnosis of TOF with a figure of "8" appearance between the trachea and the oesophagus.

3-D reconstruction images as well as the VE demonstrated the tracheoesophageal fistula.

Diagnosis: Tracheoesophageal fistula (TOF).

The patient was planned for further bronchoscopy evaluation and repair by TOF (kindly refer to Chap. 10, Movie 10.5).

12.2.4 Case Reference Number 4

A 34-year-old (air hostess) was brought to the emergency department (ED) due to increasing difficulty with breathing that followed a direct trauma to her neck due to a baggage dislodgement from the overhead compartment in the airplane.

The patient was then intubated.

CT of the neck was done which showed the following:

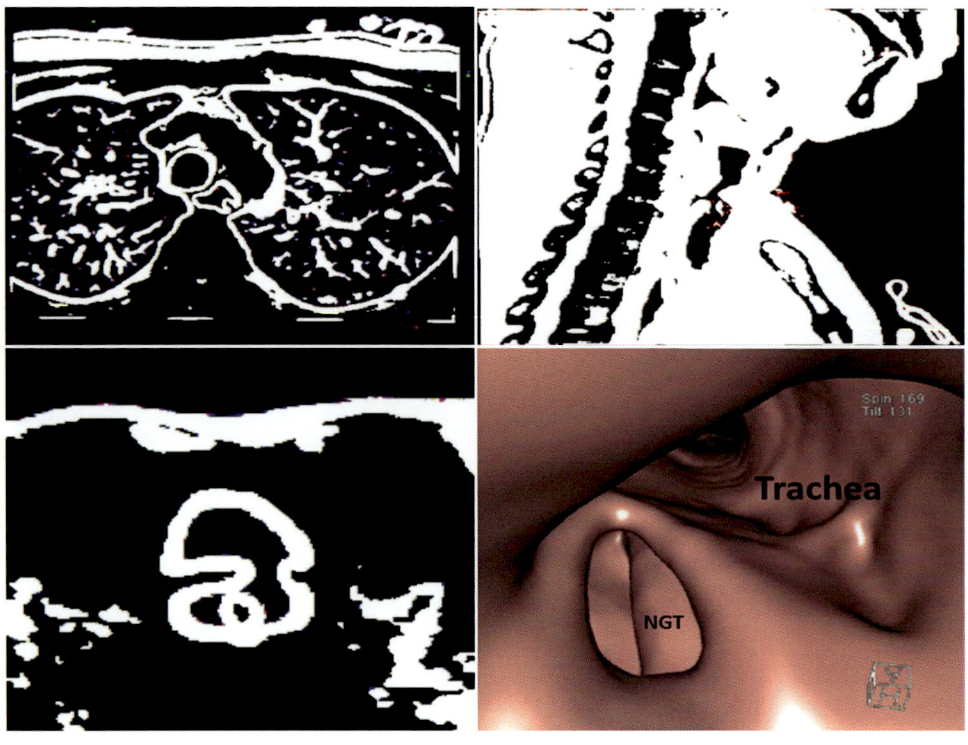

Fig. 12.7 Figure-of-8 TOF fistula with the NGT seen within the oesophagus. Right-side picture shows VB with TOF

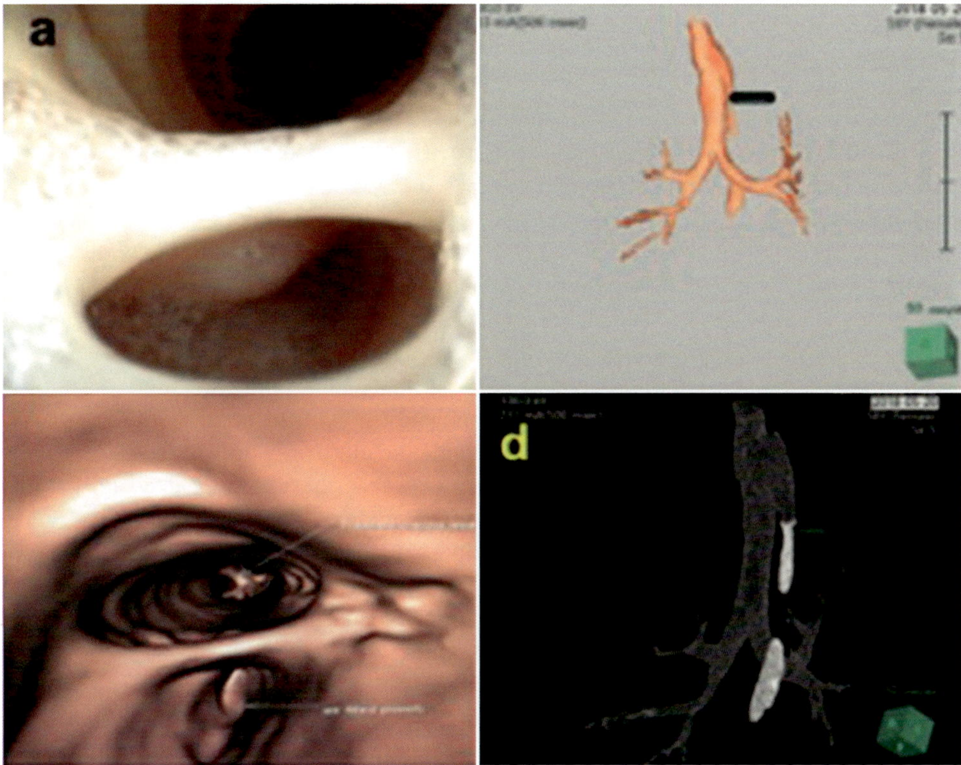

Fig. 12.8 A second case of TOF nicely demonstrated by virtual endoscopy and VRT and SSD techniques. The virtual endoscopy images and findings were identical and in accordance with the conventional endoscopy images; however, without the need for a local anaesthetic, and risk of aspiration which is considered a breakthrough in safe patients' management (kindly refer to Chap. 10, Movie 10.4)

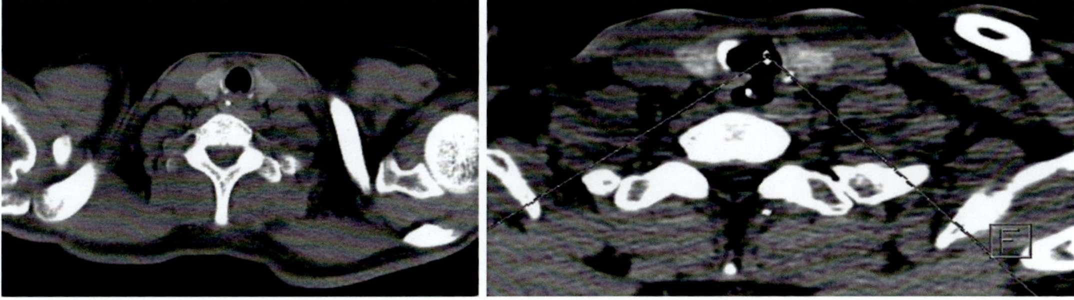

Fig. 12.9 Cross-sectional images at the level of the thyroid gland on the left at rest and on the right using modified Valsalva manoeuvre which nicely demonstrated the TOF with figure of "8"

Extensive surgical emphysema around the airway column and extending up to the superior mediastinum.

Thickening of the aryepiglottic folds noted more on the right side.

An irregular defect noted in the larynx anteriorly at the region of the thyroid cartilage on the right side.

Incidental finding of a well-defined lucent lesion with sclerotic margins noted in the D2 vertebral body extending to the left pedicle likely representing a benign lesion.

She was then taken to the operating room and had examination of the larynx and trachea under general anaesthesia.

During surgery, examination showed a dislocated arytenoid cartilage which was widely separated from the vocal cord.

The dislocated arytenoid was then repaired by suturing. The postoperative course was uneventful, and patient was extubated and sent home.

Three months later, the patient gradually developed difficulty in breathing on exertion, which progressively worsened to difficulty in breathing at rest.

She went to the ENT clinic for assessment.

ENT examination, including fibre-optic naso-endoscopy, was done which showed a glottic web.

A plan was made to surgically repair it by balloon dilatation.

She refused to have awakened intubation, as she was apprehensive due to her previous procedure.

She also refused to consent to the possibility of a tracheotomy to be done during surgery, as the neck scarring could possibly interfere with her future employment.

Preoperative CT showed evidence of vocal cord asymmetry, with a triangle-shaped structure (web) seen in the right vocal cord. The lesion measured approximately 3 × 3 mm, and it was best seen in both coronal and axial views. The thyroid cartilage was also asymmetric, which was most probably a result of trauma.

The epiglottis, arytenoids, and cricoid cartilages appeared grossly normal.

There was no obvious cervical lymphadenopathy.

ENT and anaesthesiology airway evaluation based on clinical and naso-endoscopy assessment revealed a web formation at the level of the glottis extending from the anterior commissure to the junction between the anterior two-thirds and posterior one-third of the vocal cord (glottic area) (Fig. 12.10) (Chap. 8, Movie 8.7) [1].

Virtual endoscopic evaluation was done which showed the web to be at a supraglottic region, while the glottic region was clear.

The anaesthesiologist's decision based upon the VE findings was to give the patient light sedation in addition to topical surface spray airway anaesthesia.

As the patient started to relax and become sedated; a (TCI) Propofol and Remifentanil infusion was given intravenously (as for awaken fibre-optic intubation technique).

The procedure was done using a microlaryngeal endotracheal tube size 4.5.

The supraglottic web was excised, and the postoperative course was smooth.

Kindly refer to the conventional and virtual endoscopy videos (kindly refer to Chap. 8, Movies 8.7–8.9).

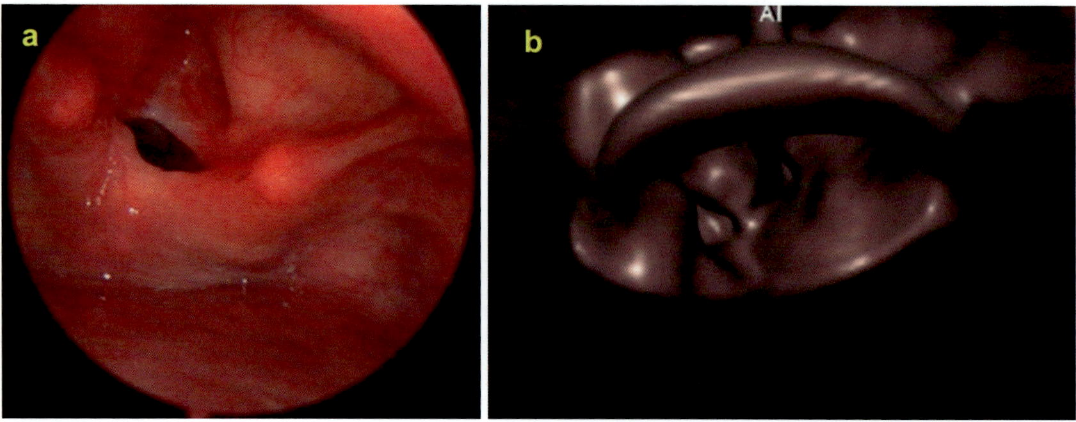

Fig. 12.10 Identical conventional (**a**) and VB (**b**) images showing the narrowed airway with web formation

12.2.5 Case Reference Number 5

A 32-year-old male was referred from the primary care clinic who had complaints of difficulty in swallowing and abnormal "pin-prick" sensation in his neck for 1.5 years.

There was no history of change in voice, fever, headache, allergy, or loss of weight.

Examination showed a deviated nasal septum to the left side.

A fibre-optic naso-endoscopy evaluation showed prominent corniculate cartilages and a left vocal cord polyp.

Other physical examinations were within normal.

Lab investigation of complete blood count and serum creatinine showed within normal limits.

A CT larynx revealed normal vocal cords and a thick abnormal hyoid bone causing oropharyngeal narrowing and indenting on the posterior upper hypopharyngeal wall.

3-D reconstruction, TTP, curved MPR, and VRT as well as virtual bronchoscopy (VE) were done which confirmed the abnormal hyoid bone shape and narrowing of the pharyngeal area (Figs. 12.11 and 12.12) (Movies 12.1 and 12.2).

Diagnosis: Abnormal hyoid bone configuration

Treatment planned: Microlaryngoscopy with excision of part of the abnormal hyoid bone on the left side with a CO_2 laser [2].

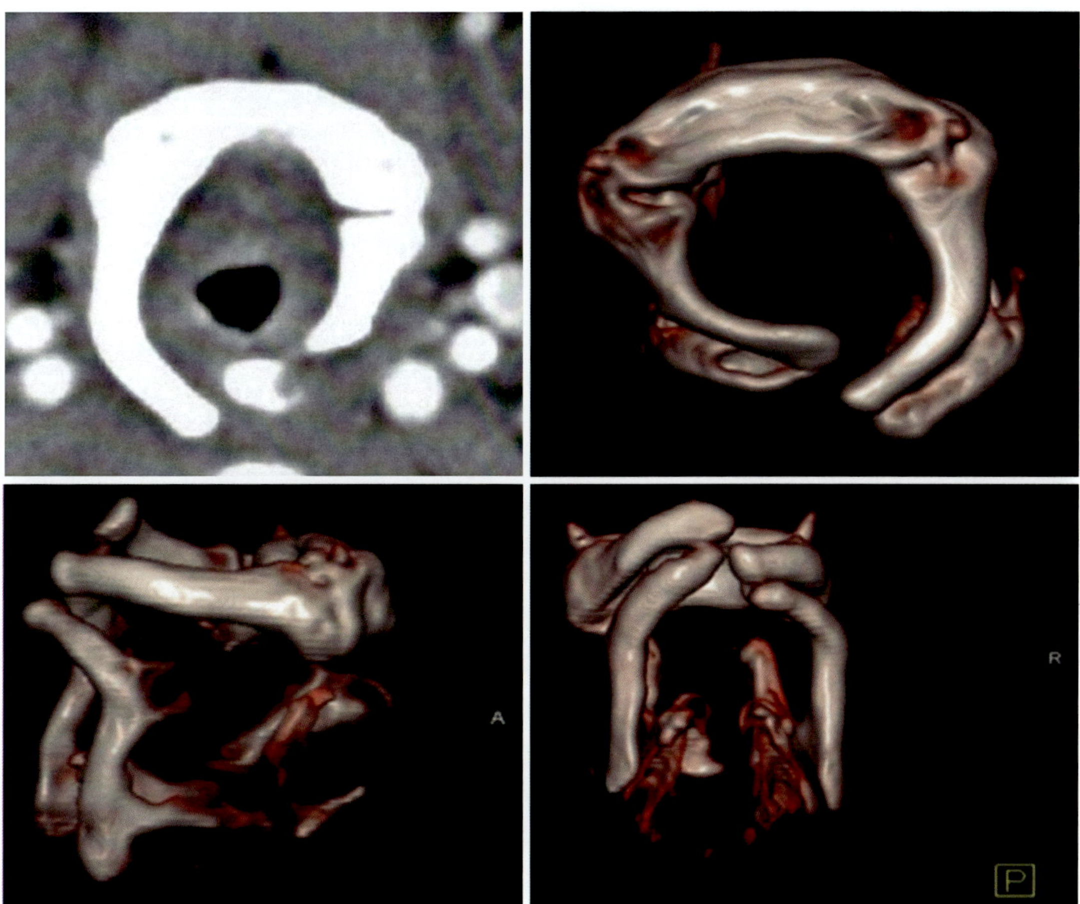

Fig. 12.11 Cross section at the level of the hyoid bone showing increased girth (thickness) with incomplete circular configuration and over-riding of its posterior aspects. The superior thyroid cornu share the same process which was demonstrated by the 3-D images of VRT

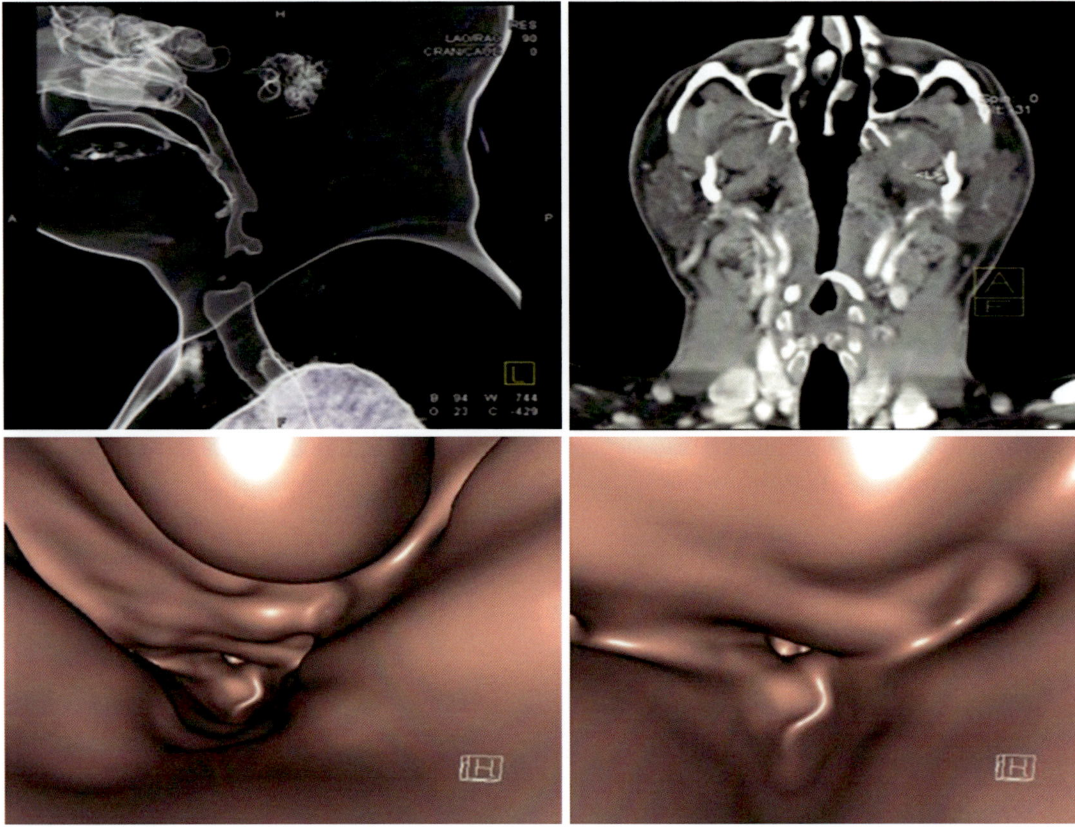

Fig. 12.12 Lateral view of the TTP showing the appreciable encroachment and narrowing of the related airway, and curved MPR demonstrates that the over-riding hyoid bone significantly violates the airway. Virtual bronchoscopy shows the significant airway narrowing

12.2.6 Case Reference Number 6

A 40-year-old lady presented with chief complaints of difficulty in breathing when she walks for 300 meters or more or during any form of exercise.

She had a past history of an acquired tracheal stenosis for which she was treated by balloon dilatation, after which she had improved.

Her presenting history is otherwise unremarkable.

Examinations are all within normal.

Lab workup including complete blood count, serum urea, and electrolytes is within normal limits.

CT of the neck and thorax was done (Figs. 12.13 and 12.14) which shows the following:

A 1.5 cm short-segment tracheal luminal narrowing of around 50% at the level of the thyroid gland and opposite to C5 vertebral body, corresponding to the previous tracheostomy site.

Diagnosis: Recurrent subglottic and tracheal stenosis.

Treatment planned: Microlaryngoscopy and balloon dilatation of the stenotic segment.

12.2.7 Case Reference Number 7

The patient has a history of CA maxilla with destructive osseous lesion within the right side of the alveolar projection of the maxilla with underlying floating teeth on chemo- and radiotherapy.

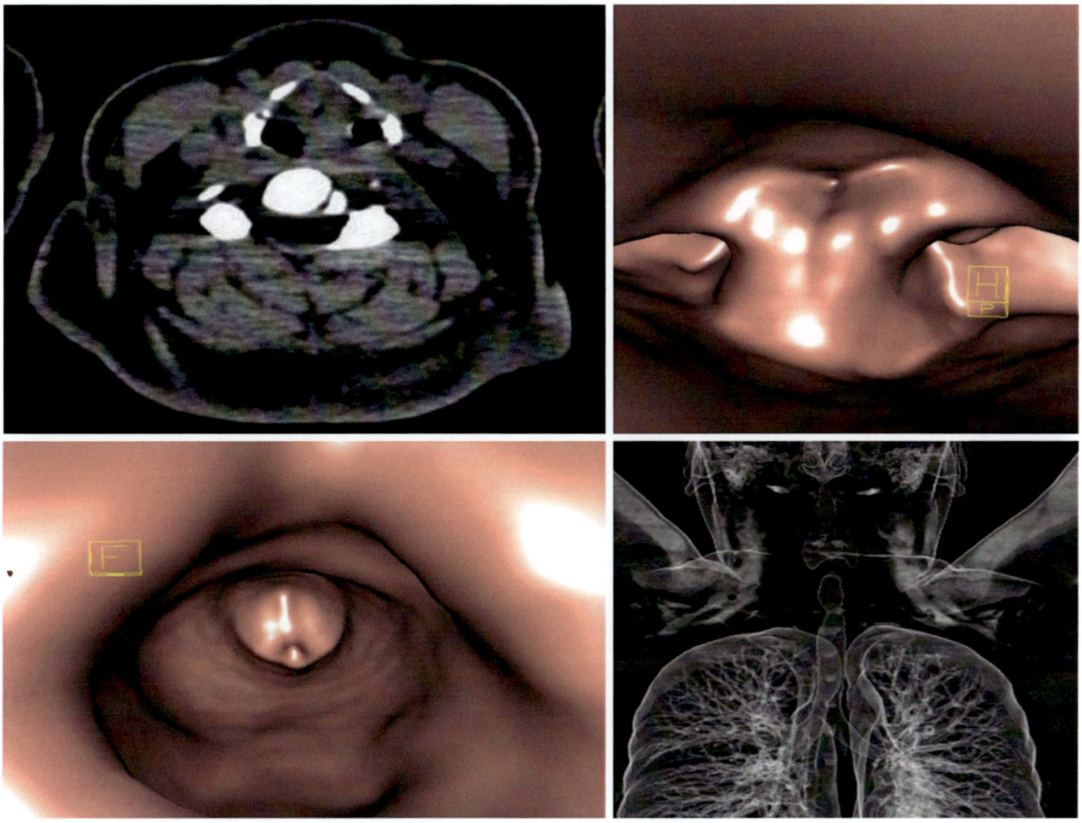

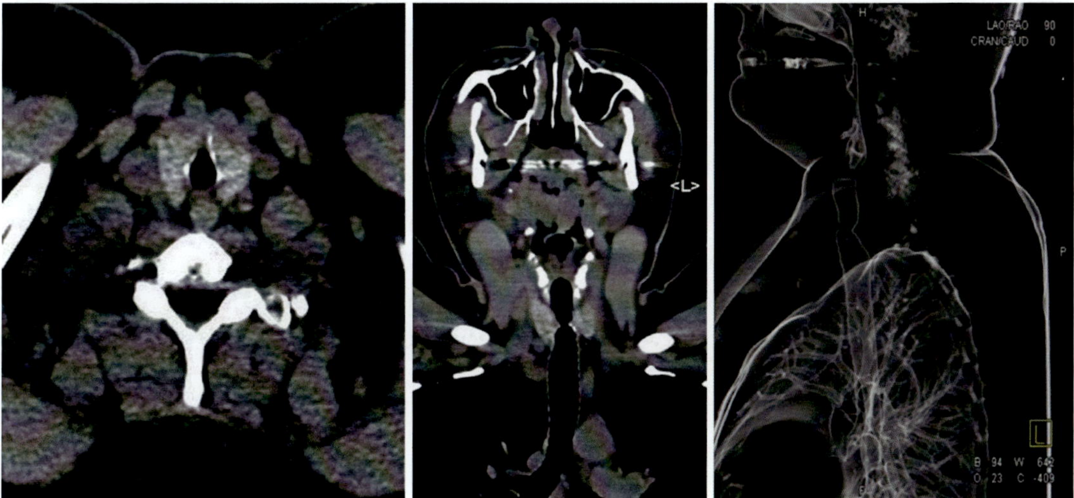

Fig. 12.13 Selected cross-section at the level of the supraglottic region showing circumferential narrowing opposite to the midlevel of the piriform sinuses with corresponding virtual endoscopy imaging. Features that correspond to none-compliance to the modified Valsalva manoeuvre that result in over-diagnosis. Frontal projection of TTP showing both levels of narrowing

Fig. 12.14 Curved MPR frontal projection showing the previously described narrow segment; TTP in lateral projection showing the narrow segment

												N. A. Shallik et al.

A year after the patient presented with sizable cervical mass lesions of different sizes causing appreciable and significant bulge contour, there were bouts of haemoptysis and difficulty in breathing.

The right-sided sizable lymph node with multiple areas of breakdown of hypervascular matrix and multiple related and surrounding malignant vascularity, violates, displaces, and encroaching upon the related airway reducing its calibre and compressing the adjacent vascular framework of the right carotid sheath.

Furthermore, the reconstruction showed evidence of right hemi-thyroidectomy with missing right thyroid lobe and isthmic portion (Movies 12.3 and 12.4) and (Figs. 12.15, 12.16, 12.17 and 12.18).

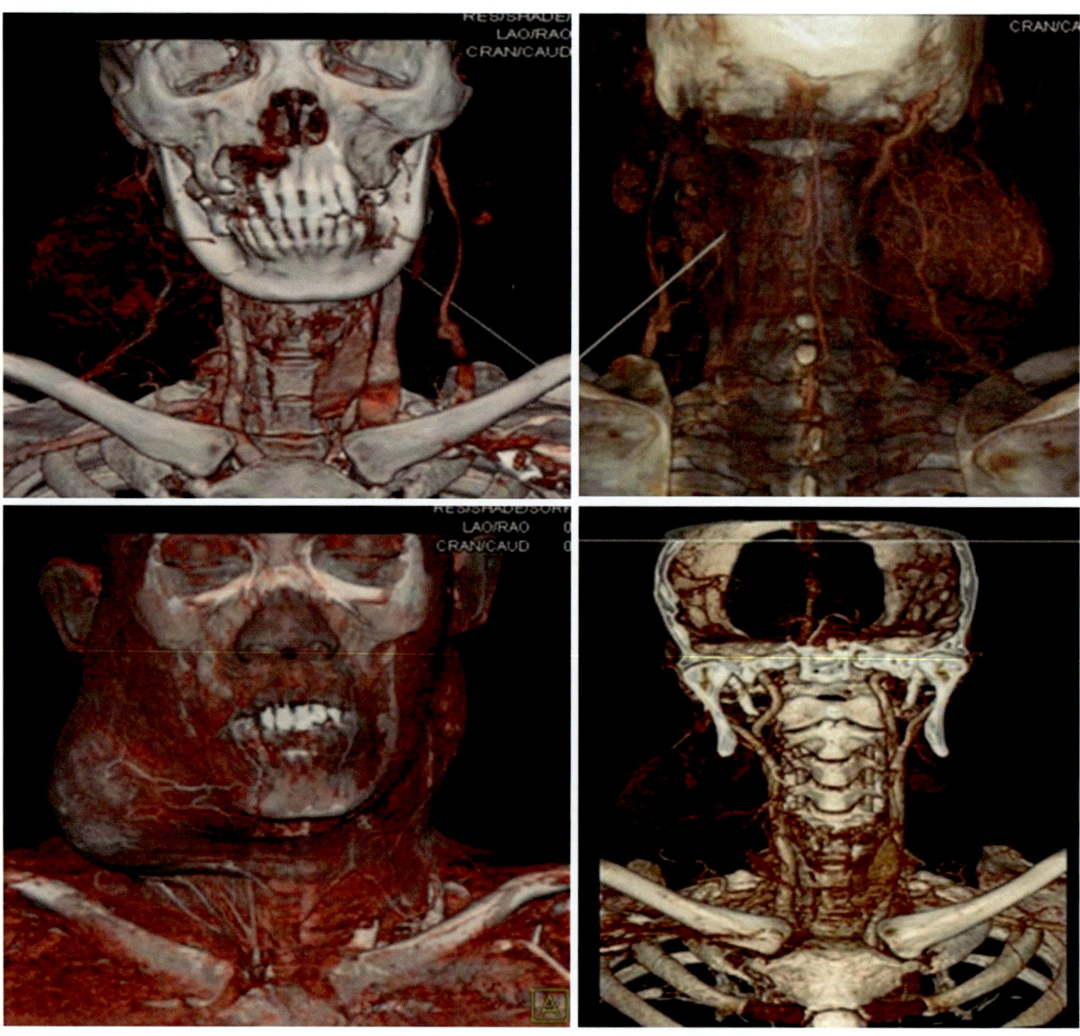

Fig. 12.15 VRT images showing the destructive osseous lesion at the right side of the maxilla with related floating teeth, sizeable hypervascular lymphadenopathy with related malignant vascular network. Evidence of right hemithyroidectomy

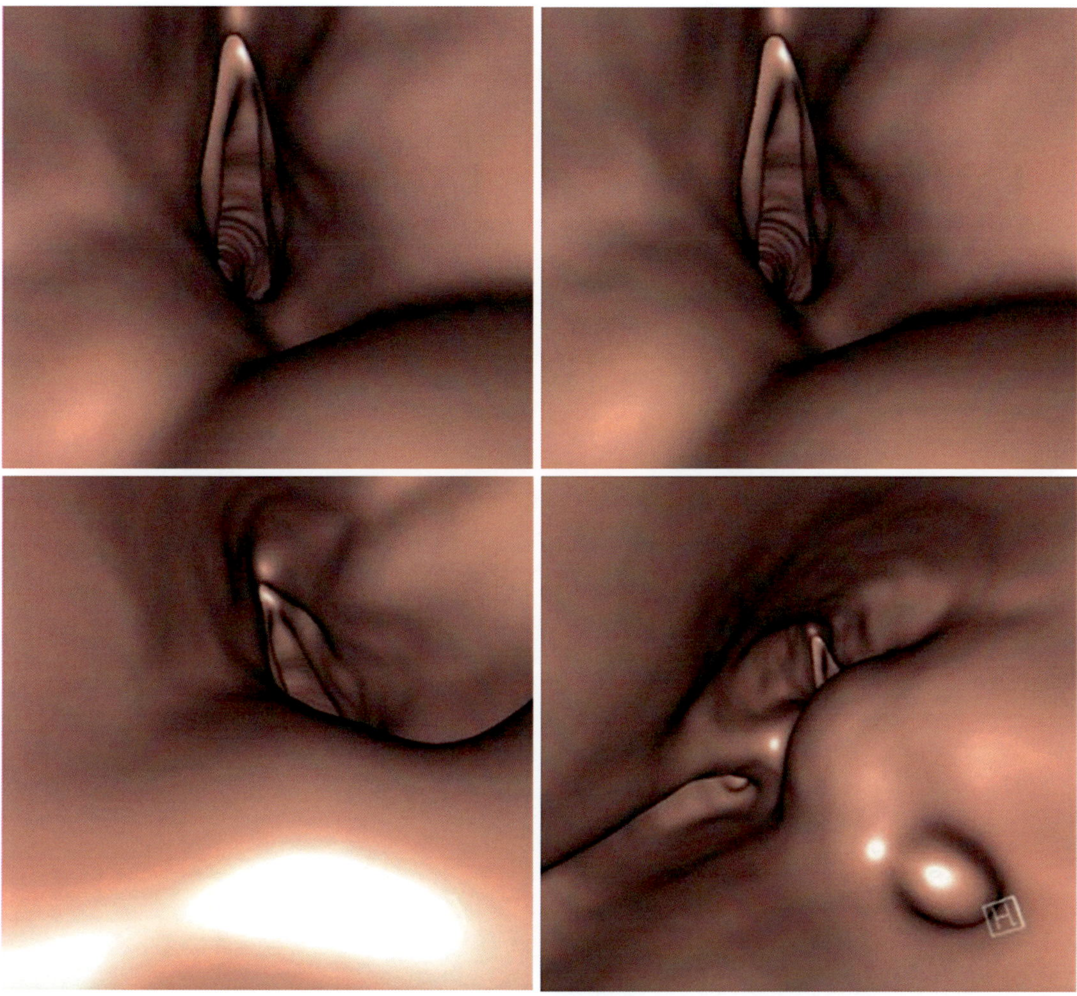

Fig. 12.16 VB at different levels showing normal laryngeal airway with displacement and relative narrowing of the infraglottic and proximal trachea to the left by the extrinsic mass effect of the lymphadenopathy

12.2.8 Case Reference Number 8

A 36-year-old male who has a history of Wegener's granulomatosis with tracheal stenosis and multiple previous surgical correction of the tracheal narrowing, presents for follow-up.

A CT scan of the neck with contrast was done and shows irregular subglottic and upper cervical tracheal narrowing.

The 3-D TTP images and VE examinations show evidence of appreciable circumferential airway narrowing noted at the infra-glottic area of mild to moderate degree (Fig. 12.19).

He is scheduled for endoscopic evaluation and balloon dilatation.

12.2.9 Case Reference Number 9

An adult female patient presented with huge thyroid swelling.

The patient was obese with short neck and a history of asthma.

Difficult intubation was expected (the clinical, radiological, and anaesthesiological from the Mallampati scoring).

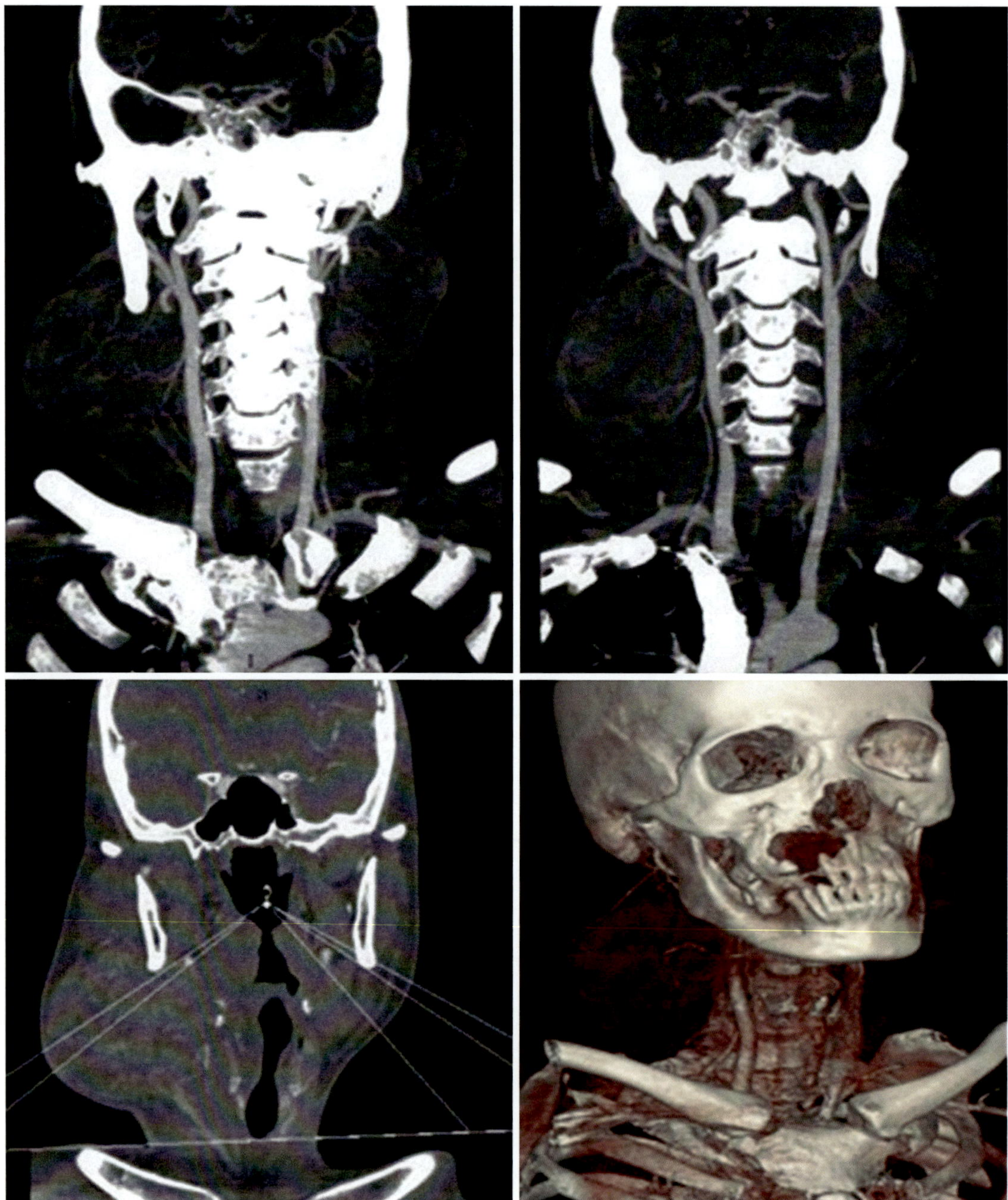

Fig. 12.17 MIP and VRT of the neck vessels showing the rich vascular and malignant circulation surrounding the lymphadenopathy more on the right side

CT of the neck was done, which shows thyroid gland swelling with mediastinal extension, which displaces the trachea and compresses the airway of the proximal trachea at the thoracic inlet.

3-D evaluation and VE highlighted the way for intubation (Figs. 12.20 and 12.21).

Diagnosis: Thyroid swelling.

Planned for surgical removal.

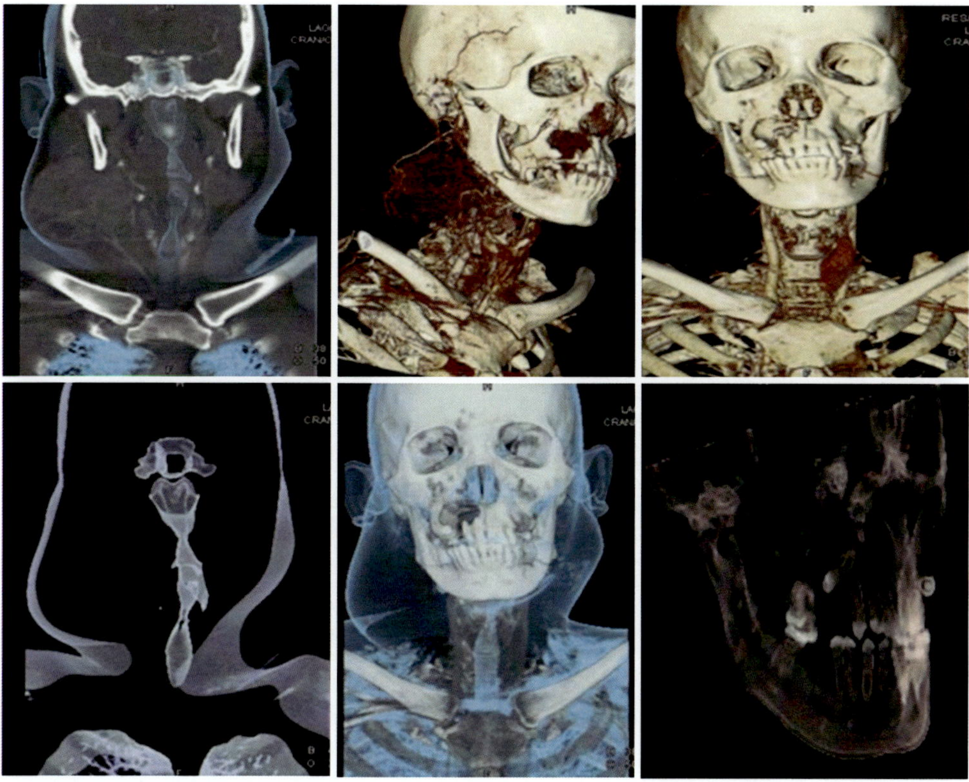

Fig. 12.18 VRT and TTP images showing the displacement and encroached upon airway by the extrinsic mass effect exerted by the rich vascular metastatic lymphadenopathy

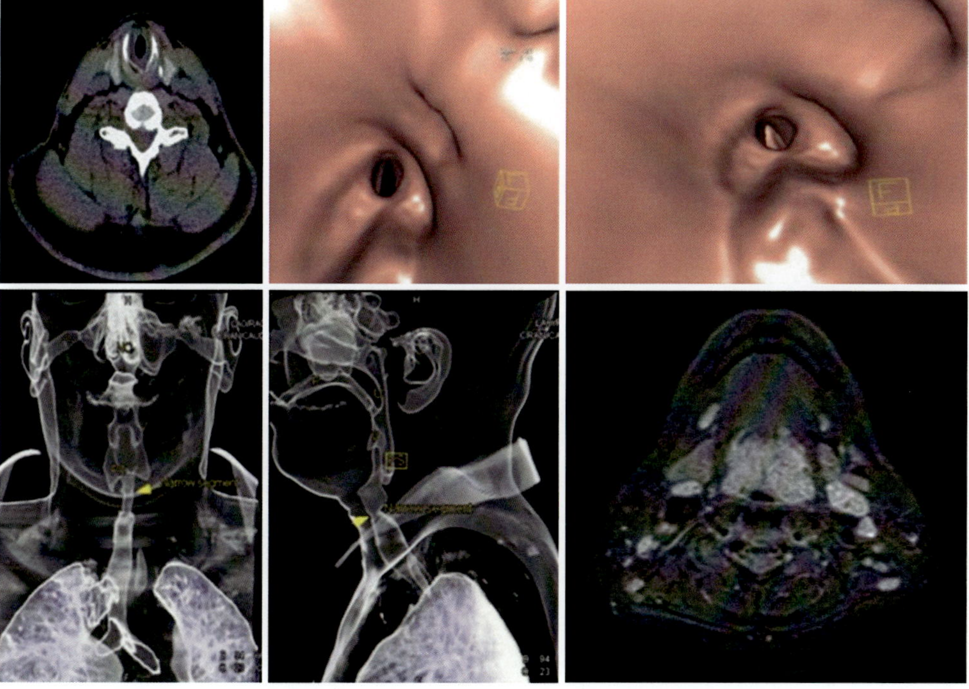

Fig. 12.19 Evidence of appreciable circumferential narrowing "arrow" noted at the infraglottic airway proper to a mild to moderate degree as appreciated from the 3-D TTP images and the VE examinations

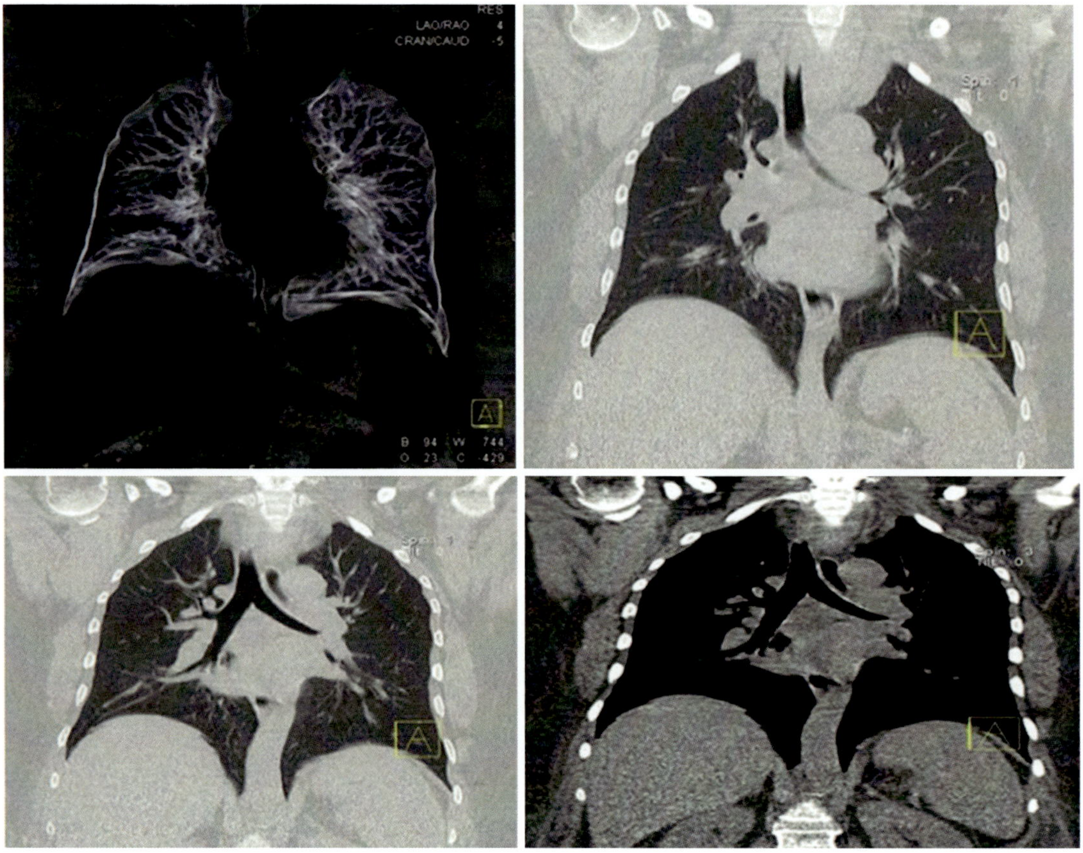

Fig. 12.20 TTP showing encroachment, displacement, and violation upon the proximal tracheal lumen caused by the enlarged thyroid gland

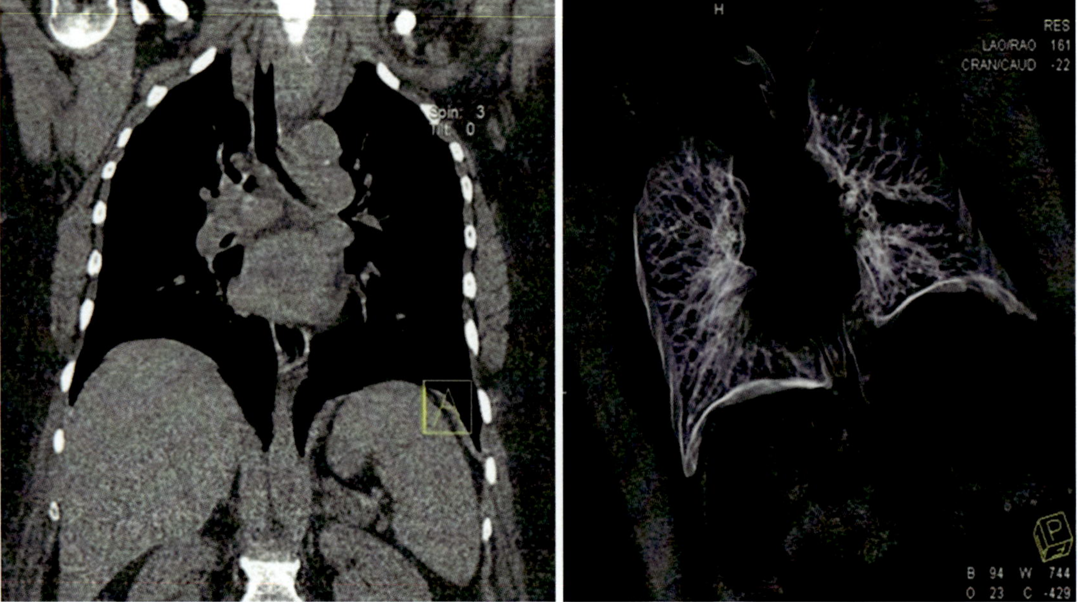

Fig. 12.21 Coronal reformatted image of the neck and thorax as well as TTP showing encroachment, displacement, and violation upon the proximal tracheal lumen caused by the enlarged thyroid gland

12.2.10 Case Reference Number 10

An adult female referred from the emergency department with a history of foreign body ingestion described as a "duck bone" few days back.

The patient was vitally stable.

Endoscopic evaluation as well as the ENT evaluation was unremarkable.

MDCT scan of the neck was carried out, which shows an angulated metallic density foreign body embedded within the left sternocleidomastoid muscle in the transverse direction. Its edges caused metallic artefacts and were seen abutting the related portion of the internal jugular vein (IJV) with inadequate opacification probably due to sluggish circulation due to partial compression.

A small fleck of air density was seen adjacent to the left side of the aerodigestive tract at the corresponding level.

No evidence of abscess formation and implication of the airway proper at its different levels of the pharynx (nasal, oral, or hypopharynx), as well as the laryngeal airway and proximal trachea.

In the 3-D reconstruction of the airway, muscles, and vessels, the foreign body was nicely demonstrated (Figs. 12.22 and 12.23).

External incision and extraction of the FB was carried out (photo), which is identified as an angulated needle, about 3 cm in length with a bevelled end on one side.

On further discussion with the patient, she claimed visiting her dentist few weeks back for dental treatment under local anaesthesia.

The needle was identified by our dentist and a maxillofacial colleague, which was identical to the one used for dental and oral local anaesthesia procedures.

The question remains is how the needle pierced the aerodigestive tract and became embedded in the muscles of the neck and how the patient related this to alleged duck bone ingestion?

CT study, which is very sensitive in discrimination between different densities of bone versus metallic objects, enables easy picking of the FB (for more foreign bodies of the upper airway, please refer to Chap. 8, Movies 8.1–8.4).

12.2.11 Case Reference Number 11

Subglottic stenosis

A 38-year-old female presented with a 1-year history of increasing difficulty in breathing, small neck swelling, and difficulty in swallowing solids.

She has no weight loss.

She is known asthmatic with a history of chronic rhinosinusitis.

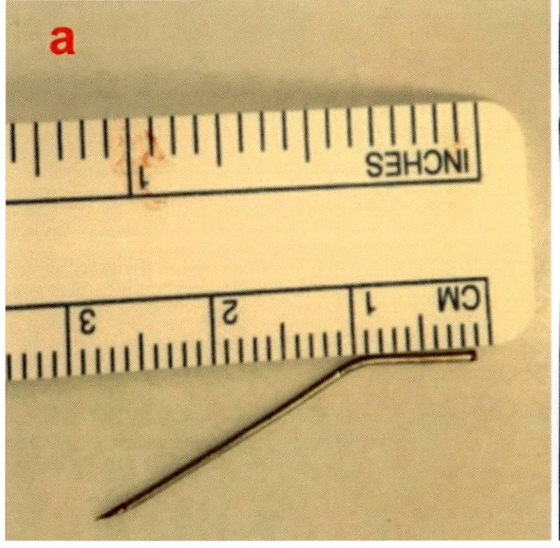
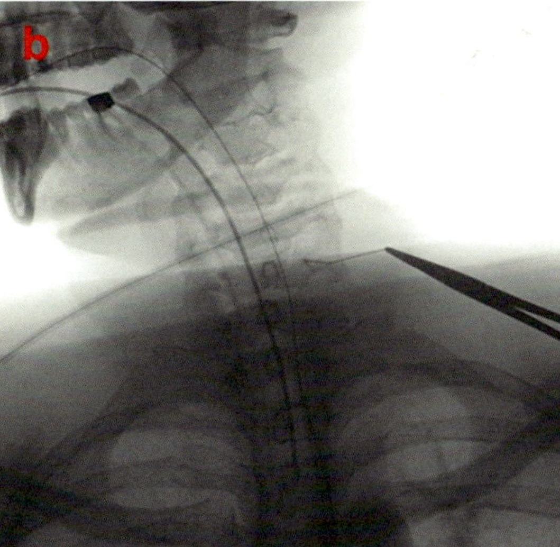

Fig. 12.22 Intraoperative and after extraction of the curved metallic bevelled needle averaging about 3 mm

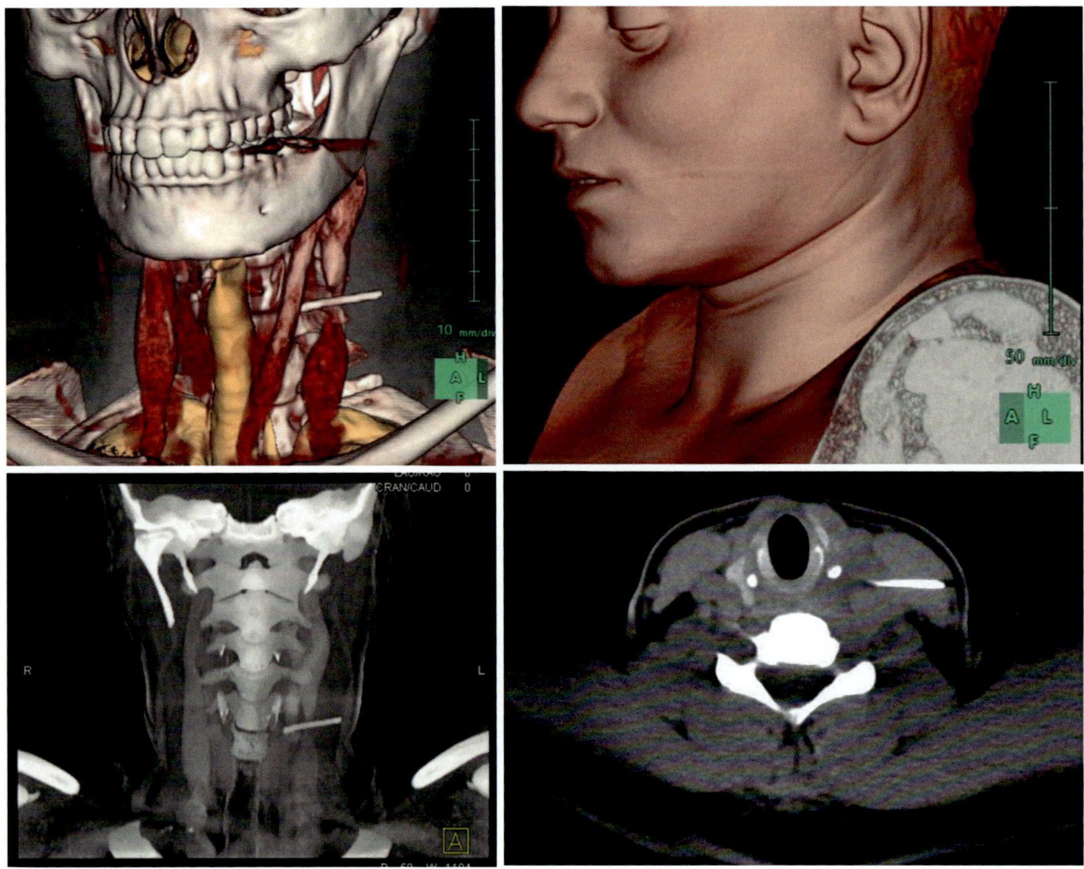

Fig. 12.23 VRT images of bony/vascular and skin reconstruction showing the metallic FB embedded with the sternocleidomastoid muscle on the left and abutting the apparently intact left carotid sheath vessels

Examination: Noisy breathing during both inspiration and expiration.

Fibre-optic naso-endoscopy examination shows subglottic stenosis and red tissue in the subglottic area, causing 60% narrowing of the airway.

Lab investigation was done which include ESR 55, CRP-9, and ANCA-negative.

CT of the neck with contrast, with multi-planar reformats, and volume-rendering VRT-negative VE and 3-D airway reconstruction shows the following:

Evidence of circumferential narrowing of the subglottis, and irregular circumferential narrowing of the upper cervical trachea, with significant encroachment on the air column as seen in the RT inguinal reconstruction. Length of the narrowed segment average 15 mm on coronal reconstruc-

tion and (between 12 and 18 mm on VRT allowing for rotational/flying VRT variation) (Figs. 12.24 and 12.25).

Normal other aspects of upper airway in the digestive tract.

Unremarkable sinonasal cavities and orbits. Incidentally noted mildly asymmetric smaller right maxillary sinus, with thickened bony walls suggestive of congenital hypoplastic sinus.

Multifocal inhomogeneity of thyroid lobe enhancement may be suggestive of possible diffuse thyroid disease versus multinodular goitre, for clinical correlation and ultrasound of the thyroid.

Final Impression: Features in keeping with subglottic and upper tracheal stenosis with circumferential soft tissue thickening, differential

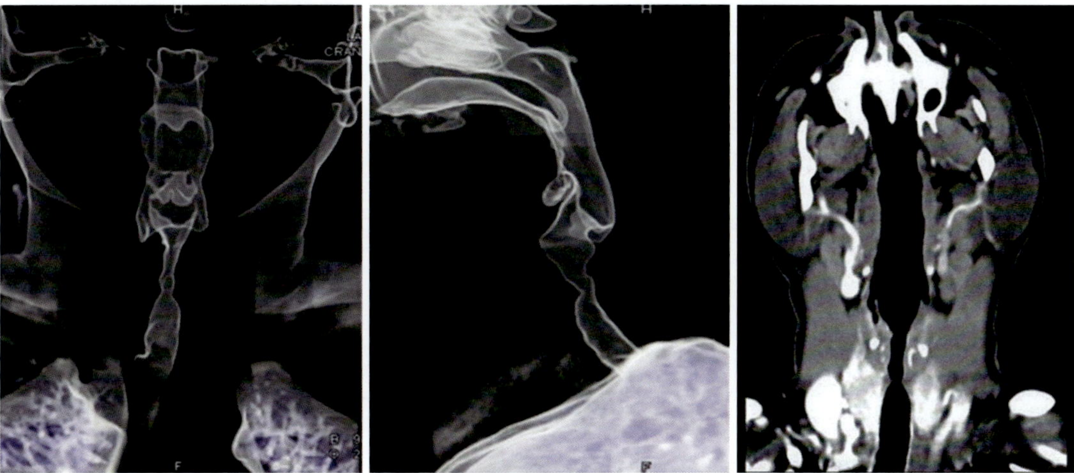

Fig. 12.24 Subglottic stenotic smooth segment as evidenced by TTP and C-MPR. Kindly compare the calibre of the normal proximal airway with the reduced one on the right-side image of the VB

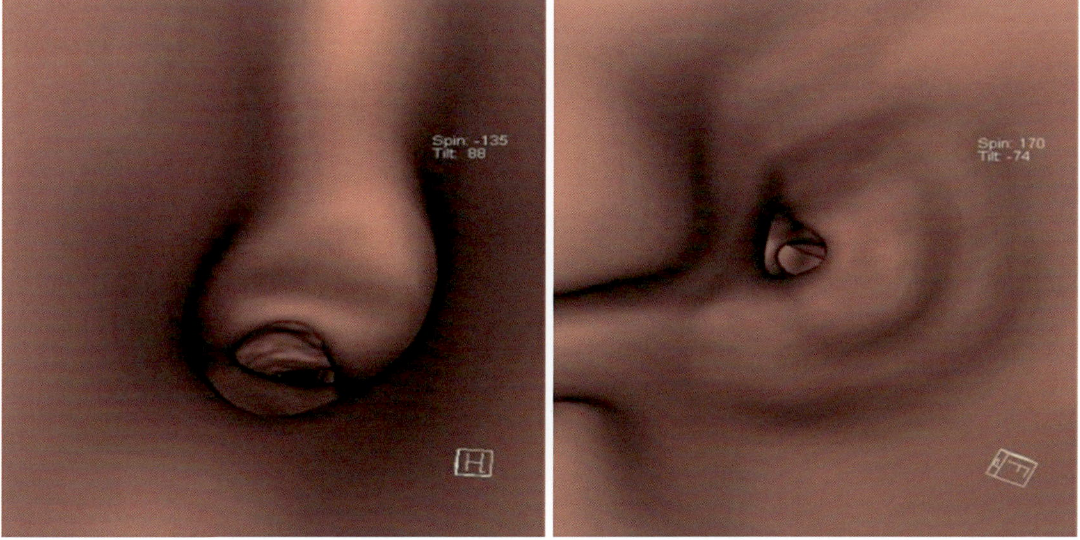

Fig. 12.25 Subglottic stenotic smooth segment as evidenced by VB. Kindly compare the calibre of the normal proximal airway with the reduced one on the right-side image of the VB

consideration include chronic inflammatory process/granulomatous disorders/amyloid deposition/post-prolonged intubation, extent as above described, for further clinical correlation.

Inhomogeneous enhancement of thyroid lobes for further clinical correlation and ultrasound evaluation.

Diagnosis of subglottic stenosis was done.

Plan: As the patient's symptoms are worsening, the patient was planned surgical intervention (tracheostomy, microlaryngoscopy, tracheoscopy, and dilatation of the subglottic stenosis) [3].

The surgery was done successfully.

12.3 Conclusion and Recommendations

Thanks for the technology that allowed us to give more comprehensive extraordinary valuable data that ultimately give accurate confident diagnosis; help in better patient's management and open the gate for further more bright future for the sake of our precious patients and Mankind. Our junior radiologists and colleagues kindly apply the volume rendering techniques and follow the protocol addressed in this book for airway assessment which may be of help in facilitating image's interpretation and reach a definitive diagnosis which is our all main goal.

References

1. Shallik N, Zaghw A, Dogan Z, Rahman A. The use of virtual endoscopy for diagnosis of traumatic supraglottic airway stenosis. JCAO. 2017;2(1):103.
2. Shallik N, .Haidar H, Dogan Z, H. Enezi, W. Rahman, N. Arun, N. Ishac, A. Moustafa. Circular hyoid bone: The first reported case in literature. Trends Anaesth Crit Care 16, 2017: 27–28. Poster Presentation https://doi.org/10.1016/j.tacc.2017.10.040.
3. Shallik N, Soliman M, Aboelhassan A, Hammad Y, Haidar H, Moustafa A. Does the surgical airway still the gold standard step in securing the airway in patients with obstructing laryngeal tumors? Trends Anaesth Crit Care. 2018;23:42–3. https://doi.org/10.1016/j.tacc.2018.09.085.